The Millennium Development Goals for Health

RISING
TO THE CHALLENGES

RISING
TO THE CHALLENGES

by Adam Wagstaff and Mariam Claeson

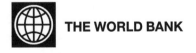 THE WORLD BANK

ISBN 0-8213-5767-0

Library of Congress Cataloging-in-Publication Data

The millenium development goals for health : rising to the challenges / The World Bank.
    p. cm.
Includes bibliographical references and index.
ISBN 0-8213-5767-0
  1. Health promotion. 2. Health promotion—Cross-cultural studies. 3. Medical policy. 4.
Medical policy—Cross-cultural studies. 5. Health planning. 6. Health
Planning—Cross-cultural studies. I. World Bank.

RA427.8.M556 2004
362.1—dc22

2004047781

Cover photo from the World Bank Photo Library
Cover design by Chris Lester of Rock Creek Creative

CONTENTS

Boxes

Figures

Tables

Foreword

The extent of premature death and ill health in the developing world is staggering. In 2000 almost 11 million children died before their fifth birthday, an estimated 140 million children under five are underweight, 3 million died from HIV/AIDS, tuberculosis claimed another 2 million lives, and 515,000 women died during pregnancy or child birth in 1995, almost all of them in the developing world.

Death and ill health on such a scale are matters of concern in their own right. They are also a brake on economic development. It was these twin concerns that led the international community to put health firmly at the center of the Millennium Development Goals when adopting them at the Millennium Summit in September 2000.

This report focuses on the health and nutrition Millennium Development Goals agreed to by over 180 governments. It assesses progress to date and prospects of achieving the goals. The report argues that where progress has been slow, the reason is not lack of technical solutions but that effective interventions are not used. The report reviews the determinants to low access and use of these interventions at household and health systems levels, and shows the role that policies and institutions play.

The report argues that low coverage of MDG-related interventions reflects in part the low level of government health spending but more fundamentally the numerous policy and institutional weaknesses across the entire health system. It shows that additional spending on health would accelerate progress toward the MDGs in countries with good policies and institutions, while progress in countries where they are weak, requires a more targeted approach. It requires first and foremost a focus on households—not only as users of services but as producers of health—and on providers and their accountability. Accelerating progress toward the MDGs in those contexts requires strengthening of input markets, such as people and pharmaceuticals, and

of core public health functions: monitoring, evaluation, surveillance, regulation, social mobilization, and concerted action beyond the health sector.

The report identifies what developing country governments can do to accelerate the pace of progress while ensuring that benefits accrue to the poorest and most disadvantaged households. It also pulls together the lessons of development assistance and country initiatives and innovations to improve the effectiveness of aid, based on a number of country case studies. It highlights some of the principles of effective development assistance: country driven coordination; strategic coherence expressed in comprehensive poverty reduction strategies, which fully address the issues of health, nutrition, and population; financial coherence embodied in medium term expenditure framework; pooling of donor funds; and a common framework for reporting and assessing progress.

A process has begun that we hope will lead to more coordinated donor actions to accelerate country level progress. This report aims to inform this process at the global level, resulting in actions to which the international community is firmly committed. But more importantly, we hope that this report will stimulate and inform policy dialogue and actions at national and sub-national levels, involving the many stakeholders—households foremost among them—that are critical for achieving the health and population MDGs. Ultimately, this report will have served its purpose if it generates action and change, and if it contributes to accelerate the pace toward achieving the MDGs. Many lives are at stake. We know what needs to be done. It is time to act.

JEAN-LOUIS SARBIB
Senior Vice President
Human Development Network

JACQUES BAUDOUY
Director
Health Nutrition and Population
Human Development Network

Acknowledgments

This report was prepared by a team led by Adam Wagstaff and Mariam Claeson. Jumana Qamruddin and Henrik Bjorn Axelsson served as research analysts. The team from within and outside the World Bank—Alexandre V. Abrantes, Anita Alban, Henrik Bjorn Axelsson, Florence Baingana, Ousmane Bangoura, Amie Batson, Eduard Bos, Logan Brenzel, Flavia Bustreo, Jillian Cohen, Isabella Anna Danel, Monica Das Gupta, François Decaillet, Pablo Gottret, Davidson Gwatkin, April Harding, Robert Hecht, Eva Jarawan, Timothy A. Johnston, Rachel Kaufmann, Peyvand Khaleghian, Rudolph Knippenberg, Christoph Kurowski, Rama Lakshminarayanan, Benjamin Loevinsohn, Elizabeth Lule, Joan MacNeil, Tonia Marek, Milla McLachlan, Julie Mclaughlin, Saul Morris, Joseph Naimoli, Tawhid Nawaz, Kjeld Pedersen, Alexander Preker, Jumana Qamruddin, Sangeeta Raja, G.N.V. Ramana, Pablo Ribera, Juan Rovira, Nicole Schwab, Meera Shekar, Agnes Soucat, Susan Stout, Eldaw Suliman, Emi Suzuki, Juan Pablo Uribe, Diana Weil, Harvey Whiteford, and Alan Wright—contributed in various ways to the background analysis, country case studies, and review of operational experiences. They also played a part in drafting and reviewing the manuscript. The work was carried out under the general direction of Jacques Baudouy.

The peer reviewers of the report were Shantayanan Devarajan, Deon Filmer, Jonathan Halpern, Daniel Kress, Samuel Lieberman, George Schieber, and Eric Swanson. An external panel provided advice and technical inputs in the early drafting of the report. Bruce Ross-Larson and Meta de Coquereaumont were the principal editors, with the assistance of Elizabeth McCrocklin, Thomas Roncoli, Christopher Trott, and Elaine Wilson. Book and cover design, copyediting, production, and printing were coordinated by the Production Services Unit of the World Bank's Office of the Publisher, under the supervision of Susan Graham and Monika Lynde.

Several consultations with partners provided helpful guidance for the report: an external and internal technical consultation with bilateral partners, agencies, and nongovernmental organizations to review the messages of an early draft, held in Washington in January 2003; a high-level policy consultation on the framework for accelerated progress toward the health-related Millennium Development Goals, cohosted by the Canadian International Development Agency, the U.K. Department for International Development, and the World Bank, held in Ottawa in May 2003; and the High-Level Forum on the Health MDGs, cohosted by the World Health Organization and the World Bank, held in Geneva in January 2004. Extensive comments were provided by partners, including the Canadian International Development Agency, the U.K. Department for International Development, the Netherlands Ministry of Foreign Affairs, the Swedish International Development Cooperation Agency, the United Nations Children's Fund, and the World Health Organization. The analytical work was also informed by the team leaders' participation in the Bellagio study group, which reviewed the evidence for child mortality and published the results in the *Lancet* series on child survival in July 2003. A consultation on the costing and financing of the health-related Millennium Development Goals was cohosted by the World Bank and the Disease Control Priorities project, in Washington in November 2003. Some team members also participated in the Millennium Project taskforces, and the analysis has benefited from interactions with them.

The work was supported in part by Dutch Trust Funds.

At the United Nations Millennium Summit in September 2001, 147 heads of state endorsed the Millennium Development Goals, half of which concern different aspects of health—directly or indirectly. This report assesses progress to date toward these goals and analyzes prospects for the future. The report argues that faster progress can be made with existing health interventions. It argues that extra government health spending is not enough, and that policies and institutions within and beyond the health sector need to be strengthened if faster progress toward the health millennium development goals is to be made. On these and other issues the report reaches clear-cut conclusions. These are summarized below.

Progress toward the Millennium Development Goals for health has been mixed.

- Some good news: nearly 80 percent of the world's people live in a country that is on track to hit the malnutrition target. In the 1990s, 38 percent of countries accelerated the rate of decline for under-five mortality despite HIV/AIDS. And in two regions—East Asia and Pacific and the Middle East and North Africa—maternal mortality appears to have fallen swiftly in the 1990s.
- But plenty of bad news, too. On under-five mortality, progress has been much too slow—and has been getting even slower. Sub-Saharan Africa is lagging behind badly across all the Millennium Development Goals for health but especially on under-five mortality, for which no Sub-Saharan country is on track to hit the target. All regions face challenges on at least some Millennium Development Goals, including regions with many middle-income countries. Overall, however, the poorest countries are progressing the slowest. And at least for under-five mortality, poor communities within countries are progressing the slowest.

Progress in the second half of the 1990–2015 window will not necessarily be swifter.

- There will be some stimuli for faster progress outside the health sector. Economic growth is set to increase in all regions except East Asia and Pacific. The Millennium Development Goal agenda may well speed up progress toward universal primary enrollment, the elimination of gender gaps in secondary education, and increased access to safe drinking water. But even on the most optimistic calculations, the combined effects of these stimuli will be insufficient for most countries to make the difference between hitting and missing the Millennium Development Targets.
- Developments within the health sector will tend to slow down progress. Many countries cannot sustain the rate of increase of coverage of attended deliveries they saw during the 1990s—the inevitable slowdown will lead to a slower rate of decline for maternal mortality.

Accelerating progress toward the Millennium Development Goals for health is possible in all regions and countries.

- Effective interventions exist for malnutrition, child mortality, maternal mortality, and communicable diseases. But they are being used too little by the people who can benefit from them—especially poor people. If universal coverage rates were achieved for a handful of key child health interventions, the number of under-five deaths worldwide would fall by nearly two-thirds—the Millennium Development Target. A three-quarters reduction in the rate of maternal mortality—the Millennium Development Target—could be achieved by scaling up coverage rates of a handful of key maternal mortality interventions, including improved access to comprehensive essential obstetric care. The technology is available—it just needs to be used by all.

Additional resources are required but will not be sufficient to reach the Millennium Development Goals.

- Increased government spending on health is a part of the answer to getting effective interventions used more widely. But it is not the whole story. In countries with very poor policies and institutions, across-the-board increases in government spending will have little if any impact on Millennium Development Indicators. In these countries, improved policies and institutions—within and beyond the health sector—are crucial if progress toward the Millennium Development Goals is to be accelerated. Even in countries with relatively good policies and institutions, additional government health spending needs to be targeted. Preliminary estimates suggest the returns to targeted spending—in reduced mortality—are much higher than the returns to across-the-board increases in government health spending.

Strengthening policies and institutions in the health sector requires working across several interrelated areas.

- Stronger policies and better institutions for health require lowering the financial and nonfinancial barriers that households face in their dual roles as producers of health and users of health services. Price is key, especially for the poor, but knowledge and geographic access are also important.
- Better policies and institutions within the health sector also entail improving the performance of health providers—on their quality, their responsiveness, and their efficiency—through greater accountability. Within provider organizations, stronger management involves increasing the accountability of frontline providers to the organization. But their performance can also be improved by making them more accountable to the public, whether along the direct route (for example, enabling community organizations to exercise oversight of providers) or the indirect route (making providers more accountable to policymakers through, for example, contracts or agreements, and making policymakers in turn more accountable to the public through greater democracy and openness). Reaching the poor requires new thinking about the most effective service delivery for the different kinds of basic services: outreach, fixed facilities, and referral.
- Human resource challenges face most developing countries, and policymakers need to work along several dimensions. Wages and monetary benefits are important elements of recruitment and retention efforts. But there are other avenues that can usefully be explored, such as increasing training opportunities, enhancing promotion prospects, and so on.
- For medicines and essential supplies, governments have to ensure that medicines reach and are affordable for people who need them most. Again, working along a variety of dimensions is required, including improved logistics, but also better incentives, more strategic procurement arrangements, and a more responsible role for industrial governments in making existing drugs available at affordable prices and providing the appropriate incentive environment for research and development into diseases that disproportionately affect poor countries.

Many governments lack credible and resource-backed strategies for the prevention, treatment, and control of communicable diseases.

- Too little effort is devoted to surveillance, monitoring and evaluation, learning the lessons of such exercises,

and incorporating the lessons into policymaking. And all too often intersectoral issues are poorly handled. Yet, as is becoming increasingly clear, investments outside the health sector (in water and sanitation, and roads and transport) do not achieve their full impact on health unless they are accompanied by well designed programs that aim to change people's behavior (for example, hand-washing) or accessing services.

Some countries appear to spend less than they can afford.

- In these countries, governments should consider raising the share of government spending in GDP, or increasing the health share of total government spending. Such reforms take time and may require technical and financial assistance from donors. Governments need also to play a stronger role in encouraging or arranging the pooling of out-of-pocket expenditures through insurance and prepayment mechanisms.

Donors can do better than they have done in the past.

- Development assistance to health is too unpredictable, and the transaction costs are too high. Development assistance to health—like government spending itself—is more productive in countries with sound policies and institutions. Aid can help foster good policies and facilitate transition to them, but donors cannot force policies on countries against their will. Aid is fungible, at least in part: this points toward enhanced coordination, aid pooling, and putting countries in the driver seat. Global partnerships in health add value, but contain risks.
- At the High-Level Forum on the Millennium Development Goals for health in Geneva in January 2004, there was broad agreement among a wide variety of different actors—donors, international technical agencies, philanthropists, and developing countries—on a number of points. It was agreed that the Millennium Development Goals for health pose formidable challenges and that it is vital for all to rise to them. All agreed that a greater sense of urgency is required if 2015 is not to pass by with a large number of countries having missed the targets. The forum participants agreed on actions in the mobilization of resources for health, aid effectiveness and harmonization, human resources, and in the monitoring of performance.

Why the Millennium Development Goals matter—it's the world's poor who die earlier.

Rates of mortality and malnutrition tend to be much higher among the world's poor and, with the exception of deaths from HIV/AIDS, lower among better-off sections of the world's population.

- 41 percent of children in the poorest quarter of the world's population are underweight, 3 percent in the richest quarter.
- 114 deaths among children under five per 1,000 live births for the poorest quarter, 13 per 1,000 for the richest quarter.
- 63 maternal deaths per 10,000 live births for the poorest quarter, 4 per 10,000 for the richest quarter.

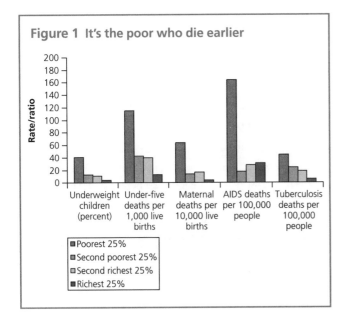

Figure 1 It's the poor who die earlier

- 164 AIDS deaths per 100,000 people for the poorest quarter, 31 for the richest quarter.

Progress toward the Millennium Development Goal targets has varied—across indicators and across regions.

Progress has been fastest for malnutrition, reflecting in part the lower target for this indicator (a halving of the rate between 1990 and 2015, compared with a two-thirds reduction in the case of maternal mortality). Progress has been slowest for under-five mortality. Progress has also var-

ied across regions—slowest in Sub-Saharan Africa, swiftest in the Middle East and North Africa.

- 60 percent of the people in the Middle East and North Africa are in countries on track to reach the goal for under-five mortality, 39 percent in Latin America and the Caribbean, 28 percent in Europe and Central Asia, 17 percent in East Asia and Pacific, 10 percent in South Asia, and 0 percent in Sub-Saharan Africa.
- 84 percent of the people in the Middle East and North Africa are in countries on track to reach the goal for

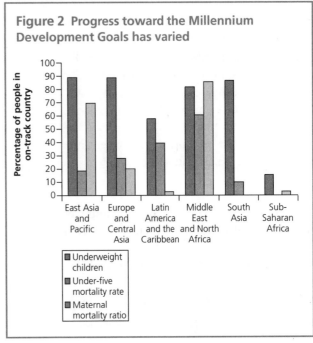

Figure 2 Progress toward the Millennium Development Goals has varied

maternal mortality, 69 percent in East Asia and Pacific, 19 percent in Europe and Central Asia, 3 percent in Sub-Saharan Africa, 2 percent in Latin America and the Caribbean, and 0 percent in Sub-Saharan Africa.

Even within a region the progress toward the Millennium Development Targets can vary tremendously.

Many countries in East Asia and Pacific reached the required annual rate of reduction to achieve the target of halving of malnutrition by 2015 in the 1990s, and the region as a whole is on track to hit the target. But several countries have not achieved the required rate of reduction.

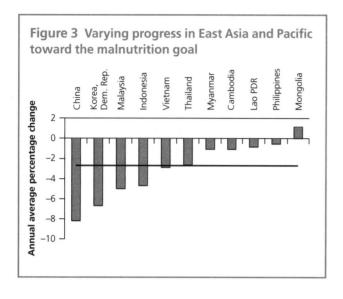

Figure 3 Varying progress in East Asia and Pacific toward the malnutrition goal

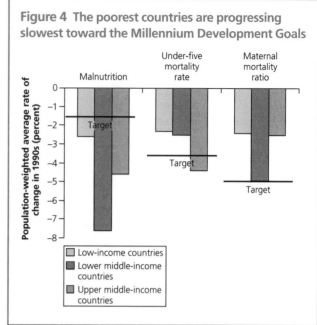

Figure 4 The poorest countries are progressing slowest toward the Millennium Development Goals

- China has been reducing malnutrition by 8.2 percent a year, Malaysia by 5 percent, Thailand by 2.7 percent (just enough to reach the goal).
- Myanmar and Cambodia have been reducing malnutrition by only 1.1 percent a year, Lao PDR by 0.9 percent, and the Philippines by 0.6 percent.
- In Mongolia malnutrition has been increasing by 1.1 percent a year.

The poorest countries are progressing slowest toward the Millennium Development Goals.

For malnutrition, under-five mortality, and maternal mortality the story is the same—the low-income countries reduced their rates least quickly in the 1990s.

- Low-income countries have been reducing malnutrition by only 2.6 percent a year, lower middle-income countries by 7.6 percent, and upper middle-income countries by 4.6 percent.
- Low-income countries have been reducing under-five mortality by 2.3 percent a year, lower middle-income countries by 2.5 percent, and upper middle-income countries by 4.9 percent.
- Low-income countries have been reducing maternal mortality by 2.4 percent a year, lower middle-income countries by 4.9 percent, and upper middle-income countries 2.5 percent.

These figures are culled from the text. Please see the text for source material.

Most of the world lives in a country where under-five mortality fell slower in the 1990s than it did in the 1980s.

Under-five mortality typically fell slower during the 1990s than it did in the 1980s.

- In South Asia only 11 percent of the people lived in a country where the rate of decline quickened in the 1990s, in East Asia and Pacific 20 percent, in Middle East and North Africa 34 percent, in Europe and Central Asia 36 percent, in Latin America and the Caribbean 38 percent, and in Sub-Saharan Africa 51 percent.

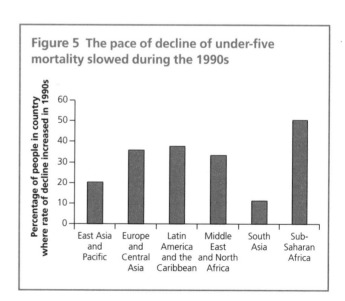

Figure 5 The pace of decline of under-five mortality slowed during the 1990s

ABBREVIATIONS

BASICS   Basic Support for Institutionalizing Child Survival

BCG   bacillus Calmette-Guerin (vaccine for tuberculosis)

DOTS   directly observed treatment, short-course (treatment regimen for tuberculosis)

DPT   diphtheria, pertussis, and tetanus

GAMET   Global HIV/AIDS Monitoring and Evaluation Support Team

GAVI   Global Alliance for Vaccines and Immunization

GDP   gross domestic product

IDA   International Development Association

IMF   International Monetary Fund

NGO   nongovernmental organization

OECD   Organisation for Economic Co-operation and Development

PAHO   Pan American Health Organization

SARS   severe acute respiratory syndrome

SEWA   Self-Employed Women's Association

TRIPS   Trade-Related Aspects of Intellectual Property Rights

UN   United Nations

UNAIDS   Joint United Nations Programme on HIV/AIDS

UNDP   United Nations Development Programme

UNICEF   United Nations International Children's Emergency Fund

USAID   United States Agency for International Development

WHO   World Health Organization

Rising to the Challenges

The scale of death and ill health in the world is staggering. In 2000 more than 11 million children died before their fifth birthday.[1] Among the world's 613 million children under five, 140 million are underweight.[1] In 1998, 843 million people were classified as undernourished on the basis of their food intake. In 2001, 3 million people died from HIV/AIDS.[2,3] Tuberculosis claimed 2 million lives, and in 1995 half a million women died during pregnancy or childbirth.

This heavy burden of death and suffering is heavily concentrated in the world's poorest countries (figure 1). Just 1 percent of the world's 11 million under-five deaths occurred in high-income countries, with 42 percent occurring in Sub-Saharan Africa alone. Almost half the world's underweight children—65 million children—live in South Asia. And 98 percent of the world's half million maternal deaths took place in the developing world—252,000 in Sub-Saharan Africa alone.[1] Within countries, too, it is the poor who shoulder the lion's share of the disease burden.

Death and disease matter in their own right, but they also act as a brake on poverty reduction. As Nobel laureate Amartya Sen recently put it, "health is among the most important conditions of human life and a critically significant constituent of human capabilities which we have reason to value."[4] But health also matters because it affects living standards—of households and countries. Health expenses can easily become burdensome for households: in Vietnam alone they are estimated to have pushed some 3 million people into poverty in 1993.[5]

Beyond its direct impact on a household's living standards through out-of-pocket expenditures, ill health has an indirect effect on labor income, through productivity and the number of hours people can spend working. The effects of illness on income may take time to appear and be long lasting. If children are malnourished, they are less likely to be in school, and they learn less when they are in school. As a result, they are less productive later in life.

The devastating economic consequences of illness and death are evident at the macroeconomic level, too. Demographic variables account for an estimated half of the difference in growth rates between Africa and the rest of the world over 1965–90.[6] Children require teachers to learn, and in some parts of Africa deaths from HIV/AIDS are making a major dent in the stock of teachers—Zambia now loses half as many teachers as it trains to HIV/AIDS.[7] The AIDS epidemic has been estimated to knock 0.3–1.5 percentage points off rates of economic growth.[8]

During the 1990s the international community became more alarmed about the scale of ill health and death in the developing world and at the growth of HIV/AIDS and tuberculosis. The decade also saw major new global health initiatives and partnerships, including UNAIDS (the Joint United Nations Programme on HIV/AIDS); the Global Alliance for Vaccines and Immunization; the Stop TB Partnership; the Global Fund to Fight AIDS, TB and Malaria; and many others. With the 1990s drawing to a close the international community decided that even more needed to be done. At the UN Millennium Summit in September 2001, 147 heads of states endorsed the Millennium Development Goals (MDGs), nearly half of which concern different aspects of health—directly or indirectly (box 1).★

★ Throughout the report, "health" is interpreted broadly. For example, nutrition is both a key aspect of health in its own right and a key influence on other aspects of health.

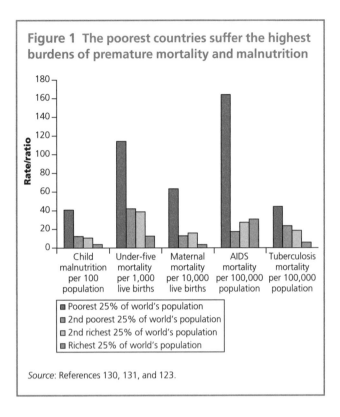

Figure 1 The poorest countries suffer the highest burdens of premature mortality and malnutrition

Child malnutrition per 100 population; Under-five mortality per 1,000 live births; Maternal mortality per 10,000 live births; AIDS mortality per 100,000 population; Tuberculosis mortality per 100,000 population

- Poorest 25% of world's population
- 2nd poorest 25% of world's population
- 2nd richest 25% of world's population
- Richest 25% of world's population

Source: References 130, 131, and 123.

Box 1 The health-related Millennium Development Goals

- Goal 1: Eradicate extreme poverty and hunger. The target is to cut in half the proportion of people who suffer from hunger between 1990 and 2015, with progress measured in terms of the prevalence of underweight children under five. The target implies an average annual rate of reduction of 2.7 percent.

- Goal 4: Reduce child mortality. The target is to reduce the under-five mortality rate by two-thirds between 1990 and 2015, equivalent to an annual rate of reduction of 4.3 percent.

- Goal 5: Improve maternal health. The target is to reduce the maternal mortality ratio by three-quarters between 1990 and 2015, equivalent to an annual rate of reduction of 5.4 percent.

- Goal 6: Combat HIV/AIDS, malaria, and other diseases. The target is to have halted and begun to reverse the spread of these diseases by 2015.

- Goal 7: Ensure environmental sustainability. The target is to cut in half the proportion of people without sustainable access to safe drinking water by 2015.

- Goal 8: Develop a global partnership for development. The target is to provide access to affordable essential drugs in developing countries.

Source: Reference 9.

The health Millennium Development Goals: Progress and prospects

Tracking progress toward the health goals is not straightforward. Good-quality trend data are available for most countries only for under-five mortality. Poorer-quality trend data are available for a limited set of countries for child malnutrition. Limited trend data are available for maternal mortality, so this study used a model to forecast rates in the 1990s and beyond. Trend data are also limited for communicable diseases, and no modeling was undertaken for the report.

A mixed score at half-time

Of the Millennium Development Goals for which trend data are available or estimated, the fastest progress has been on malnutrition (table 1). The following factors are important in interpreting the mixed score at half time:

- *The number of people living in on-track countries, not just the number of countries, matters.* Worldwide 77 percent of the people living in the developing world live in countries that are on track to meet the malnutrition target. In Sub-Saharan Africa only 15 percent of the people live in an on-track country.

- *Different indicators show different levels of improvement.* For under-five mortality the developing world managed only a 2.5 percent average annual reduction in the 1990s, well short of the target of 4.2 percent. For maternal mortality the average population-weighted decline was just 3.2 percent, far from the 5.4 percent target.

- *Health targets are relevant for middle-income countries as well as low-income countries.* Two of the most affluent regions—Europe and Central Asia and Latin America and the Caribbean—have the smallest shares of countries on track for the child mortality target (22 percent and 10 percent). Only 4 percent of countries in Latin America and the Caribbean are on track to meet the maternal mortality target.

- *Evidence on how the poor are faring within countries is mixed.* For malnutrition, within countries the poorest 20 percent of the population appears, on average, to have been experiencing broadly similar rates of reduction as the population as a whole. But for under-five mortality the rate has been falling more slowly among the poor.

Table 1 Progress toward selected health Millennium Development Goals (percent)

Region/income group	Underweight prevalence			Under-five mortality rate						Maternal mortality ratio		
	Population-weighted average, 1990s (yearly percentage change)	Share of countries on track for Millennium Development Target	Share of population living in on-track country	Population-weighted average, 1990s (yearly percentage change)	Share of countries on track for Millennium Development Target	Share of people living in on-track country	Population-weighted average, 1980s (yearly percentage change)	Share of countries with faster rate of decline in 1990s	Share of population living in country with faster rate of decline in 1990s	Population-weighted average, 1990s (yearly percentage change)	Share of countries on track for Millennium Development Target	Share of population living in on-track country
Millennium Development Target	-2.7	n.a.	n.a.	-4.3	n.a.	n.a.	n.a.	n.a.	n.a.	-5.4	n.a.	n.a.
East Asia and the Pacific	-6.7	45.5	88.7	-2.7	26.1	17.4	-2.7	56.5	20.2	-4.5	14.3	68.5
Europe and Central Asia	-9.6	37.5	88.2	-2.5	22.2	27.8	-2.8	33.3	35.8	-4.3	25.0	18.8
Latin America and the Caribbean	-4.1	50.0	57.6	-3.7	10.0	38.7	-4.4	33.3	37.7	-1.5	4.2	1.6
Middle East and North Africa	-6.3	62.5	81.5	-3.6	46.7	60.0	-5.6	26.7	33.5	-6.9	64.3	84.4
South Asia	-3.5	33.3	86.4	-2.6	25.0	9.7	-3.2	37.5	11.4	-2.9	12.5	0.0
Sub-Saharan Africa	-0.2	27.6	15.2	-0.3	0.0	0.0	-1.1	41.7	50.6	-1.6	7.3	2.7
Low income	-2.6	30.2	69.1	-2.3	6.3	14.4	-2.5	39.7	31.3	-2.4	10.3	1.3
Lower middle income	-7.6	53.8	87.3	-2.5	22.2	20.9	-3.3	40.7	19.8	-4.9	32.6	67.0
Upper middle income	-4.6	45.5	65.0	-4.4	23.5	34.2	-4.4	35.3	28.9	-2.5	5.6	2.1
High income (non–OECD)	n.a.	n.a.	n.a.	-5.7	34.4	58.6	-5.2	21.9	37.0	-1.9	10.0	1.3
High income (OECD)	n.a.	n.a.	n.a.	-4.1	62.5	41.3	-4.7	54.2	31.5	-2.5	0.0	0.0
Developing countries	-5.0	40.0	77.0	-2.5	15.9	18.7	-3.0	39.1	25.8	-3.2	17.4	32.0
Industrial countries	n.a.	n.a.	n.a.	-4.1	46.4	41.9	-4.7	35.7	31.7	-2.5	4.5	0.0
World	n.a.	n.a.	n.a.	-2.8	24.2	22.3	-3.2	38.2	26.7	-3.1	15.6	28.3

n.a. Not applicable.

Source: World Bank staff calculations; see chapter 2.

Will the second half go better?

As a comparison of the child mortality experiences in the 1980s and 1990s demonstrates, past performance is not necessarily a good predictor of future performance. The fact that a country is on track on the basis of its performance in the 1990s does not guarantee that it will maintain the required annual rate of reduction of malnutrition or mortality during 2000–15. It is also possible that countries currently off track may get on track in the second half of the Millennium Development Goal "window."

STIMULI FROM OUTSIDE THE HEALTH SECTOR CAN BE EXPECTED The World Bank estimates that economic growth will fall somewhat in East Asia and the Pacific in 2000–15, turn from negative to positive in Europe and Central Asia and Sub-Saharan Africa, and increase somewhat in Latin America and the Caribbean, the Middle East and North Africa, and South Asia.[10] Primary education completion rates will also probably grow faster in the new millennium as a result of the "Education For All" and "Fast Track" initiatives. But higher rates of educational attainment among women of childbearing age will not show up until 2005 or so, and even then the first full round of effects on under-five mortality will not be felt until 2010. More relevant is the fact that gender gaps in secondary education may well narrow more quickly in the new millennium than in the 1990s as a result of the gender Millennium Development Goal. To achieve parity with boys by 2015 in the proportion of the population 15 and over who have completed secondary education, girls' completion rates will have to grow faster in the new millennium than in the 1990s in most regions, especially in South Asia and East Asia and the Pacific. And if the water Millennium Development Goal is to be reached, access rates will need to grow much faster in 2000–15, especially in Sub-Saharan Africa.

EVEN WITH ECONOMIC GROWTH AND FASTER PROGRESS ON THE NONHEALTH GOALS, MANY REGIONS WILL STILL MISS MANY OF THE HEALTH TARGETS The combined contributions to the decline in malnutrition and mortality of faster economic growth and achieving the gender and water goals could be significant. In Europe and Central Asia progress on these fronts might add as much as 1.4 percentage points to the rate of decline of under-five mortality, 1.1 percentage points to the rate of decline of maternal mortality, and just under 1 percentage point to the annual rate of reduction in underweight children. In South Asia they might add as much as 2.6 percentage points to the annual rate of reduction in maternal mortality, taking it from 2.9 percent a year to 5.5 percent. While these contributions will push countries and regions firmly toward the targets, they will for the most part not get them there (figure 2). The picture is bleakest for under-five mortality—and for Sub-Saharan Africa. Even with Sub-Saharan Africa's extra percentage point in annual reductions in under-five mortality coming from economic growth and achievement of the gender and water goals, its projected rate of reduction of under-five mortality for 2000–15 is still only 1.6 percent a year.

WHY THE PICTURE MAY BE BLEAKER The assumptions underlying these calculations are probably overoptimistic. The gender and drinking water targets may well be missed. And contrary to what has been assumed, it is unlikely in the absence of these stimuli that the pace of decline of the Millennium Development Indicators achieved in the 1990s will continue. The three variables used to forecast maternal mortality in the model are likely to be less conducive to reductions in maternal mortality in the new millennium than in the 1990s.

The goals matter for all countries

Given the likelihood that many countries will miss several of the goals, why should they be taken seriously? The goals matter for several reasons.

- *Faster progress is important even if targets are missed.* A key message of this report is that progress can be accelerated through a judicious mix of spending and policy and institutional reform.

- *The goals facilitate benchmarking.* By focusing on a limited set of outcomes, the Millennium Development Goals show what is achievable and where faster progress can be made.

- *The poor risk being left behind.* One weakness of the Millennium Development Targets is that they are national averages and so do not remind us automatically that progress needs to be for everyone, not just the better off. Progress has been uneven, with the poorer countries lagging behind the rest. For under-five mortality, the poor within countries are lagging behind the rest of the population. Progress needs to be monitored and analyzed by income—and efforts directed toward population groups that are being left behind.

Effective interventions exist—they need to reach more people

Lack of interventions is not the obstacle to faster progress toward the goals. It is the low levels of use—especially among the poor—of interventions that work.

Figure 2 Faster economic growth and other changes outside the health sector will help move regions toward the targets, but in most cases it will not get them there

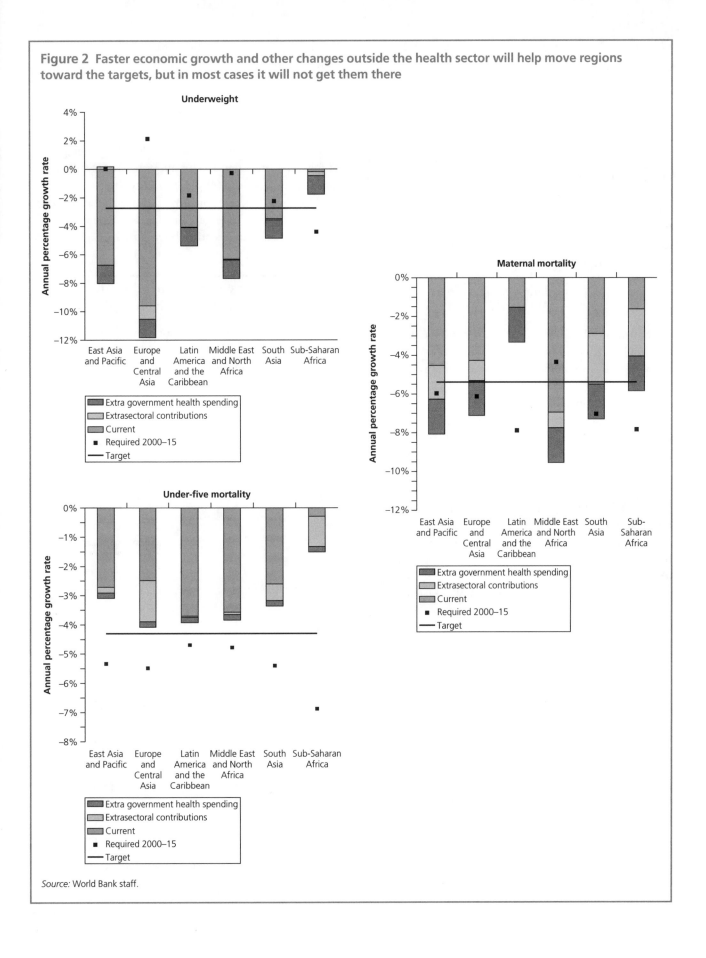

Source: World Bank staff.

The array of existing effective interventions is impressive

The available interventions constitute a powerful arsenal for preventing and treating the main causes of malnutrition and death (see chapter 3, table 3.1). Diarrhea, pneumonia, and malaria account for 52 percent of deaths among children worldwide. For each of these causes, there is at least one proven effective preventive intervention and at least one proven effective treatment intervention, each capable of being delivered in a low-income setting. In most cases, several proven effective interventions exist. For diarrhea—the second-leading cause of child deaths—there are no fewer than five proven preventive interventions and three proven treatment interventions.

Effective interventions are underused, especially by the poor

Why, then, are the high rates of malnutrition and death in the developing world so high? For one reason or another, people do not receive the effective interventions that could save their lives or make them well nourished. In upper middle-income and high-income countries, 90 percent of children receive DPT3 vaccinations, more than 90 percent of babies are delivered by a medically trained person, and more than 90 percent of pregnant women make at least one antenatal visit. In South Asia less than 50 percent of pregnant women have antenatal checkups, and only 20 percent of babies are delivered by a medically trained person. The story is similar for other childhood interventions—and for interventions for other goals. Of the estimated 6 million people in low-income and middle-income countries currently needing antiretroviral therapy, only 300,000 receive it. In Asia, where more than 7 million people are living with HIV/AIDS, no country has exceeded 5 percent antiretroviral therapy coverage.

Just as shortfalls in coverage vary across countries, they vary within countries, with the poor and other deprived groups invariably lagging behind. These groups are less likely to receive full basic immunization coverage, have their deliveries attended by a medically trained person, or make at least one antenatal care visit to a medically trained person. On the positive side, the poor for the most part are making faster progress in coverage, reflecting that the better off already have high coverage rates for many interventions. Progress has been more propoor in professionally delivered interventions.

Underuse of effective interventions costs lives

The low use of effective interventions—in the developing world in general and among the poor in particular—translates into rates of mortality, morbidity, and malnutrition that are far higher than they need be.

If use of all the proven effective childhood preventive and treatment interventions were to rise from current levels to 99 percent (95 percent for breastfeeding), the number of under-five deaths worldwide could fall by as much as 63 percent.[11] Deaths from malaria and measles could be all but eliminated. And deaths from diarrhea, pneumonia, and HIV/AIDS could be dramatically reduced. If coverage rates of the key maternal mortality interventions were increased from current levels to 99 percent, 391,000 maternal deaths worldwide—74 percent of current maternal deaths—might be averted. One intervention stands out as especially important: access to essential obstetric care, which accounts for more than half the deaths averted (figure 3).

What countries need to do to rise to the challenges

If the lack of interventions is not keeping countries from achieving the goals, what is? What do countries need to do to accelerate progress toward them?

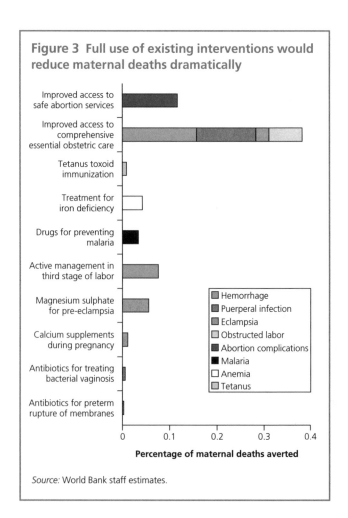

Figure 3 Full use of existing interventions would reduce maternal deaths dramatically

Source: World Bank staff estimates.

Extra government health spending is needed, but it is not enough

Some argue that the cause of slow progress is the lack of government health spending.[12] The evidence presented in support of this view is not altogether compelling. Arbitrary assumptions are made about the links between scaling up expenditures and intervention coverage rates, and no explicit assumptions are made about the links between coverage levels and health outcomes. There is no assurance that incurring the extra government health spending claimed to be necessary would reduce mortality at all—let alone by the proportions required to reach the goals.

In fact, some writers have argued that government health spending has little impact at the margin on health outcomes, once the effects of other determinants have been accounted for. The reason? The many weak links in the chain running from government spending to health outcomes.[13–15] Their evidence has limitations. It refers simply to child mortality, not to health outcomes in general. It indicates what happens to child mortality among the whole population, in an average country, and therefore hides significant spending effects among specific subpopulations and in well-governed countries.[16–19] And it indicates what would happen to child mortality if additional government spending were to take the form of a proportional scaling up of all government health programs, not what would happen if extra spending were focused on specific subpopulations or specific programs.

Policies and institutions mediate the impact of government health spending

In countries with good governance, additional government health spending does reduce child mortality.[19] This result is consistent with recent studies that find that the elasticity of infant mortality to development assistance depends on the quality of a country's policies and institutions. Development assistance has a stronger effect in countries with strong policies and institutions than in countries with only average quality policies and institutions—and an insignificant effect in countries where policies and institutions are weak.[20,21] The assertion is also consistent with the findings of a study undertaken for this report, which includes other outcomes alongside child mortality and uses the Bank's Country Policy and Institutional Assessment index[†] to measure the quality of policies and institutions.

How much would reaching the goals cost in well-governed countries?

Well-governed countries with good policies and institutions could, in principle, achieve the goals simply by scaling up their expenditures on existing programs in proportion to current allocations. In practice, however, the amount of extra spending required would likely be prohibitive. Take East Asia and the Pacific. If economic growth proceeds as expected and the other relevant Millennium Development Targets are hit, the region would achieve the required rates of reduction of underweight and maternal mortality even without additional government health spending. But it would miss the under-five mortality target. To hit this target, a minimum of five percentage points would need to be added to the rate of growth of the government health share of GDP. That would take the projected share of GDP spent on government health programs to 3.7 percent in 2015—more than twice what it would be if the 1990s pattern of growth continues.

In Sub-Saharan Africa the conclusions are even starker. Even if faster economic growth materializes and the other targets are hit, the share of government health spending in GDP would need to grow by an additional 12.3 percentage points a year, taking the share to 12.2 percent in 2015. Compare that with a 2000 figure of 1.8 percent and a 2015 forecast of 2.2 percent based on the 1990s annual growth of just 1.2 percent in the government health share of GDP.

Poorly governed countries cannot expect to make much progress toward the Millennium Development Goals simply by scaling up their expenditures on existing programs in proportion to current allocations. And while well-governed countries could in principle simply scale up existing spending to reach the targets, this is unlikely to be affordable—for them or for their donors.

What are the implications for health spending? The first is that targeting additional government spending is important for both sets of countries. The second is that building good policies and institutions is important for all countries: it increases the productivity not just of additional spending but also of existing spending commitments. But what do better policies and institutions entail in the health sector? Health systems are very broad—far broader than many people think. Weak policies and institutions can arise at several points along the pathway from government health spending to health outcomes (figure 4). The report uses this framework to tackle the difficult question of how to build stronger policies and institutions.

---

† The Country Policy and Institutional Assessment is an annual assessment by World Bank staff of the quality of International Bank for Reconstruction and Development and International Development Association borrowers' policy and institutional performance in areas relevant to economic growth and poverty reduction. It consists of 20 equally weighted criteria representing policy dimensions of an effective poverty reduction and growth strategy, such as economic management, structural policies, policies for social inclusion and equity, and public sector management.

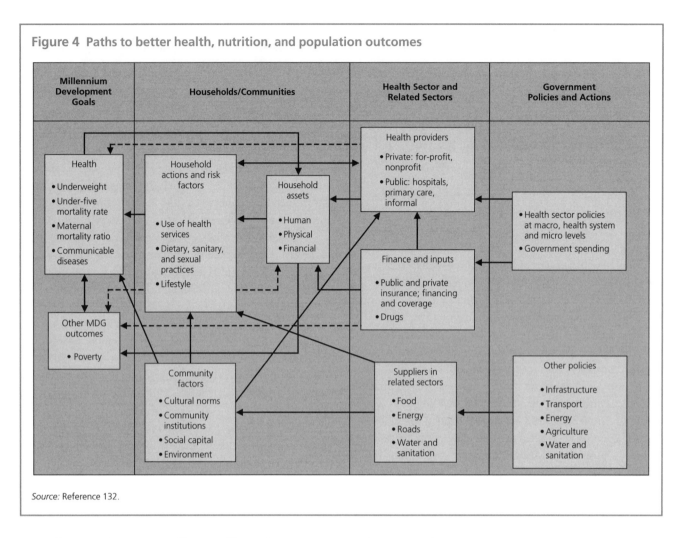

Figure 4 Paths to better health, nutrition, and population outcomes

| Millennium Development Goals | Households/Communities | Health Sector and Related Sectors | Government Policies and Actions |

Health
• Underweight
• Under-five mortality rate
• Maternal mortality ratio
• Communicable diseases

Household actions and risk factors
• Use of health services
• Dietary, sanitary, and sexual practices
• Lifestyle

Household assets
• Human
• Physical
• Financial

Health providers
• Private: for-profit, nonprofit
• Public: hospitals, primary care, informal

Health sector policies at macro, health system and micro levels
• Government spending

Finance and inputs
• Public and private insurance; financing and coverage
• Drugs

Other MDG outcomes
• Poverty

Community factors
• Cultural norms
• Community institutions
• Social capital
• Environment

Suppliers in related sectors
• Food
• Energy
• Roads
• Water and sanitation

Other policies
• Infrastructure
• Transport
• Energy
• Agriculture
• Water and sanitation

Source: Reference 132.

Improving expenditure allocations and targeting

Geographic targeting

In most countries, governments spend most of their money in cities, and spending disproportionately benefits the better off.[22,23] Resource allocation formulas can be used to reduce government spending gaps across regions.[24] In Bolivia, which has used such formulas since 1994 as part of its decentralization efforts, some fairly large—and propoor—improvements in maternal and child health indicators have occurred. Targeting resources to poor regions and provinces may benefit from nontraditional mechanisms for priority-setting and implementation, such as social investment funds. A recent impact evaluation in Bolivia concluded that such funds were responsible for a decline in under-five mortality from 88.5 per 1,000 live births to 65.6.[25]

Changing the allocation of spending across levels of care

Developing country spending on health is characterized by a surprisingly high concentration of spending on secondary and tertiary infrastructure and personnel—despite low bed occupancy rates. Some governments have tried to scale back the share of hospital spending. Tanzania, for example, reduced the share from 60 percent in 2000 to 43 percent in 2002.

Simply reallocating the budget toward primary care need not result in higher payoffs to government health spending in lower malnutrition and child and maternal mortality, however.[14,15] In many instances service providers have failed to deliver good-quality care and use resources efficiently. The trick is to couple expenditure reallocations with measures to improve the performance of primary care facilities and district hospitals—and measures to ensure that households actually demand relevant interventions.

Targeting specific programs

Programs such as the directly observed treatment, short-course for tuberculosis (DOTS) and Integrated Management of Childhood Illness for child health are good examples of programs that may yield high returns to government spending at the margin. Both are the subject of ongoing evaluation, but early results are encouraging.[26,27] A recent World Bank study[28] in India provides further support for the idea that the way government spending is allocated across programs makes a difference to its impact on the Millennium Development Indicators.

Targeting specific population groups

Many countries subsidize all government health services for everyone. These blanket subsidy schemes fail to target interventions that give rise to externalities, and they fail to disproportionately benefit the poor—this, despite the stronger equity case for subsidizing their care and the fact that they tend to bear a disproportionate burden of malnutrition and child and maternal mortality.

Targeting spending to remove bottlenecks

Another approach is to assess the health sector impediments to faster progress in a country, identify ways to remove them, and estimate both the costs of removing them and the likely impacts of their removal on Millennium Development Goal outcomes.[29] Work along these lines—sometimes referred to as marginal budgeting for bottlenecks—has begun in several African countries and India.[30] In Mali key bottlenecks were identified for supporting home-based practices and delivering periodic and continual professional care. These included low access to affordable commodities and the need for community-based support for home-based care; low geographical access to preventive professional care (immunization, vitamin A supplementation, and antenatal care); shortages of qualified nurses and midwives; and an absence of effective third-party payment mechanisms for the poor for professional continuous care.

Combining estimates of the costs of measures to remove these bottlenecks with estimates of the mortality reduction on their removal gives an elasticity of mortality to government health spending that compares very favorably with the elasticities for untargeted government health spending—even those for well-governed countries with good policies and institutions. Only time—and careful monitoring and evaluation—will tell whether these estimates turn out to be accurate.

Better policies toward households—as producers and demanders of care

Improving people's health is the overarching aim of the health sector. But households are not just the endpoint of the sector's activity.[‡] They are major actors. Indeed, they play a dual role: as users of health services delivered by professional

providers (if patients don't demand care, providers cannot deliver it) and as producers of health through the delivery of home-based interventions and in their everyday health behaviors (this is especially important for child health). In both roles they face barriers. Policymakers need to be aware of those barriers and to formulate appropriate policies.

Lowering financial barriers

Low income is a barrier to the use of most health interventions. Economic growth is therefore an important weapon in the war against malnutrition and mortality.[31,32] But social protection programs are also important. South Africa's old-age pension scheme increased the height of under-five black children by eight centimeters, half a year's growth.[33,34] Also important are informal community solidarity schemes, which often substitute for formal social protection programs.[35]

The other part of the affordability equation is price. Higher money prices tend to reduce demand—especially among the poor—unless accompanied by improvements in service quality.[36] In many cases out-of-pocket payments are informal rather than formal.[37] And it is not just the payments to health providers that matter—users of health services incur other money costs in using health facilities, including transportation costs.

User charges for Millennium Development Goal interventions are to be discouraged. Why? Many of these interventions involve benefits that spill over to people who do not receive the intervention (immunization is a classic example). But an equity case can also be made for reducing prices facing the poor and near-poor, even where there are no spillovers. Subsidies should thus be targeted to services with spillovers and to the poor. In practice, they are often badly targeted in at least one respect if not both. There are exceptions, however. In Ifakara, Tanzania, a voucher program for mosquito nets was launched successfully for pregnant women and children under five.[38–40] And in Indonesia a health card introduced during the economic crisis increased use among the poor.[41]

Some recent programs, especially in Latin America, have not simply made health care affordable for the poor—they have made it profitable. Rather than simply reducing the cost of using specific interventions these programs provide cash payments to users, linked to specific interventions and restricted to certain groups—often poor mothers and their children. The experience with these programs, in targeting and impact, is encouraging.[42–47]

There is another reason for limiting user charges. Risk aversion coupled with the unpredictability of illness provides a motivation for pooling risks through an insurance scheme. Lack of insurance and the consequent exposure to the risk of medical expenses cause households to hold more wealth (and more of their wealth in liquid form) than they

---

‡ The term "household" is used here to refer to whatever grouping of people share responsibility for health. It is not limited to parents (caregivers of children might be grandparents, aunts, stepparents) and can encompass the broad array of kinship and household patterns around the world.

otherwise would in the hope that they can smooth their consumption when health shocks occur.[48] Evidence from rural China suggests that households fail in these efforts and that the poor have the least success in self-insuring against income shocks.[49] Insurance in the developing world is very limited, and those who are least able to smooth consumption without insurance are the least likely to have insurance coverage.[50] Governments have a role to play here. In Egypt a school health insurance program for all children attending school resulted in larger increases in coverage among the poor than among other groups and achieved considerable impact on use and out-of-pocket expenditures.[51]

Empowering women

Women exercise little control over household resources in many countries. All else constant, such women are less likely to receive antenatal care, to have antenatal visits, and to have visits in the first trimester of pregnancy.[52] Microcredit programs aimed at poor women are thought to be one way of increasing women's financial autonomy. Whether they increase the use of maternal and health services is less clear.[53] Also important is a woman's ability to make decisions more generally. In India, although contraceptives are readily available in retail shops, community pressure or disapproval by husbands often prevent women from using them.

Providing information—enhancing knowledge

Lack of knowledge is a major factor behind poor health. It results in people not seeking care when they need it, despite the absence of price barriers. In Bolivia a large fraction of poor babies are not delivered by a trained attendant even though the mothers are eligible for free care under the Maternal and Child Health Insurance program.[54] Lack of knowledge also results in people, especially poor people, seeking and receiving inappropriate care—and paying for it.[55] Ignorance may also result in people not getting the maximum health gain out of inputs they have available to them for use. Many people do not know that piped water in many countries requires further purification or that hand-washing confers much of the health benefit of piped water. Not surprisingly, piped water has a much greater impact on the prevalence of diarrhea among the children of the better off and better educated.[56]

Better-educated women—especially those with a secondary education—achieve better health outcomes for themselves and their children.[57] They do this not by using health-specific knowledge that they acquire at school but by using general numeracy and literacy skills learned at school to acquire health-specific knowledge later in life.[58] So, while better-educated girls will mean healthier women and healthier children in years to come, a shorter and more direct route to increasing health-specific knowledge

and skills is through information dissemination and counseling in the health sector.

One venue for delivering health messages is the public facility. A lactation clinic at the Children's Hospital in Islamabad, Pakistan, promoted exclusive breastfeeding by altering women's perceptions of its importance and by counseling them on techniques.[59] But a focus on public health facilities is far from ideal, since many people, including many poor people, do not use them when they fall ill—and may not even seek care at all. Programs in the community—where the conveyers of knowledge seek out target groups—seem likely to have a better chance of reaching a broader group and reaching the poor.

There are several success stories here. In Brazil health knowledge among mothers and feeding practices improved after health workers trained by the Integration of Childhood Management Illness provided information and counseling at health facilities and in the community.[30] After only 18 months the nutritional status of children in the area improved as well. Social marketing and media campaigns have also proved effective in some circumstances.[38,39,60]

Reducing time costs

Transportation systems, road infrastructure, and geography influence the demand for care delivered by formal providers through their impact on time costs, which can be substantial.[61–65] In rural communities, where roads are poor and transport unreliable, the time spent waiting for transport is also a major cost. Time costs tend to be a major issue for maternal mortality. Health centers are unable to provide essential obstetric care for a complicated delivery, and hospitals, which could provide the needed care, are hard to reach. Road rehabilitation and other transport projects are important here.[66] But so are subsidies linked to the use of health services. Malaysia and Sri Lanka provide free or subsidized transportation to hospitals in emergencies.[67] Other options to tackle inaccessibility include engaging in outreach, building new public facilities in underserved areas, and establishing partnerships between government and nongovernmental organizations (NGOs), private providers, or community organizations.

Providing access to water and sanitation

The availability of plenty of water and improved sanitation are associated with better maternal and child health outcomes, at least among the better educated, even after controlling for other influences.[61,63,68–74] This isn't altogether surprising. Hand-washing is easier if the household has piped water that provides readily available quantities of safe water. And the safe disposal of feces is easier if the household has an improved form of sanitation. The developing world lags well behind the industrial world in both—and poor people fare especially badly. They are less likely to be connected to a network, and the sources they rely on tend to be more costly per liter than the networked services used by the better off.[75]

The two challenges from a health perspective are to increase access to water and sanitation infrastructure and to ensure that people know how to get the maximum health benefits from such investments. The first was addressed extensively in the World Bank's 2004 *World Development Report: Making Services Work for Poor People*.[75] The second is addressed in chapter 8 of this volume.

Improving health service delivery

Health providers—in both the public and private sectors, and in both the formal and informal sectors—deliver interventions of relevance to the Millennium Development Goals. Many are efficient, deliver high-quality care, and are responsive to their patients. But many are not. As a result, resources—public and private—are wasted and facilities sit underused. Patients often receive care—and pay for it, out of very limited means—that is inappropriate to their needs. They may also receive downright dangerous care.

Two things can make a difference. One is the quality of management. Better management means a clearer delineation of responsibilities and accountabilities inside organizations, a clearer link between performance and reward, and so on. Management means getting accountabilities right within an organization. The other thing that can make a difference is getting accountabilities right between the organization and the public.[75] Some strategies work along a "short route" leading directly from the patient to the provider (figure 5). Others work along a "long route"

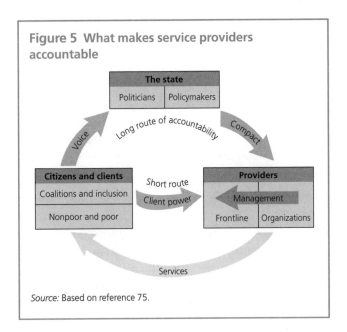

Figure 5 What makes service providers accountable

Source: Based on reference 75.

leading from the citizen to the policymaker and thence to the provider. Still others work along both routes simultaneously.

Improving management—increasing accountability within provider organizations

Much of the world's public sector is managed through what is, in effect, a command-and-control structure. Initiative and decisionmaking are exercised only at the highest level. Problems at lower levels are passed up to higher levels for decisions. There are few managers in the true sense of the word. Instead, administrators execute decisions according to previously agreed protocols and rules, with little or no scope for autonomous decisionmaking at facilities.

Management styles have recently begun to change, though the impact is not altogether clear. Responsibility for tasks and decisionmaking is delegated to specific parts of the organization and to specific individuals. Individual accountability is emphasized, and there is a focus on performance—not inputs or processes but outputs and outcomes. Good performance is rewarded, financially or in some other way. There is also a focus on clients and a belief that an organization is ultimately accountable to its clients. A client-oriented strategy emphasizes customer choice and satisfaction. Business techniques enhance performance and are a standard part of strategic planning.

The new approach is evident in several countries, including Malaysia. Elements of the approach are also evident in successful nutrition and child health programs. In the Tamil Nadu Integrated Nutrition Program, in India, community nutrition workers were given clearly defined duties. Information on outputs enabled the community to keep them accountable, but it also enabled the nutrition workers to see how their program was working. In the Programa de Agentes de Saude, in Céara, Brazil, health agents and nurse-supervisors were assigned clear tasks and given clear responsibilities. The program has been credited with substantially reducing child mortality.[76] The intended outcomes of the program were emphasized to health workers and members of the public. Good team performance was rewarded with a prize. And health agents were held accountable through community-based monitoring.

Increasing the accountability of provider organizations to the public

GOVERNANCE PARTICIPATION Having community representatives participate in the governance and oversight of providers can improve the productivity and quality of public sector providers. Relatively little is known about the impact, and several governments have had difficulty establishing meaningful participation. But where it has been established, the changes have been for the better. In Burkino Faso participation of community representatives in public primary healthcare clinics increased immunization coverage, the availability of essential drugs, and the percentage of women with two or more antenatal visits.[77] In Peru comparisons of primary healthcare clinics with and without governance participation indicated that governance was associated with decreases in staff absenteeism and waiting times and increases in perceived quality by patients.[22,78] The approach probably works best for primary care and when strong technical and advisory support is provided to community representatives.

CONTRACTING Contracting can take the form of internal contracts within the public sector or external contracts between the public sector and the private sector, whether nonprofit or for-profit. Contracts are between the policymaker and the provider, specifying remuneration for the delivery of certain types of service, with or without a quality threshold. Payment is tied to some measurable aspect of performance. Some contracting arrangements also strengthen the short route of accountability—by encouraging patients to choose between providers and having the payment follow the patient, for example. Contracts with NGOs commonly include outreach in urban slums for health promotion or education, services for stigmatized or hard-to-reach groups, and social marketing of priority health goods or services, such as condoms and oral rehydration salts. In the for-profit private sector, contracting often focuses on primary care services and services for which the public sector lacks capacity, such as diagnostic and high-tech services.

Evidence on the impact of contracting within the public sector is mixed, but such contracting seems to work best in middle-income countries. In several countries in Europe and Central Asia, there is evidence of positive impact from performance-based payment at the primary care level.[79–82] In Argentina and Nicaragua social security institutes have increased productivity by establishing capitation-based payments for an integrated package of inpatient and ambulatory services.[83] In several countries in Europe and Central Asia the introduction of capped case-based payments for inpatient services was followed by an increase in services and a reduction in average length of stay.[79] Quality has not deteriorated because of skimping on costly unobservable aspects of quality. In the former Soviet republics and in Latin America, however, the results are more ambiguous. Key influences on the success of contracts within the public sector include whether the provider has the ability to respond, whether service commitments are congruent with funding levels, whether output and key components of performance expectations are easily measurable (as in primary health care), and how far capacity-strengthening of the payer or funder is addressed as a central part of the initiative.

Contracting with nonprofits is most common in low-income countries. Most cases have had positive impacts on target outcome or output variables. In Bangladesh contracts with nonprofits for the planning and implementation of an expanded program on immunization was credited with a dramatic increase in immunization. In Haiti contracting for a primary healthcare package also significantly increased immunization coverage.[84] In Bangladesh, Madagascar, and Senegal significant reductions in nutrition rates were attributed to contracting initiatives.[85] Only a few cases assess efficiency. Contracting with nonprofits works best when the contractors have well-functioning accountability arrangements and strong intrinsic motivation. The government needs to be capable of assessing, selecting, and managing the ongoing relationship with contractors. It must be able to fulfill its side of the deal (contractual agreements on funding are genuine) and not interfere with the running of the services.

Results on contracting with for-profits are mixed. Efficiency gains were achieved in contracting for high-tech diagnostic services in Thailand.[86] But experience from the hospital sector warns that weak government contracting capacity often allows the provider to capture efficiency gains or expand volume to generate more income. In Zimbabwe the cost per service decreased, but the lack of volume control led to an increase in total cost.[87] Other adverse outcomes are also possible. In Brazil contracting with for-profit hospitals led to increases in access but also to false billing and cream-skimming to avoid costly patients.[88] These problems seem less pronounced in primary health care. In Peru and El Salvador contracting with private primary healthcare providers increased access, choice, and consumer satisfaction.[89] Contracting with for-profit providers seems to work best when the government invests in the development of capacity to manage the contracting process,[90] when quality is at least as high in the private sector as in the public sector (ability to monitor quality is usually low), and when it involves primary care or other relatively observable services (diagnostic services).

DECENTRALIZATION Decentralization can increase patient leverage because local governments are more easily pressured than central ones. It strengthens policymaker-provider accountability because the government supervisor gets closer to the provider. But the impact of decentralization on the health sector has been mixed in low-income countries. In Tanzania it improved the efficiency of and access to primary healthcare services, but in Ghana efficiency declined.[91] There is less evidence on the impact in middle-income countries, though in Colombia it has improved both responsiveness and equity.[92] One important factor influencing the success of decentralization is whether the other arm of the long route of accountability (the voter-policymaker link) is functioning well. Also important are building local government capacity—planning, supervision, budgeting, expenditure and financial management—and setting up mechanisms to ensure continuing capacity to cover core public functions.

Ensuring adequate human resources for health

A common lament in international health is that faster progress toward the health-related Millennium Development Goals is being impeded by a variety of human resources problems.

The issues

Human resource stocks in health are often low, and in some countries they are falling. In Europe and Central Asia there are on average 3.1 physicians per 1,000 population, in Sub-Saharan Africa just 0.1. Tanzania is projected to see its health workforce fall from 49,000 in 1994 to 36,000 in 2015.[93] Many developing countries appear to face the double burden of low personnel inflows and high personnel outflows.[94–98]

Skills are often woefully inadequate, with misdiagnosis and mistreatment commonplace.[99] Even if the correct treatment is administered, there is no assurance that it will be administered successfully. In the public sector in India in the early 1990s less than 45 percent of patients diagnosed with tuberculosis were successfully treated.[100]

It is not just the level of skills that matter—it is also the skill mix. A recent study in Tanzania found an excess of unskilled labor of 5,000 full-time equivalents and a shortage of skilled labor of 8,000.[93]

Low application to the job is another concern. Recent random surveys of primary health facilities in six developing countries found absenteeism rates of between 19 percent (Papua New Guinea) and 43 percent (India).[75] In Tanzania time-and-motion studies showed overall staff productivity in public facilities as low as 57 percent, with only 37 percent of staff time spent on patient care and as much as 10 percent spent on irregular breaks and social contacts.[101]

Narrowing compensation differentials

Low wages in the medical professions relative to wages in other professions discourage people from entering training institutions, completing their studies, and joining the profession if they graduate. They also encourage people in the profession to think about leaving—to exit from the labor force, join another profession, or leave for another country.[102] And they encourage absenteeism, which makes for higher workloads for those left behind, further reducing motivation and prompting further absenteeism and exits. Low rates of compensation in rural settings help explain rural-urban imbalances. And compensation differentials between the public and private sectors influence transitions from the public sector to the private—and occasionally back again.

Narrowing compensation differentials is clearly an important potential policy tool. Thailand has attracted back medical professionals through a reverse brain-drain program offering generous research funding and monetary incentives.[103] Zambia more than doubled nursing salaries with the support of 16 development partners. Several countries have experimented with bonus schemes for health workers working in rural areas, some successfully.

There are, however, limits to what can be achieved through changes in compensation alone. Fortunately, research suggests that nonpecuniary aspects of jobs also matter to people. A recent study from India shows what public and private health workers hope to get from their job and the extent to which they get it (figure 6).[104] It shows that in the public sector, health workers want—and have—good working relationships with colleagues, freedom from political interference, and absence of bribes. What they lack are the tools and materials they need to apply their skills, training opportunities and opportunities to advance, employment benefits, good physical working conditions, income, and time for personal and family life. A recent study in Uganda found that medical staff working in religious nonprofit institutions work for a wage below the market rate but that these institutions provide more propoor services than other providers and more services with a public good element—dimensions of the job that the underpaid staff presumably derive some satisfaction from.[105] There would seem to be much scope for using the results of such studies to build feasible and better human resource policies.

Refining recruitment and training

People raised in rural areas are more likely to practice in rural locations and to choose family medicine.[106] In Thailand rural recruitment and training yielded some success. Evidence suggests that rural service of graduates lengthened, with two-thirds of the graduates continuing their rural placement after their compulsory years.[103]

Training opportunities are clearly valued by health workers. But training makes health workers more marketable and

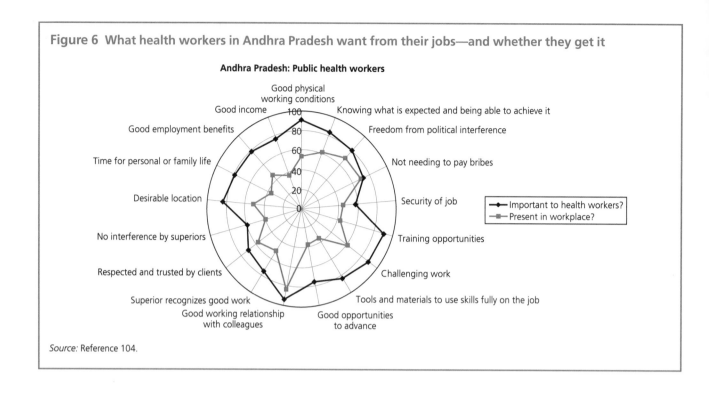

Figure 6 What health workers in Andhra Pradesh want from their jobs—and whether they get it

Andhra Pradesh: Public health workers

Good physical working conditions

Good income

Good employment benefits

Time for personal or family life

Desirable location

No interference by superiors

Respected and trusted by clients

Superior recognizes good work

Good working relationship with colleagues

Good opportunities to advance

Tools and materials to use skills fully on the job

Challenging work

Training opportunities

Security of job

Not needing to pay bribes

Freedom from political interference

Knowing what is expected and being able to achieve it

—◆— Important to health workers?
—■— Present in workplace?

Source: Reference 104.

more likely to leave the public sector for the private sector or foreign countries. One way around this is to focus government spending on the development of specific skills and to leave health workers themselves to pay—in the form of lower wages—for any general training. This seems sensible in the light of the emerging evidence on the poaching and international migration of health workers. The countries that have emulated the training standards of industrial countries (such as Ghana) are those that have been most vulnerable to poaching by them.[75] Training in areas of special relevance to the goals—such as Integrated Management of Childhood Illness[107,108]—provides a good example of specific training unlikely to be especially valued in industrial countries.

Realigning the skills mix represents another option. Many interventions for the Millennium Development Goals can be delivered by relatively low-skilled providers, such as community health workers. In addition to being cheaper, these providers are more likely to be willing to work in rural areas and less likely to lured away by the private sector, urban provider organizations, or foreign health sectors.

Ensuring appropriate and affordable medicines and other health supplies

Medicines and other commodities are key components of the arsenal of effective interventions against child and maternal mortality, and against communicable disease mortality. Here, too, are major concerns.

Getting drugs to the frontline

Some countries have succeeded in improving the supply chain through better logistics. In Ghana, as part of the "Strategies for Enhancing Access to Medicines" initiative funded by the Bill and Melinda Gates Foundation, part of the drug distribution system has undergone innovative reforms to improve mission hospitals' use of medicines, with good results. Better management is important. But without institutional arrangements that give the right incentives to the different actors involved in drug distribution and prescription, drug availability will improve only marginally.

Where drugs are not in facilities, part of the reason—sometimes a major reason—is that providers have little incentive to have them there. Surveys in Uganda suggest that on average about 70 percent of medical supplies and drugs in public facilities were appropriated by staff for use in their private work.[109–111] Where providers have an incentive to have the drugs available, they often are. The concern then is that they will prescribe inappropriate or poor-quality drugs. Limiting this through regulation and behavior change is not impossible, but it is not easy either. There may be scope in changing the incentive arrangements in the distribution of drugs—by contracting out the distribution of medicines to the private sector, for example.

Information asymmetries and drug regulation

Health education in various forms (providing information on dosages and how to administer to patients) and building trust between patients and prescribers have helped increase patient compliance and reduce high levels of self-medication.[112] A mix of interactive group discussions with mothers, training seminars for various providers at the community level, and districtwide monitoring has reduced the "irrational" use of injections for children.[113] But behavior change programs directed at providers and retailers will have only limited effects if they have strong economic incentives not to be responsible in their prescribing behavior.

All countries require some form of drug regulatory framework. It is unreasonable and largely inappropriate to expect developing countries to set up a drug regulatory authority with the resources and capacity of, say, the U.S. Food and Drug Administration or the European Medicines Agency. Policymakers can, however, usefully explore, identify, and set up a drug regulatory authority that implements the most essential functions in an efficient, transparent, and affordable way.

Policies toward drug prices and drug spending

Drug costs are often not covered by insurance at all, or they are covered only partially. This reflects both the lack of insurance in the developing world and the tendency to exclude at least some (usually outpatient) drug costs from schemes that do exist. The exclusion of outpatient drug costs makes little sense, since it deters people from both taking preventive care and seeking care from a low-level provider as soon as they fall ill. They may well get even sicker later and end up in the hospital, where they incur large inpatient bills against which they are fully covered.

Governments have ways of influencing drug prices—both the prices they (and ultimately taxpayers) pay when they subsidize the cost and the prices consumers pay out of pocket. They can exert a direct influence over retail prices by regulating them (through fixed prices, risk-sharing agreements, and reference-based pricing schemes). They can also influence retail prices indirectly through their policies toward the domestic pharmaceutical industry. And they can make large bulk purchases from manufacturers and then sell drugs at wholesale prices to the private non-profit sector. Whether governments sell the drugs they purchase or keep them for use or sale in their own facilities, they can exert a major influence over drug prices by engaging in strategic purchasing—purchasing from abroad, pooling procurement efforts with other groups (including international agencies), and focusing on generics.

Research and development and intellectual property

The lengthening of patents under the Trade-Related Aspects of International Property Rights agreement led to concerns that new drugs would become even less affordable to developing countries. In August 2003 it was agreed that countries facing public health emergencies without the capacity to manufacture medicines could still use the Doha compulsory licensing opportunities by contracting with foreign firms. So far, the provision has been cited to increase the supply only of antiretroviral therapy. An additional route to making antiretrovirals affordable is the Accelerating Access Initiative, launched by five UN agencies and five pharmaceutical companies to reduce the high cost of antiretroviral drugs and increase access to HIV/AIDS care and treatment. One way out of the impasse on neglected diseases is to separate research and development from drug manufacturing and sales.[114] Industrial countries, donors, or foundations would commit to purchasing—for a sizable fee—the patent resulting from the development of a major new vaccine or drug and then make the patent available freely to drug manufacturers. Another innovative idea is the global public-private partnership known as the International AIDS Vaccine Initiative, a public-private partnership supporting and speeding vaccine development in order to expand the number and quality of new vaccines.

Strengthening core public health functions

Vulnerable populations need to be informed, educated, and protected from risks and damages. Public health regulations need to be established and enforced. Infrastructure needs to be in place to reduce the impact of emergencies and disasters on health. All this needs to be done through a public health system that is transparent and accountable.

Developing country governments generally recognize that these public health functions are important, but they often lack the capacity and financial resources to implement them. Indeed, few low-income countries invest in these public health functions.

National strategies for disease prevention, treatment, and control

By employing skilled public health professionals, the government can develop and enforce standards, monitor the health of communities and populations, and emphasize health education, public information, health promotion, and disease prevention. Public action can help improve consumer knowledge and change attitudes so that private markets can operate effectively to meet the needs of the poor—through, for example, the social marketing of insecticide-treated bednets to reduce transmission of malaria or condoms to reduce transmission of HIV.

Government-led monitoring and evaluation

Integrated disease surveillance, program assessment, and collection and analysis of demographic and vital registration data are essential if governments and donors are to ascertain whether policies and programs are having an impact on the health goals. Chapter 2 presents a list of intermediate indicators and "proxies" for the goals that can help monitor progress, test the impact of policies, and adjust programs going forward. There is a need for much greater investments in systems to monitor these intermediate indicators. Disease surveillance then helps determine whether health outcomes are improving.

Some good practices in surveillance are being developed, in Brazil and elsewhere. But not all developing countries can afford to invest in the infrastructure required for strong surveillance systems. Most rely on alternative short- to medium-term solutions for data gathering, such as intermittent household surveys, health facility surveys, and simplified facility-based routine reporting. A few countries have made special efforts to improve the surveillance of a specific intervention, such as tuberculosis treatment or immunization, while others attempt to monitor progress toward a specific Millennium Development Goal. Some governments are explicitly developing or modifying their monitoring and evaluation framework to focus on the goals.

Intersectoral actions—going beyond the ministry of health

Significant potential exists for intersectoral synergies in meeting the Millennium Development Goals. Roads and transport are vital for health services, especially for reducing maternal mortality. But it is not just physical infrastructure that matters. Also important are the availability of transportation and the affordability of its use.[115] Transport and roads are complementary to health services. A 10-year study in Rajasthan, India, found that better roads and transport helped women reach referral facilities, but many women died anyway because there were no corresponding improvements at household and facility levels.[116]

Improved hygiene (hand-washing) and sanitation (using latrines, safely disposing of children's stools) are at least as important as drinking water quality in shaping health outcomes, specifically on reducing diarrhea and associated child mortality.[117] Constructing water supply and sanitation facilities is not enough to improve health outcomes—sustained human behavior change must accompany the infrastructure investment. In collaboration with other sectors, the health sector can develop public health promotion and education strategies and implement them in collaboration with agencies that plan, develop, and manage water resources. The health sector can also work with the private sector to manufacture, distribute, and promote affordable in-home water purification solutions and safe storage vessels—and advocate for water, sanitation, and hygiene interventions in poverty-reduction strategies.

Indoor air pollution is caused by the use of low-cost, traditional energy sources, such as coal and biomass (wood and cow dung) for cooking and heating, the main source of energy for about 3.5 billion people. Indoor air pollution is a major risk factor for pneumonia and associated deaths in children and for lung cancer in women who risk exposure during cooking. Projects in China, Guatemala, and India are under way to improve access to efficient and affordable energy sources through local design, manufacturing, and dissemination of low-cost technologies, modern fuel alternatives, and renewable energy solutions.[118] The community-based project in China was initiated by the health sector, troubled by the leveling off of child mortality reductions among the rural poor.

Agricultural policies and practices influence food prices, farm incomes, diet diversity and quality, and household food security. Policies that focus on women's access to land, training, and agricultural inputs; on their roles in production; and on their income from agriculture are more likely to have a positive impact on nutrition than policies that do not specifically focus on women, particularly if combined with other strategies, such as women's education and behavior change.[119,120]

Financing additional spending for the goals—in a sustainable way

Additional health spending will be required in many countries to accelerate progress toward the health goals. But how should this extra spending be financed?

Encouraging risk-pooling and private spending

Health spending can be broken down into private (out-of-pocket expenditures and private insurance), public (expenditures financed out of general revenues and social insurance contributions), and external sources (development assistance).

Private spending absorbs a larger share of income in poorer countries. In low-income countries it absorbs a larger share of GDP, on average, than domestically financed public spending. And in low-income and lower middle-income countries, private spending invariably means out-of-pocket expenditures, not private insurance.[50] This leaves many near-poor households heavily exposed to the risk of impoverishing health expenses. The risk is clearly greater the poorer the country, since poorer countries tend to have larger shares of poor people.[121] A country's private share of health spending in GDP may not in practice be related to its per capita income. But on poverty-reduction grounds, there are good reasons to wish that it were. Governments thus have a major role to play in helping shape effective risk-pooling mechanisms.

Getting governments to spend what they can afford

Government spending as a share of GDP is higher in richer countries. But at any given per capita income, there is a surprising amount of variation across countries in the share of GDP allocated to government health programs. Countries that appear able to spend similar shares of GDP on government health programs end up spending quite different amounts.

How can extra domestic resources be mobilized where countries are spending less than they can afford to? Domestically financed government health spending comes from general revenues, social insurance contributions, or both. The amount of general revenues flowing into the health sector is the product of the amount of general (tax and nontax★★) revenues collected by the government (the general revenue share) and the share of general revenues allocated to the health sector (the health share of government spending).[122] Low government health spending could be due to either or both being low. In poorer countries both shares are typically lower than they are in richer countries. But there are differences across countries that cannot be explained by per capita income alone.

Countries need to ascertain whether their low spending is due to unduly low general revenues or to unduly low allocations to health and explore ways of making appropriate adjustments. Bolivia managed to raise its general revenue share in the 1990s, as the result of a sustained reform process begun in 1983. The health sector there has been one of the beneficiaries of this growth of tax revenues: government health spending as a share of GDP grew at an annual rate of nearly 10 percent in the 1990s.[123]

Raising domestic resources takes time. This does not mean, though, that countries that can apparently afford to spend more out of their own resources should not be encouraged to start the process. Development agencies have a role to play here—by providing technical support of tax reform, helping develop government commitment to health in public expenditure allocations, and providing financial assistance, both to ease the adjustment costs and to provide support while the gap between current and affordable spending is being closed.

Recognizing the limits of development assistance

Official development assistance tends to account for a larger share of government health spending in poorer

★★Some countries with large public sector companies, especially in the Middle East and North Africa, South Asia, and Sub-Saharan Africa regions, have important nontax revenues, which can represent as much as 9 percent of GDP. Increasing revenues from this source would require consideration of the competitive environment in which the companies operate and the need for reinvestment in the companies.

countries. Development assistance for health is especially important in Sub-Saharan Africa: in all countries in the region, external funding exceeded 35 percent of total health expenditures in 2000.[124]

Development assistance is not, however, without its drawbacks. There is no assurance that development assistance to the health sector will continue to grow. Many donors require that assistance be kept in parallel budgets outside the ministries of finance, which eliminates the possibility of appropriate planning and targeting of expenditures. Such off-budget expenditures make it impossible to properly target resources to particular interventions, geographic locations, or population groups. Yet such targeting may be essential to improving the impact of expenditures on outcomes and the probability of reaching the health goals. Last and most important, commitments of expenditures in health must be permanent, implying that any external financing must at some point be substituted by additional domestic revenues or expenditure reallocations.

What the development community needs to do to rise to the challenges

With the advent of new funding sources for health in 2000–02—including the Gates Foundation; the Global Fund to Fight AIDS, Tuberculosis and Malaria; the special U.S. financing for HIV/AIDS; and the use of World Bank International Development Association (IDA) grants—development assistance to health from all external sources rose from an average of $6.4 billion in 1997–99 to about $8.1 billion in 2002. What has this money achieved in recent years? Can it be spent in a way that will achieve a greater impact on the Millennium Development Goals? What are some of the lessons that can be carried forward as the external financing envelope expands?

Learning the lessons of development assistance for health

Development assistance to health works— in a good policy environment

Recent research suggests that development assistance to health does lead to better health outcomes.[20,21] But it does not do so in countries where the policy environment is poor.[21] The productivity of aid is not a black and white issue—there are gradations of good policy, and as policy gets better, the productivity of aid increases. This finding, corroborated by the World Bank's experience with projects, is influencing IDA allocations.

Aid can help improve health policies— but only under certain conditions

Tying aid to the adoption of policy changes through conditions is widely used, but recent studies cast doubt on its wisdom.[125] If governments are committed to reform, conditions can help by enabling governments to publicly commit to certain reforms and thereby persuade private investors of their seriousness. But if governments are not committed to reform, conditions will not make them reform, not least because disbursements often continue even when the conditions are not met. Donors cannot force policies on governments, but they can help in policy design.

Donors have recently begun to use innovative financing mechanisms to improve performance by linking disbursements to specific performance measures, including better policies. This is the tack taken by the Global Fund to Fight AIDS, Tuberculosis and Malaria and by the Global Alliance for Vaccines and Immunization, which disburses funds to countries using a per capita payment for each additional child fully vaccinated against a target schedule. Recent programmatic social adjustment loans to Brazil and Peru by the World Bank link the disbursement of large single tranches of funding to changes in key policies in the health sector to improve the targeting of public spending toward the poor. Performance-based lending is also at the heart of the new scheme for IDA credit buy-downs for polio.

There is substantial fungibility in development assistance for health

Recent research suggests that aid is fungible—across sectors and within sectors.[125] This implies that when aid is earmarked for primary health services and excludes tertiary care, governments simply focus their resources on health services for the population served by public hospitals—a wealthier, urban population in many poor countries. This suggests that donors should not try to channel their external funding to specific programs without engaging in a dialogue with the government on basic changes in the overall patterns of public spending for health. If these changes occur, donors may be able to transfer their financial assistance to the health sector as a whole, knowing that they are likely to have a positive impact on Millennium Development Goal outcomes.

The transactions costs of aid are still too high

More than 20 donors involved in health—including bilaterals, multilaterals, global programs, foundations, and large NGOs—can operate in a single low-income country. Donors are starting to acknowledge that the demands on recipient countries can be huge and that individual project management units have not made sustainable contributions. Donor-funded units have sometimes run parallel to local structures, fostered a sense that the project staff were accountable to the financier rather than the government, and redirected the most qualified human resources away from government employment toward employment in development assistance agencies.

There is need to enhance coordination, explicitly pool aid, and put countries in the driver seat

There is a growing view that if aid is indeed fungible and earmarking imposes transaction costs on recipient countries, donors should dispense with the fiction that they can identify what their money buys. This view has encouraged a search for broader development assistance mechanisms that recognize the importance of the entire expenditure program. These mechanisms range from the Multi-Country AIDS Program in Africa to sectorwide approaches in health and Poverty Reduction Support Credits that back a broad public spending agenda.

Several key principles are emerging:

- Countries, not donors, need to drive the coordination.

- Poverty Reduction Strategy Papers and the health sector analysis that feeds into them can help achieve strategic coherence.

- Medium-term expenditure frameworks and agreements that all donor funding will respect the overall spending plans and limits of the government can help achieve financial coherence.

- Donor funds are best pooled into a single account, and aid is best untied from procurement only from the donor country.

- Programs have greater impact when the number of country coordination bodies is limited and when a common reporting and progress assessment framework is used, with a strong focus on countries doing the monitoring and evaluation, learning from it, and using the information to make their programs more effective.

Global partnerships can add value, but they involve risks

The many global initiatives and partnerships in the health sector speak different technical languages, have vastly different resource bases, and target different risk groups. But they all seek to add value through a common array of functions, including national and global coordination, strategy development and evaluation, global financing and delivery mechanisms and new tools, and resource mobilization, social mobilization, and advocacy.

Recent external evaluations of some of the major health partnerships, such as Stop TB and the Global Alliance for Vaccines and Immunization, suggest that these collaborations are adding significant value in these areas. But several challenges call for caution in embarking on new global partnerships for health instead of concentrating on improving the effectiveness of some of the existing partnerships. Some partnerships lack strategic focus and try to do too much. Others fail to engage adequately with country processes. Partnerships can easily ignore or even exacerbate the problems afflicting the entire health system, such as the lack of human resources for service delivery and weaknesses in integrated monitoring and evaluation.

Getting funds to the frontline

Central government funds can easily leak as they move through the system to the periphery of the country. And in the absence of local initiative and the right incentives, service provision can fail to reflect the views of local people. Effective development assistance for health needs to channel technologies, ideas, finance, and technical assistance closer to households, health providers, and supervisory officials in ways that are consistent with national policies and amenable to monitoring and reporting. Assistance is likely to be more successful if the following are in place:

- decentralized systems of fiduciary and technical management in the public sector

- financially sound NGOs and private providers

- a government body equipped and charged with regulating the quality of public and private providers

- a balanced approach to community-driven development in health, to ensure that social fund–type financing for community health initiatives is sustainable

Development assistance for health remains unpredictable

Development assistance for health depends on donor budgets, which are subject to the usual business and political cycles. Assistance may go up or down yearly as a result of decisions by legislative bodies during budgetary processes. Further work is needed in designing mechanisms that provide greater assurance of sustained long-term financial support. The challenges are to overcome the factors that result in interruptions in long-term assistance, including those stemming from changes in political leadership and aid agency management that can lead to reneging on earlier agreements.

Applying the lessons to the World Bank's work

A review of recent trends and changes in the Bank's principal instruments suggests some encouraging developments in the way the institution is responding to the Millennium Development Goal challenge. While much more needs to be done in the coming years, some positive signs are already visible.

Analyzing Millennium Development Goal trends, prospects, and challenges

A study of the causes of the large interstate disparities in Millennium Development Goal outcomes in India concludes that the impact of additional public spending for improved child health and nutrition would be greatest in the poorer Indian states.[28] It recommends steps to improve the efficiency of public expenditures, by targeting immunization and community-based nutrition activities and villages and districts in the poorer states, where health and nutrition indicators are the worst. In Egypt a recent Millennium Development Goal analysis also found that targeting publicly financed services and involving civil society in implementing programs and monitoring progress for the health goals are critical for success.[126]

The World Bank has collaborated with local analysts and policymakers in Africa over the past two years to conduct studies on the causes of health trends, especially among the poorest households. Country status reports have been completed for nine countries—Burkina Faso, Chad, the Gambia, Guinea, Malawi, Mauritania, Mozambique, Niger, and Tanzania—and are under way in several others.

Helping incorporate the Millennium Development Goals in government policies and budgets

The findings of the country status reports have fed into country-led processes—for the Poverty Reduction Strategy Papers and the medium-term expenditure frameworks—changing key policies in the health sector and reallocating public spending toward health-related services likely to have an impact on the health goals. In Mauritania the results of the country status report and the linked marginal budgeting for bottlenecks exercise shaped the Poverty Reduction Strategy Paper and resulted in important policy shifts. Success in promoting policy change and increasing spending for the health goals requires awareness and buy-in from the ministries of health and finance, a strong donor coalition, involvement of the International Monetary Fund in budget discussions, high-quality technical assistance, and information campaigns and the mobilization of local government and civil society.

Using the goals to assess World Bank country assistance

To better align the Bank's country assistance strategies with the goals, informal assessments have been carried out in several regions. A portfolio ranking in Benin found that the Bank's activities were weakly related to the goals. It concluded that the Bank needed to do more—through Poverty Reduction Support Credits and other projects—to have a substantial impact on the health-related Millennium Development Goals.[127]

Bank staff in the European and Central Asia region drafted a Millennium Development Goal "business plan," including a country-by-country analysis showing that official data on child mortality and malnutrition are questionable and that many countries in the region are unlikely to meet the goals for 2015. The business plan called for special efforts to strengthen capacity for monitoring and evaluation, align Bank projects to support achievement of the goals, and expand multisectoral linkages.

Integrating the goals in sectorwide and programmatic instruments

The goals are increasingly providing the strategic underpinning of Bank assistance to countries in programs in health and multisectoral budget support. A recent health project in the Dominican Republic used Millennium Development Goal intermediate and outcome indicators to monitor progress. The health information system was designed to capture data on these indicators, augmented by periodic household surveys. In Bolivia performance indicators for the Bank-financed health project include coverage and quality of key child and maternal health and disease control services, as well as changes in mortality and disease incidence. Monitoring will be at the municipal and national levels, with the involvement of civil society, to increase local participation and make local politicians and health care providers more accountable for results. Some sectorwide health operations in Africa embody a strong focus on the goals.

Reorienting and increasing Bank loans and grants to achieve Millennium Development Goal outcomes

To underpin national efforts to improve health outcomes—through projects focused on specific diseases and population groups or through broader health sectorwide approaches and other multisectoral operations—the Bank has expanded its financial commitments in health significantly over the past four years, consistent with the stated goal of systematically increasing health lending from $1 billion in fiscal 2001 to $2.2 billion in fiscal 2005. New lending commitments grew from $0.95 billion in fiscal 2000 to $1.7 billion in fiscal 2003.

An important feature in health lending is that much of it is being incorporated as health components in other sectors, such as transport, social protection, and water supply and sanitation. Of the $1.7 billion committed in fiscal 2003, some 44 percent was in projects and programs outside the health sector. This pattern is consistent with the lessons of development assistance, but it also raises new issues. The Bank's organizational structure and incentives make it difficult to bring health specialists into project teams led by staff from other fields, and a different inhouse skills mix is required to work along these lines. Monitoring and evaluation also need to be improved in order to assess such cross-sectoral projects.

Using the Millennium Development Goals to build monitoring and evaluation capacity

Effective national programs to pursue the health goals depend on intermediate indicators to track progress—and on national monitoring and evaluation systems. The Bank convened a meeting of technical experts in November 2001 to review and agree on a framework of intermediate determinants. Those determinants were published in a booklet now being used in identifying indicators for Millennium Development Targets in Poverty Reduction Strategy Papers and other national strategies and in developing monitoring and evaluation systems.[128]

Strengthening the capacity for monitoring and evaluation is taking different forms. In Albania a monitoring and evaluation template has been prepared to help four ministries, including health, develop their own systems, and a specialized advisory body on monitoring has been established. In Mali a health card has been developed to give government officials and the public access to a snapshot of policy actions, health service indicators, and health outcomes for the country and for income groups. One of the most important efforts to improve monitoring and evaluation for the Millennium Development Goals is in HIV/AIDS, and the World Bank has been asked to take the lead role in coordinating the support to country monitoring.

Coordinating donor actions to accelerate progress toward the goals

The Framework for Action to Accelerate Progress on the health, nutrition, and population Millennium Development Goals, endorsed at the high-level policy meeting in May 2003 in Ottawa, Canada, holds promise for all stakeholders in coordinating their efforts.[129] An important part of this framework is building stronger national health systems as a platform for delivering essential services to the poor in pursuit of the goals. The framework lays out common principles and describes a process for countries and donors to work together in expanding and improving the effectiveness of their investments in health systems. The framework requires country actions, such as incorporating analysis of Millennium Development Goal challenges and policy and funding gaps in Poverty Reduction Strategy Papers and simplifying donor coordination arrangements. It also calls for stronger efforts at the global level to invest in key public goods with multicountry benefits, such as supporting research and development on new drugs and vaccines for AIDS, tuberculosis, and malaria and documenting and sharing successful national efforts to achieve the goals for malnutrition and maternal and child health.

The top issues identified in Ottawa included increasing human resource and related system capacity; improving management and strategic planning; creating efficient health information systems; providing safe, affordable, and predictable supplies of drugs; understanding the social and cultural determinants of health, illness, and care-seeking behaviors and the related policy responses; and moving beyond the traditional public sector service delivery mode to work with NGOs and the private sector in extending the coverage of the interventions for core health, nutrition, and population. It was decided to establish a High-Level Forum on health MDGs to review progress on health goals, to monitor changes in donor commitments and behaviors in moving toward better harmonization, and to act on issues holding back progress.

The first High-Level Forum for health MDGs, held in January 2004 in Geneva, addressed several of these issues. Heads of development agencies, bilateral agencies, global health initiatives, and ministers of finance and health met to informally discuss concrete actions to accelerate and monitor progress toward the MDGs for health and nutrition. They agreed on actions in four areas:

- *Resources for health and poverty reduction strategy papers.* Countries should have a single process leading to one "MDG-responsive" Poverty Reduction Strategy Paper. Participants agreed on the importance of incorporating explicit reference to progress toward the MDGs in joint assessments of Poverty Reduction Strategies.

- *Aid effectiveness and harmonization.* A working group would follow up on country pilots in budget support for health and link with other broader development efforts on harmonization, drawing out lessons on common methods and instruments for health.

- *Human resources.* Participants agreed to assess expenditures on human resources and conduct in-depth human resources, and learning by doing studies in selected countries.

- *Monitoring performance.* Participants agreed on the need for a common set of intermediate indicators and measures of policy and institutional performance to gauge short- and medium-term progress toward the MDGs.

References

1. UNICEF. 2001. *Progress Since the World Summit for Children: A Statistical Review.* New York: UNICEF.

2. Food and Agricultural Organization of the United Nations. 2000. *The State of Food Security in the World.* Rome: FAO.

3. UNAIDS. 2002. *Report on the Global HIV/AIDS Epidemic.* Geneva: UNAIDS.

4. Sen, A. 2002. "Why Health Equity?" *Health Economics* 11 (8): 659–666.

5. Wagstaff, A., and E. Van Doorslaer. 2003. "Catastrophe and Impoverishment in Paying for Health Care: With Applications to Vietnam 1993–1998." *Health Economics* 12 (11): 921–34.

6. Bloom, D., and J. Sachs. 1998. "Geography, Demography and Economic Growth in Africa." *Brookings Papers on Economic Activity* 2: 207–295.

7. Grassly, N.C., K. Desai, E. Pegurri, A. Sikazwe, I. Malambo, C. Siamatowe, and D. Bundy. 2003. "The Economic Impact of HIV/AIDS on the Education Sector in Zambia." *AIDS* 17 (7): 1039–1044.

8. Bell, C., S. Devarajan, and H. Gersbach. 2003. "The Long-Run Economic Costs of AIDS: Theory and an Application to South Africa." World Bank, Washington, DC.

9. United Nations. 2004. Millennium Development Goals. www.un.org/millenniumgoals.

10. World Bank. 2003. *Global Economic Prospects and the Developing Countries.* Washington, DC: World Bank.

11. Jones, G., R.W. Steketee, R.E. Black, Z.A. Bhutta, and S.S. Morris. 2003. "How Many Child Deaths Can We Prevent This Year?" *Lancet* 362 (9377): 65–71.

12. World Health Organization. 2001. *Macroeconomics and Health: Investing in Health for Economic Development.* Report of the Commission on Macroeconomics and Health. Geneva: WHO.

13. Filmer, D., and L. Pritchett. 1999. "The Impact of Public Spending on Health: Does Money Matter?" *Social Science and Medicine* 49 (10): 1309–1323.

14. Filmer, D., J. Hammer, and L. Pritchett. 2000. "Weak Links in the Chain: A Diagnosis of Health Policy in Poor Countries." *World Bank Research Observer* 15 (2): 199–224.

15. Filmer, D., J. Hammer, and L. Pritchett. 2002. "Weak Links in the Chain II: A Prescription for Health Policy in Poor Countries." *World Bank Research Observer* 17 (1): 47–66.

16. Bidani, B., and M. Ravallion. 1997. "Decomposing Social Indicators Using Distributional Data." *Journal of Econometrics* 77 (1): 125–139.

17. Gupta, S., M. Verhoeven, and E.R. Tiongson. 2003. "Public Spending on Health Care and the Poor." *Health Economics* 12 (8): 685–696.

18. Wagstaff, A. 2003. "Child Health on a Dollar a Day: Some Tentative Cross-Country Comparisons." *Social Science and Medicine* 57 (9): 1529–1538.

19. Rajkumar, A., and V. Swaroop. 2002. "Public Spending and Outcomes: Does Governance Matter?" Policy Research Working Paper 2840, World Bank, Washington, DC.

20. Feyzioglu, T.N., V. Swaroop, and M. Zhu. 1996. "Foreign Aid's Impact on Public Spending." Policy Research Working Paper 1610, World Bank, Washington, DC.

21. Burnside C., and D. Dollar. 2000. "Aid, Growth, the Incentive Regime and Poverty Reduction." In *The World Bank: Structure and Policies,* eds. C.L. Gilbert and D. Vines, 210–227. Cambridge: Cambridge University Press.

22. World Bank. 1999. *Peru: Improving Health Care for the Poor.* Washington, DC: World Bank.

23. Ensor, T., A. Hossain, Q. Ali, S. Begum, and A. Moral. 2001. "Geographic Resource Allocation in Bangladesh." Research Paper 21, Ministry of Health and Family Welfare, Health Economics Unit, Dhaka.

24. Diderichsen, F., E. Varde, and M. Whitehead. 1997. "Resource Allocation to Health Authorities: The Quest for an Equitable Formula in Britain and Sweden." *British Medical Journal* 315 (7112): 875–878.

25. Newman, J.L., M. Pradhan, L. Rawlings, G. Ridder, R. Coa, and J.L. Evia. 2002. "An Impact Evaluation of Education, Health, and Water Supply Investments by the Bolivian Social Investment Fund." *World Bank Economic Review* 16 (2): 241–274.

26. Lambrechts, T., J. Bryce, and V. Orinda. 1999. "Integrated Management of Childhood Illness: A Summary of First Experiences." *Bulletin of the World Health Organization* 77 (7): 582–594.

27. Santos, I., C.G. Victora, J. Martines, H. Goncalves, D.P. Gigante, N.J. Valle, and G. Pelto. 2001. "Nutrition Counseling Increases Weight Gain among Brazilian Children." *Journal of Nutrition* 131 (11): 2866–2873.

28. World Bank. 2003. "Attaining the Millennium Development Goals in India: How Likely and What Will It Take?" Washington, DC.

29. Soucat, A., W. Van Lerberghe, F. Diop, S. Nguyen, and R. Knippenberg. 2002. "Marginal Budgeting for Bottlenecks: A New Costing and Resource-Allocation Practice to Buy Health Results." World Bank, Washington, DC.

30. UNICEF and World Bank. 2003. *Marginal Budgeting for Bottlenecks: How to Reach the Impact Frontier of Health and Nutrition Services and Accelerate Progress towards the MDGs: A Budgeting Model and Application to Low Income Countries.* New York: UNICEF; Washington, DC: World Bank.

31. Pritchett, L., and L.H. Summers. 1996. "Wealthier Is Healthier." *Journal of Human Resources* 31 (4): 841–868.

32. Haddad, L., H. Alderman, S. Appleton, L. Song, and Y. Yohannes. 2003. "Reducing Child Malnutrition: How Far Does Income Growth Take Us?" *World Bank Economic Review* 17 (1): 107–131.

33. Case, A. 2001. "Does Money Protect Health Status? Evidence from South African Pensions." Center for Health and Wellbeing Working Paper, Woodrow Wilson School, Princeton University, Princeton, NJ.

34. Case, A. 2001. "Health, Income, and Economic Development." Paper presented at the Annual World Bank Conference on Development Economics, Washington, DC.

35. Aye, M., F. Champagne, and A.P. Contandriopoulos. 2002. "Economic Role of Solidarity and Social Capital in Accessing Modern Health Care Services in the Ivory Coast." *Social Science and Medicine* 55 (11): 1929–1946.

36. Alderman, H., and V. Lavy. 1996. "Household Responses to Public Health Services: Cost and Quality Tradeoffs." *World Bank Research Observer* 11 (1): 3–22.

37. Lewis, M. 2000. "Who Is Paying for Health Care in Europe and Central Asia?" Report 20940, World Bank, Washington, DC.

38. Schellenberg, J.R., S. Abdulla, R. Nathan, O. Mukasa, T.J. Marchant, N. Kikumbih, A.K. Mushi, H. Mponda, H. Minja, H. Mshinda, M. Tanner, and C. Lengeler. 2001. "Effect of Large-Scale Social Marketing of Insecticide-Treated Nets on Child Survival in Rural Tanzania." *Lancet* 357 (9264): 1241–1247.

39. Abdulla, S., J.A. Schellenberg, R. Nathan, O. Mukasa, T. Marchant, T. Smith, M. Tanner, and C. Lengeler. 2001. "Impact on Malaria Morbidity of a Programme Supplying Insecticide-Treated Nets in Children Aged under 2 Years in Tanzania: Community Cross-Sectional Study." *British Medical Journal* 322 (7281): 270–273.

40. Armstrong Schellenberg, J., A. Mushi, H. Mponda, and C. Lengeler. 2002. "Discount Vouchers for Treated Nets in Tanzania: Targeted Subsidy for Malaria Control." Presentation at meeting on malaria and equity organized by the World Bank and the London School of Hygiene and Tropical Medicine, London School of Hygiene and Tropical Medicine, London.

41. Saadah, F., M. Pradhan, and R. Sparrow. 2001. "The Effectiveness of the Health Card as an Instrument to Ensure Access to Medical Care for the Poor During the Crisis." World Bank, Washington, DC.

42. Mesoamerica Nutrition Program Targeting Study Group. 2002. "Targeting Performance of Three Large-Scale, Nutrition-Oriented Social Programs in Central America and Mexico." *Food Nutrition Bulletin* 23 (2): 162–174.

43. International Food Policy Research Institute. 2002. *Final Report: Nicaragua Social Protection Network, Pilot Evaluation System, Impact Evaluation.* Washington, DC: IFPRI.

44. International Food Policy Research Institute. 2003. *Sexto Informe. Proyecto PRAF/BID Fase II: Impacto Intermedio.* Washington, DC: IFPRI.

45. International Food Policy Research Institute. *Estudo De Avaliação De Impacto Para O Programa Bolsa Alimentação. Relatório 3: Análise De Impacto Final.* Washington, DC: IFPRI.

46. Gertler, P., and S. Boyce. 2001. "An Experiment in Incentive-Based Welfare: The Impact of PROGRESA on Health in Mexico." University of California, Berkeley CA.

47. Morris, S., R. Flores, P. Olinto, and J. Medina. 2003. "A Randomized Trial of Conditional Cash Transfers to Households and Peripheral Health Centers: Impact on Child Health and Demand for Health Services." Paper presented at the Fourth International Health Economics Association World Congress, San Francisco.

48. Jalan, J., and M. Ravallion. 2001. "Behavioral Responses to Risk in Rural China." *Journal of Development Economics* 66 (1): 23–49.

49. Jalan, J., and M. Ravallion. 1999. "Are the Poor Less Well Insured? Evidence on Vulnerability to Income Risk in Rural China." *Journal of Development Economics* 58 (1): 61–81.

50. Musgrove, P., R. Zeramdini, and G. Carrin. 2002. "Basic Patterns in National Health Expenditure." *Bulletin of the World Health Organization* 80 (2): 134–142.

51. Yip, W., and P. Berman. 2001. "Targeted Health Insurance in a Low Income Country and Its Impact on Access and Equity in Access: Egypt's School Health Insurance." *Health Economics* 10 (3): 207–220.

52. Beegle, K., E. Frankenberg, and D. Thomas. "Bargaining Power within Couples and Use of Prenatal and Delivery Care in Indonesia." *Studies in Family Planning* 32 (2): 130–146.

53. Pitt, M.M., S.R. Khandker, S.M. Mckernan, and M. Abdul Latif. 1999. "Credit Programs for the Poor and Reproductive Behavior in Low-Income Countries: Are the Reported Causal Relationships the Result of Heterogeneity Bias?" *Demography* 36 (1): 1–21.

54. Koblinsky, M.A., and O. Campbell. 2003. "Factors Affecting the Reduction of Maternal Mortality." In *Reducing Maternal Mortality: Learning from Bolivia, China, Egypt, Honduras, Indonesia,*

Jamaica, and Zimbabwe, ed. M.A. Koblinsky, Xiv, 132. Washington, DC: World Bank.

55. Das, J., and C. Sánchez–Párano. 2003. "Short But Not Sweet : New Evidence on Short Duration Morbidities from India." Policy Research Working Paper 2971, World Bank, Washington, DC.

56. Jalan, J., and M. Ravallion. 2003. "Does Piped Water Reduce Diarrhea for Children in Rural India?" *Journal of Econometrics* 112 (1): 153–173.

57. Desai, S., and S. Alva. 1998. "Maternal Education and Child Health: Is There a Strong Causal Relationship?" *Demography* 35 (1): 71–81.

58. Glewwe, P. 1999. "Why Does Mother's Schooling Raise Child Health in Developing Countries?" *Journal of Human Resources* 34 (1): 124–59.

59. Abbas, K.A. 1995. "Counselling in a Hospital Setting. Breastfeeding." *Dialogue Diarrhoea* (59): 3.

60. Heerey, M., and A. Kols. 2003. *Improving the Quality of Care: Quality Improvement Projects from the Johns Hopkins University Bloomberg School of Public Health Center for Communication Programs.* Center Publication No. 101, Johns Hopkins University, Bloomberg School of Public, Baltimore, MD.

61. Benefo, K., and T. Schultz. 1996. "Fertility and Child Mortality in Côte d'Ivoire and Ghana." *World Bank Economic Review* 10 (1): 123–158.

62. Mwabu, G., M. Ainsworth, and A. Nyamete. 1993. "Quality of Medical Care and Choice of Medical Treatment in Kenya: An Empirical Analysis." *Journal of Human Resources* 28 (4): 838–862.

63. Lavy, V., J. Strauss, D. Thomas, and P. De Vreyer. 1996. "Quality of Care, Survival and Health Outcomes in Ghana." *Journal of Health Economics* 15 (3): 333–357.

64. Thomas, D., V. Lavy, and D. Strauss. 1996. "Public Policy and Anthropometric Outcomes in the Côte d'Ivoire." *Journal of Public Economics* 61 (2): 155–192.

65. Wong, E., B. Popkin, D. Guilkey, and J. Akin. 1987. "Accessibility, Quality of Care and Prenatal Care Use in the Philippines." *Social Science and Medicine* 24 (11): 927–944.

66. Van De Walle, D., and D. Cratty. 2002. "Impact Evaluation of a Rural Road Rehabilitation Project." World Bank, Washington, DC.

67. Pathmanathan, I., J. Liljestrand, J.M. Martins, L.C. Rajapaksa, C. Lissner, A. De Silva, S. Selvaraju, and P.J. Singh. 2003. "Investing in Maternal Health: Learning from Malaysia and Sri Lanka." World Bank, Health, Nutrition, and Population Department, Washington, DC.

68. Merrick, T.W. "The Effect of Piped Water on Early Childhood Mortality in Urban Brazil, 1970 to 1976." *Demography* 22 (1): 1–24.

69. Ridder, G., and I. Tunali. 1999. "Stratified Partial Likelihood Estimation." *Journal of Econometrics* 92 (2): 193–232.

70. Lee, L–F., M. Rosenzweig, and M. Pitt. 1997. "The Effects of Improved Nutrition, Sanitation, and Water Quality on Child Health in High-Mortality Populations." *Journal of Econometrics* 77 (1): 209–235.

71. Esrey, S.A., and J.P. Habicht. 1988. "Maternal Literacy Modifies the Effect of Toilets and Piped Water on Infant Survival in Malaysia." *American Journal of Epidemiology* 127 (5): 1079–1087.

72. Jalan, J., and M. Ravallion. 2001. "Does Piped Water Reduce Diarrhea for Children in Rural India?" Policy Research Working Paper 2664, World Bank, Washington, DC.

73. Wolfe, B., and J. Behrman. 1982. "Determinants of Child Mortality, Health and Nutrition in a Developing Country." *Journal of Development Economics* 11 (1): 163–193.

74. Behrman, J., and B. Wolfe. 1987. "How Does Mother's Schooling Affect Family Health, Nutrition, Medical Care Usage and Household Sanitation?" *Journal of Econometrics* 36 (1): 185–204.

75. World Bank. 2003. *World Development Report 2004: Making Services Work for Poor People.* Washington, DC: World Bank.

76. Victora, C., F. Barros, J. Vaughan, A. Silva, and E. Tomasi. 2000. "Explaining Trends in Inequities: Evidence from Brazilian Child Health Studies." *Lancet* 356 (9235): 1093–1098.

77. Eichler, R. 2001. "Improving Immunization Coverage in an Innovative Primary Health Care Delivery Model: Lessons from Burkina Faso's Bottom Up Planning, Oversight, and Resource Control Approach that Holds Providers Accountable for Results." World Bank, Washington, DC.

78. Ewig, C. 2003. "The Contributions of Community-Based Decentralization to Democracy: Peru's Local Health Administration Committees." Paper presented at the annual meeting of the American Political Science Association.

79. Langenbrunner, J. 2003. "Resource Allocation and Purchasing in the ECA Region: A Review." World Bank, Washington, DC.

80. Chawla, M., P. Berman, A. Windak, and M. Kulis. 1999. "Provision of Ambulatory Health Services in Poland: A Case Study from Krakow." World Bank, Washington DC.

81. Cotlear, D. 1999. "Peru: Improving Health Care for the Poor." LCSHD Paper Series 57, World Bank, Human Development Department, Washington, DC.

82. Vladescu, C., and S. Radulescu. 2001. "Primary Health Services: Output-Based Contracting to Lift Performance in Romania." *Public Policy for the Private Sector* 239. http://rru.worldbank.org/viewpoint/HTMLNotes/239/239Vlade-831.pdf.

83. Bitran, R. 2001. "Paying Health Providers through Capitation in Argentina, Nicaragua and Thailand: Output, Spending, Organizational Impact and Market Structure." USAID PHR Project, Washington, DC.

84. Eichler, R., P. Auxilia, and J. Pollock. 2001. "Output-Based Health Care: Paying for Performance in Haiti." World Bank, Washington, DC.

85. Marek, T., I. Diallo, B. Ndiaye, and J. Rakotosalama. 1994. "Successful Contracting of Prevention Services: Fighting Malnutrition in Senegal and Madagascar." *Health Policy Planning* 14 (4): 382–389.

86. Tangcharoensathien, V., and N. Khongsawatt Nas. 1997. "Private-Sector Involvement in Public Hospitals: Case-Studies in Bangkok." In *Private Health Providers in Developing Countries: Serving the Public Interest?* ed. A. Mills. London: Zed Books.

87. Mcpake, B., and C. Hongoro. 1995. "Contracting Out of Clinical Services in Zimbabwe." *Social Science and Medicine* 41 (1): 13–24.

88. Slack, K., and W. Savedoff. 2001. "Public Purchaser-Private Provider Contracting for Health Services: Examples from Latin America and the Caribbean." Sustainable Development Department Technical Paper Series 111, Inter-American Development Bank, Washington, DC.

89. Fiedler, J.L. 1996. "The Privatization of Health Care in Three Latin American Social Security Systems." *Health Policy Planning* 11 (4): 406–417.

90. Mills, A., S. Bennett, and S. Russell. 2001. *The Challenge of Health Sector Reform: What Must Governments Do?* New York: St Martin's Press.

91. Gilson, L., and A. Mills. 1995. "Health Sector Reforms in Sub-Saharan Africa: Lessons of the Last 10 Years." *Health Policy* 32 (1–3): 215–243.

92. Londoño, B, I. Jaramillo, and J.P. Uribe. 1999. "Decentralization and Reforms in Health Services: The Colombian Case." World Bank, Washington, DC,

93. Oliveira-Cruz, V., C. Kurowski, and A. Mills. 2003. "Delivery of Priority Health Services: Searching for Synergies within the Vertical Versus Horizontal Debate." *Journal of International Development* 15 (1): 67–86.

94. Raufu, A. 2002. "Nigeria Concerned over Exodus of Doctors and Nurses." *British Medical Journal* 325: 65.

95. Federation for American Immigration Reform. 2002. "Brain Drain." http://www.Fairus.Org/Immigrationissuecenters/ Immigrationissuecenters.Cfm?ID=1242&C=17.

96. Marcelo, R. 2003. "Hospital 'Angels' Look for Heaven Elsewhere." *Indian Financial Times,* October 13.

97. Padarath, A., C. Chamberlain, D. Mccoy, A. Ntuli, M. Rowson, and R. Loewenson. 2003. "Health Personnel in Southern Africa: Confronting Maldistribution and Brain Drain." EQUINET Discussion Paper 3.

98. Upadhyay, A. 2003. "Nursing Exodus Weakens Developing World." Inter Press Service News Agency. http://www. Ipsnews.Net/Migration/Stories/Exodus.Html.

99. World Health Organization. 1998. *CHD 1996–97 Report.* Geneva: WHO.

100. Ministry of Health and Social Welfare. 2002. *RNTCP Performance Report: India. 3rd Quarter.* Central TB Division, Delhi.

101. Kurowski, C., S. Abdulla, and A. Mills. 2003. "Human Resources for Health: Requirements and Availability in the Context of Scaling-Up Priority Interventions. A Case Study from Tanzania." London School of Hygiene & Tropical Medicine, London.

102. Holmas, T.H. 2002. "Keeping Nurses at Work: A Duration Analysis." *Health Economics* 11 (6): 493–503.

103. Wilbulpoprasert. 2002. "Integrated Strategies to Tackle Inequitable Distribution of Doctors in Thailand: Four Decades of Experience."

104. Peters, D.H., A.S. Yazbeck, R.R. Sharma, G.N.V. Ramana, L.H. Pritchett, and A. Wagstaff. 2002. *Better Health Systems for India's Poor: Findings, Analysis, and Options.* Washington: World Bank.

105. Reinikka, R., and J. Svensson. 2003. "Working for God? Evaluating Service Delivery of Religious Not-for-Profit Health Care Providers in Uganda." Policy Research Working Paper 3058, World Bank, Washington, DC.

106. Rabinowitz, H. 1999. "A Program to Increase the Number of Family Physicians in Rural and Underserved Areas: Impact after 22 Years." *Journal of the American Medical Association* 281 (3): 255–260.

107. Tulloch, J. 1999. "Integrated Approach to Child Health in Developing Countries." *Lancet* 354 (Suppl. 2): SII16– SII20.

108. Gove, S. 1997. "Integrated Management of Childhood Illness by Outpatient Health Workers: Technical Basis and Overview." WHO Working Group on Guidelines for Integrated Management of the Sick Child. *Bulletin of the World Health Organization* 75 (Suppl. 1): 7–24.

109. Reinikka, R. 1999. "Using Surveys for Public Sector Reform." *PREM Notes.* World Bank, Washington, DC.

110. Mcpake, B., D. Asiimwe, F. Mwesigye, M. Ofumbi, L. Orthenblad, P. Streefland, and A. Turinde. 1999. "Informal Economic Activities of Public Health Workers in Uganda: Implications for Quality and Accessibility of Care." *Social Science and Medicine* 49 (7): 849–865.

111. Ablo, E., and R. Reinikka. 1998. "Do Budgets Really Matter? Evidence from Public Spending on Education and Health in Uganda." Policy Research Working Paper 1926, World Bank, Washington, DC.

112. Cruz, O., K. Hanson, and A. Mills. 2001. "Approaches to Overcoming Health Systems Constraints at the Peripheral Level: A Review of the Evidence." WG5 15, CMH Working Paper Series. World Health Organization, Geneva.

113. Santoso, B., S. Suryawati, and J.E. Prawaitasari. 1996. "Small Group Intervention vs. Formal Seminar for Improving Appropriate Drug Use." *Social Science and Medicine* 42 (8): 1163–1168.

114. Weisbrod, B. 2003. "Solving the Drug Dilemma." *Washington Post,* August 22.

115. Eissen, E., D. Efenne, and K. Sabitu. 1997. "Community Loan Funds and Transport Services for Obstetric Emergencies in Northern Nigeria." *International Journal of Gynecology and Obstetrics* 59 (Suppl. 2): 48.

116. Pendse, V. 1999. "Maternal Deaths in an Indian Hospital: A Decade of (No) Change?" *Reproductive Health Matters.*

117. Esry, S., J. Potash, and L. Roberts, and C Schiff. 1991. "Effects of Improved Water Supply and Sanitation on Ascariasis, Diarrhea, Dracunculiasis, Hookworm Infection, Schistosomiasis, and Trachoma." *Bulletin of the World Health Organization* 69 (5): 609–621.

118. World Bank. 2003. "Public Health at a Glance Fact Sheet: Indoor Air Pollution." Health, Nutrition, and Population Department, Washington, DC.

119. Quisumbing, A.R. 1995. "Gender Differences in Agricultural Productivity: A Survey of Empirical Evidence." *FCND Discussion Paper* 5: 1–71. International Food Policy Research Institute, Washington, DC.

120. Johnson-Welch, C. 1999. "Focusing on Women Works: Research on Improving Micronutrient Status through Food-Based Interventions." International Center for Research on Women/Opportunities for Micronutrient Interventions Project, Washington, DC.

121. World Bank. 2000. *World Development Report 2000/2001: Attacking Poverty.* Washington, DC: World Bank.

122. Hay, R. 2003. "The 'Fiscal Space' for Publicly Financed Health Care." Oxford Policy Institute Policy Brief.

123. World Bank. 2003. *World Development Indicators 2003.* Washington, DC: World Bank.

124. World Health Organization. 2000. *The World Health Report 2000. Health Systems: Improving Performance.* Geneva: WHO.

125. World Bank. 1998. *Assessing Aid: What Works, What Doesn't, and Why.* Oxford: Oxford University Press.

126. El-Saharty, S., E. Richardson, and S. Chase. 2003. *Egypt and the Millennium Development Goals.* Washington, DC: The World Bank.

127. Abrantes, A. 2003. Personal communication. World Bank, Washington, DC.

128. World Bank. 2002. *Annual Review of Development Effectiveness: Achieving Development Outcomes: The Millennium Challenge.* Washington, DC: World Bank.

129. Claeson, M. 2003. "A Framework for Action: Accelerating Progress to Meet the HNP MDGs." World Bank, Health, Nutrition, and Population Department, Washington, DC.

130. World Health Organization. 2003. Global Database on Child Growth and Malnutrition. www.Who.Int/Nutgrowthdb/.

131. UNICEF. 2003. Statistics: Child Mortality. www.Childinfo.Org/Cmr/Revis/Db2.Htm.

132. Claeson, M., C.G. Griffin, T.A. Johnston, and others. 2001. "Health, Nutrition and Population." In Poverty Reduction Strategy Paper Sourcebook, 2nd ed., ed. World_Bank. Washington, DC: World Bank.

CHAPTER 1

Backdrop to the Millennium Development Goals

"It started in 1999 when my brother, Geogys, went away—I mean, he died at that time. He was ill so many times with fever. He was 28 when he went away. After two months, his first-born went away too, and three months later our two sisters, Margaret and Lucy, followed them. Malaria killed all of them. And it keeps on going. Two weeks ago our aunt died from malaria. She was ill on Tuesday, complaining about a bad headache and fever, and on Wednesday she was dead. It is not unusual like that. At least with AIDS it can take you a long time to die, but malaria is quick. In the past three years, 25 of my family and friends have died in this way.

My village is in the highlands. Everyone is getting malaria nowadays. Recently, we have buried 10 people from this disease, including my aunt, because it is so bad. Everyone knows mosquitoes are the danger, but the problem is that people are poor. Even if you tell them about bednets, they are thinking about how they will eat. Nobody uses nets. Instead we build fires in our places to try to keep the mosquitoes out with smoke. But we still get infected. When the fever comes, it's better to find the doctor quickly and think about how to pay later. It can force you to sell a cow sometimes, or maybe the doctor will take some hens or a sheep. But sometimes the medicine does not work well, so maybe it is better just to pray.

Me, I am worried about my wife and my second-born, Marcy. They are always complaining of fever. I have taken them to hospital, and they have taken different medicines, but still they have the headaches and the fever. What should I do? I'm worried

that they will go away, too. And now my youngest boy, Isaac, is also starting. He is a year old now, but it's very easy with young children to see how they feel with their malaria. Their temperature rises very quickly and they start to sweat. For myself, it comes and goes. Last year, I was affected almost all year, so I could not work well. The headaches were very bad. But this year, it is better."

—GEORGE OSIGA, COBBLER, KENYA
(adapted from a supplement in the Guardian,
*"Earth: Health check for a planet and its people under pressure,"
August 22, 2002)*

The extent of premature death and ill health in the developing world is staggering. In 2000 almost 11 million children died before their fifth birthday, 99 percent of them in the developing world, 4.5 million in Sub-Saharan Africa alone. An estimated 140 million children under five are underweight, almost half of them in South Asia. In 2001, 3 million people died from HIV/AIDS, 99 percent of them in the developing world. Tuberculosis claimed another 2 million lives. And 515,000 women died during pregnancy or childbirth in 1995, 98 percent of them in the developing world.

Death and poor health on such a scale are matters of concern in their own right. But they also act as a brake on economic development. It was these twin concerns that led the international community to put health firmly at the center of the Millennium Development Goals when adopting them in 2001.

Health, interventions, poverty, and people

The Kenyan cobbler in the opening story records the deaths of no fewer than 25 family members and friends over three years—deaths that are far from atypical.

- Almost 11 million children died before their fifth birthday in 2000.[1] Less than 1 percent of these deaths (79,000) occurred in high-income countries, compared with 42 percent in Sub-Saharan Africa, 35 percent in South Asia, and 13 percent in East Asia.

- Of the estimated 140 million children under the age of five who are underweight, almost half (65 million) are in South Asia.

- In 1998 an estimated 843 million people were considered to be undernourished on the basis of their food intake.[2]

- Of the 3 million people who died from HIV/AIDS in 2001,[3] almost all (99 percent) were in the developing world—73 percent in Sub-Saharan Africa alone.

- Tuberculosis claimed 2 million lives, with the epidemic worsening during economic and social crises.

- In 1995, 515,000 women died during pregnancy or childbirth: 1,000 in the industrial world, 252,000 in Sub-Saharan Africa.[1]

Death, disease, and malnutrition on this scale are matters for concern in their own right—the first theme of this report. As Nobel laureate Amartya Sen put it, "Health is among the most important conditions of human life and a critically significant constituent of human capabilities which we have reason to value."[4] Put another way, being poor is not simply about having too little money. To be poor, as the *2001 World Development Report: Attacking Poverty* notes, is "to be hungry, to lack shelter, to be sick and not cared for, to be illiterate and not schooled."[5]

George Osiga's story illustrates a second theme of the report. For the most part, it is not the lack of effective interventions that is the principal cause of the large number of deaths in the developing world. It is that *the coverage of preventive and treatment interventions is too low.* For example, insecticide-treated nets are effective in preventing malaria, and effective antimalarials exist for treating it. The scope for reducing mortality by scaling up the coverage rates of effective interventions is considerable: if the utilization rates of childhood interventions were to rise from current levels to 99 percent, the number of under-five deaths worldwide would fall by an estimated two-thirds.[6]

This begs the question: why are effective interventions so little used in the developing world? The opening story points to one of the reasons—*the close connection between health and poverty*, a third theme of this report. Poverty makes people especially vulnerable to sickness. But it also means they have few resources to spend on preventive measures and on curative care. So they are more likely to be malnourished and to die early (box 1.1).

As George's story illustrates, people's ability to work depends on their health. As long as they remain ill, their earning capacity is reduced, and the income flow into the household remains limited. George and many like him in the developing world appear to be caught in a vicious circle: their poverty keeps them from taking appropriate preventive measures and seeking health care when sick. This keeps them sick—which keeps them in poverty. If the poor spend their limited resources on preventing disease and restoring themselves to good health when they fall sick, they risk leaving themselves and their loved ones with too little for food and other necessities.

Illness and death in a household reduce income and lead to potentially impoverishing expenses on medical care. In Vietnam health expenses are estimated to have pushed about 3 million people into poverty in 1993 and 2.7 million in 1998.[7] *Voices of the Poor* records the case of a 26-year-old man in Lao Cai, in the north of Vietnam. As a result of the high health care costs of his daughter's severe illness, he moved from being the richest man in his community to one of the poorest.[8]

The vicious circle of ill health and poverty is evident at the country level also. With a daily per capita income of $1.17 (purchasing power parity of $5.60) in 2000, it is hardly surprising that coverage levels of key preventive and treatment interventions are so low in low-income countries.[9] Barely 40 percent of the births in low-income countries take place with the assistance of a medically trained person. Barely 60 percent of children receive DPT3 immunization. And only a third of infectious patients with tuberculosis are using effective treatment. These low coverage rates translate into high rates of child and maternal mortality and low levels of nutrition. That, in turn, acts as a brake on economic growth and contributes to income poverty. Children are less likely to be in school if ill and malnourished, and they learn less when they are in school. Their productivity in later life is reduced as a result. A recent study estimates that $1 invested in an early child nutrition program in the Philippines would yield at least a $3 return in higher earnings thanks to better educational outcomes.[10] But children require teachers to learn, and in some parts of Africa deaths from HIV/AIDS are making a major dent in the stock of teachers—Zambia now loses half as many teachers as it trains to HIV/AIDS.[11]

Illness and malnutrition reduce the productivity of current workers, too—as well as the hours they can

Box 1.1 Worlds apart: The poor die earlier

Between the world's poorest and richest people are large differences in the risk of premature death and malnutrition. Box figure 1 lines countries up by their per capita income and divides the world's population into four equal groups based on the per capita income of the country they live in—the world's poorest quarter, the world's second poorest quarter, and so on. The figure does not capture the fact that people within countries vary in terms of per capita income and mortality risks. But box figure 2 does. (The scales of the denominators for the rates and ratios were chosen to ensure that each gradient is visible.)

The under-five mortality rate among the poorest quarter of the world's population is 10 times that of the richest quarter (box figure 1). The figure for tuberculosis mortality is only slightly lower. The figure for maternal mortality is 20 times that of the richest quarter. Within countries too, gaps exist—and persist—between the rich and the poor, as box figure 2 shows.[14,15]

The distribution of malnutrition and mortality between poor and rich countries is unequal

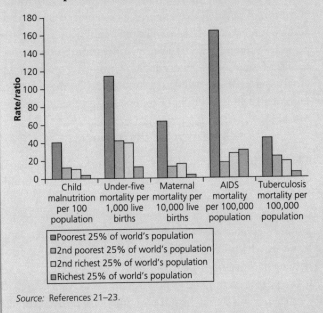

Source: References 21–23.

Poor children die earlier than other children

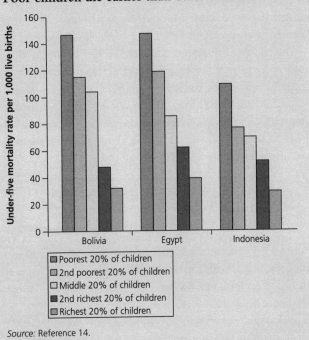

Source: Reference 14.

spend working. A recent study from Indonesia finds that the loss of the ability to undertake a typical activity of daily living leads to a loss of earnings equivalent to 10 percent of average earnings, while a loss of ability to undertake any activity of daily living wipes out earnings altogether.[12] The effects of poor health and mortality show up in macroeconomic aggregates: health and demographic variables have been estimated to account for as much as half the difference in growth rates between Africa and the rest of the world between 1965 and 1990.[13] Low rates of economic growth and low initial per capita incomes translate into low coverage of key interventions and high rates of mortality and malnutrition. And so the cycle goes on.

George Osiga's story draws attention to a fourth theme of the report: *interventions are not dropped like manna from heaven; they are demanded by people and delivered by people.* Households

decide whether to use mosquito nets or build fires, whether to seek treatment when fever comes or simply to pray. If treatment is sought, it is a health provider who makes the diagnosis and delivers the care. Households and providers are fallible, and their knowledge and skills are often lacking. Patients often request inappropriate drugs and tests in the mistaken belief that they are appropriate. And providers often knowingly administer or prescribe them, since they have a financial incentive to do so. This contributes to drug resistance, to poverty, and in the extreme to death.

Providers can also be ill informed, lacking even rudimentary diagnostic skills. In a survey in Burundi in 1992 only 2 percent of children with diarrhea taken to a health facility were correctly diagnosed, and of these only 13 percent were correctly rehydrated.[16] Households need not always be ignorant of health matters, and providers can acquire the appropriate skills. In Vietnam in 1997, 78 percent of children seeking care for diarrhea were correctly assessed, and of those 67 percent were correctly rehydrated.[16] Vietnam is also one of the few high-burden countries that have already surpassed global targets for 2005 for tuberculosis treatment and cure.

This report argues for better understanding of what prompts households to engage in preventive activities and to seek care when sick—and what makes some providers but not others deliver good-quality care. Poor households and poor countries can break out of the vicious circle linking poor health and poverty. Improving knowledge is one avenue. Lowering prices and other barriers to using effective interventions is another. Sri Lanka started to achieve dramatic reductions in its maternal mortality ratio as far back as the 1930s, when it was extremely poor.[17]

The exercise of understanding the factors behind household and provider behavior has to be done in the context of the health system, but it also has to go beyond the health system. It has to be done in the context of government policies for the health sector, but also for other sectors. And it has to be done in the context of development assistance and international initiatives and partnerships.

Health gets on the international community's radar screen—and the Millennium Development Goals are born

In the 1990s the international community recognized the importance of health in development. In a period when official development assistance (ODA) was declining, development assistance to health rose—in real terms.[18] It also doubled as a share of International Development Association (IDA) disbursements, which in turn accounted for a larger share of ODA (27 percent in 1996–98, up from 25 percent in 1990–92).*

The 1990s saw a growing clamor in the industrial world over debt in the developing world, fueled in no small measure by a perception that interest payments were constraining government health expenditures in developing countries.[19] The enhanced Highly Indebted Poor Country Initiative was explicitly geared to channeling freed resources into the health and other social sectors.[20] The Poverty Reduction Strategy Paper was introduced for developing country governments seeking debt relief or concessional IDA loans to set out their plans for fighting poverty on all fronts, including health.

The 1990s also saw the development of major new global health initiatives and partnerships, including UNAIDS, the

Global Alliance for Vaccines and Immunization, the Stop TB Partnership, Roll Back Malaria, the Global Fund to Fight AIDS, Tuberculosis and Malaria, and most recently the Global Alliance for Improved Nutrition (box 1.2). The scale of philanthropic involvement in international health also increased, with the launch of the Bill and Melinda Gates Foundation and the Packard Foundation and the greater attention to global health issues by such established foundations as the Rockefeller Foundation. These initiatives brought new funds to the fight against disease, death, and malnutrition in the developing world—as well as new ideas, new energy, and new coordination challenges and mechanisms.

With the 1990s drawing to a close, the international community decided that even more needed to be done to address the array of development challenges facing the poor. In September 2001 at the Millennium Summit, 147 heads of states endorsed the Millennium Development Goals. Later, at the UN General Assembly, the heads of state of all 189 UN member states adopted the goals.

The rest of the report

This report focuses on the Millennium Development Goals, which all governments have agreed on. Other health outcomes are equally or even more important in many countries, especially in countries going through the demographic, epidemiological, and nutritional transitions and those in which noncommunicable disease and injury contribute significantly to the burden of disease. The focus in this report is on outcomes, on households, on health system constraints and public health functions, and on investments in improving policies and institutions. The agenda is relevant for all countries, whether their targets are the Millennium Development Targets, other national and subnational targets, or some combination of the two. All countries have an interest in monitoring progress using national and context-specific intermediate indicators, in buying better results with their limited resources, and in accelerating progress toward their goals.

- Chapter 2 sets out the Millennium Development Goals for health and assesses progress to date and prospects of achieving the goals.

- Chapter 3 argues that where progress has been slow, the reason is not a lack of effective interventions but inadequate use of existing interventions.

- Chapter 4 introduces the report's second part (chapters 5–10). It argues that low coverage rates partly reflect the low levels of government health spending but more fundamentally the numerous policy and institutional weaknesses across the entire health system.

---

* The International Development Association, part of the World Bank Group, provides loans to the world's poorest countries at zero interest with a grace period of 10 years and maturities of 35–40 years.

Box 1.2 The promising (and challenging) array of health-related partnerships

This list is not comprehensive, but it gives a sense of the large number of partnerships, most of them formed in the past seven to eight years. Many involve formal governance structures with international institutions, donors, governments, industry, and civil society.

Communicable diseases

Global Fund to Fight AIDS, Tuberculosis and Malaria

UNDP/World Bank/WHO Special Program for Research & Training in Tropical Diseases

Joint United Nations Program on HIV/AIDS (UNAIDS)

Global Alliance for Vaccines and Immunization

International AIDS Vaccine Initiative

Stop TB Partnership

Global Drug Facility

Global Alliance for TB Drug Development (TB Alliance)

Fund for Investment in New Diagnostics

Roll Back Malaria

Multilateral Initiative on Malaria

Medicines for Malaria Venture

International Trachoma Initiative

International Public/Private Partnership for Health

Global AIDS Monitoring and Evaluation Team

International Treatment Acceleration Coalition

Region-specific partnerships

African Program for Onchocerciasis Control

International Partnership against AIDS in Africa

Maternal and child health and nutrition

Safe Motherhood Initiative

Research in Human Reproduction Program

Global Alliance for Improved Nutrition Partnership for Child Development

Child Health and Nutrition Research Initiative

Health systems strengthening and financing

Alliance for Health Policy and Systems Research

European Observatory on Health Care Systems

INDEPTH Health Surveillance and Experimentation Network

- Chapter 5 shows that additional government health spending would accelerate progress toward the health Millennium Development Goals only in countries with relatively good policies and institutions.

- Chapter 6 argues that poor progress toward the goals reflects weak household demand for the services of formal providers and weak household capacity to deliver key home-based interventions.

- Chapter 7 argues that slow progress also reflects the inefficiency and unresponsiveness of provider organizations, which reflects poor management and weak accountability to the public.

- Chapter 8 discusses the role of input markets in holding back progress toward the Millennium Development Goals, examining human resource shortages, inadequate skills, and unaffordable and often inappropriate drugs.

- Chapter 9 argues that many countries have a weak public health infrastructure that leaves core public health functions uncovered.

- Chapter 10 discusses the role of the World Bank and issues of interagency coordination and partnerships.

References

1. UNICEF. 2001. *Progress Since the World Summit for Children: A Statistical Review.* New York: UNICEF.

2. Food and Agricultural Organization of the United Nations. 2000. *The State of Food Security in the World.* Rome: FAO.

3. UNAIDS. 2002. *Report on the Global HIV/AIDS Epidemic.* Geneva: UNAIDS.

4. Sen, A. 2002. "Why Health Equity?" *Health Economics* 11 (8): 659–666.

5. World Bank. 2001. *World Development Report 2000/2001: Attacking Poverty.* Washington, DC: World Bank

6. Jones, G., R. W. Steketee, R. E. Black, Z. A. Bhutta, and S. S. Morris. 2003. "How Many Child Deaths Can We Prevent This Year?" *Lancet* 362 (9377): 65–71.

7. Wagstaff, A., and E. van Doorslaer. 2003. "Catastrophe and Impoverishment in Paying for Health Care: With Applications to Vietnam 1993–98." *Health Economics* 12 (11): 921–933.

8. Narayan, D., R. Patel, K. Schafft, A. Rademacher, and S. Koch-Schulte. 2000. *Voices of the Poor: Can Anyone Hear Us?* New York: Oxford University Press.

9. World Bank. 2004. *World Development Report 2004: Making Services Work for Poor People.* Washington, DC: World Bank.

10. Glewwe, P., H.G. Jacoby, and E.M. King. 2001. "Early Childhood Nutrition and Academic Achievement: A Longitudinal Analysis." *Journal of Public Economics* 81 (3):345–368.

11. Grassly, N.C., K. Desai, E. Pegurri, A. Sikazwe, I. Malambo, C. Siamatowe, and D. Bundy. 2003. "The Economic Impact of HIV/AIDS on the Education Sector in Zambia." *AIDS* 17 (7): 1039–1044.

12. Gertler, P., and J. Gruber. 2002. "Insuring Consumption against Illness." *American Economic Review* 92 (1): 51–76.

13. Bloom, D., and J. Sachs. 1998. "Geography, Demography and Economic Growth in Africa." *Brookings Papers on Economic Activity* 2: 207–295.

14. Gwatkin, D., S. Rutstein, K. Johnson, R. Pande, and A. Wagstaff. 2000. "Socioeconomic Differences in Health, Nutrition and Population." Health, Nutrition and Population Discussion Paper, World Bank, Washington, DC. http://www.worldbank.org/poverty/health/data/index.htm.

15. Wagstaff, A. 2000. "Socioeconomic Inequalities in Child Mortality: Comparisons across Nine Developing Countries." *Bulletin of the World Health Organization* 78 (1): 19–29.

16. World Health Organization. 1998. *CHD 1996–97 Report.* Geneva: WHO.

17. Pathmanathan, I., J. Liljestrand, J.M. Martins, L.C. Rajapaksa, C. Lissner, A. de Silva, S. Selvaraju, and P.J. Singh. 2003. *Investing in Maternal Health: Learning from Malaysia and Sri Lanka.* Washington, DC: World Bank.

18. OECD Development Assistance Committee. 2000. *Recent Trends in Official Development Assistance to Health.* Paris: OECD.

19. Kirby, A. 1999. "UK Archbishop Heads Debt Chain." BBC Online, June 13.

20. Gupta, S., B. Clements, M.T. Guin-Siu, and L. Leruth. 2002. "Debt Relief and Public Health Spending in Heavily Indebted Poor Countries." *Bulletin of the World Health Organization* 80 (2): 151–157.

21. World Health Organization. 2003. Global Database on Child Growth and Malnutrition. http://www.who.int/nutgrowthdb/.

22. UNICEF. 2003. Statistics: Child Mortality. http://www.childinfo.org/cmr/revis/db2.htm.

23. World Bank. 2003. *World Development Indicators 2003.* Washington, DC: World Bank.

CHAPTER 2

The Millennium Development Goals for Health: Progress and Prospects

Nearly half the Millennium Development Targets concern health—directly or indirectly. They vary in their ambitiousness, with the maternal mortality goal of a three-quarters reduction between 1990 and 2015 being the most ambitious. Progress has varied across the goals, in part reflecting the differences in ambitiousness. All World Bank regions except Sub-Saharan Africa will hit the malnutrition targets, but many countries— even in regions where malnutrition has fallen rapidly—will not. Progress on child survival has been insufficient to leave any Bank region or any Sub-Saharan country on track to hit the target, but 40 percent of Sub-Saharan countries accelerated their pace of reducing child mortality in the 1990s. All but one Bank region will miss the maternal mortality target, albeit by a smaller margin than for the child mortality target. That's the

situation at "half time" in the 1990–2015 period for the goals.

The "second half" may go better. Per capita incomes are forecast to grow faster in all but one region (East Asia and the Pacific). And reaching the targets for gender and environment would imply faster progress in girls' education and access to safe drinking water than in the 1990s for most regions. This impetus may push three regions to (or close to) the maternal mortality target. But it will still leave all regions well short of the child mortality target and Sub-Saharan Africa well short of the malnutrition target. This chapter argues that the Millennium Development Goals are useful because they focus on outcomes and remind us of what is achievable. What is important is to accelerate progress toward the targets, even if the targets will not be hit.

Health is prominent in the Millennium Development Goals

It is a reflection of the international community's concern for health in the developing world that nearly half the goals and targets concern—directly or indirectly—different aspects of health.★ Table 2.1 sets out the goals, targets, and indicators, along with key additional monitoring indicators recommended by a technical consultation in 2001.[1]

The first goal explicitly aims to improve the living standards of poor people. The other goals do not. It is statistically possible for there to be no reduction in child malnutrition among, say, the poorest 20 percent of a population but for the population as a whole to achieve the required 50 percent reduction. Achieving such a result would require a 62.5 percent reduction among the top 80 percent of the population, but it is a possibility with which policymakers need to be concerned. One bilateral aid agency recently expressed concern over this, urging that the pursuit of the goals be done through a propoor approach to ensure that the poor see gains across all goals.[2] This report presents new evidence on whether progress toward the health-related Millennium Development Goals has left the poor behind.

There are, of course, links and interdependencies among the various goals:

- Nutrition has an important influence on maternal and child health, so progress toward meeting goals 1, 4, and 5 is likely to be related.

- Nutrition also influences the severity of communicable diseases, including HIV/AIDS and tuberculosis, reducing people's ability to fight off such diseases. Similarly, diarrhea, measles, and malaria are major influences on children's nutritional status (such as anemia). Success on goals 1 and 6 is thus also likely to be linked.

- Progress in securing access to safe water and satisfactory sanitation (goal 7) and on securing access to affordable medicines (goal 8) is likely to influence progress toward goals 1 and 2.

- Progress on the health Millennium Development Goals is also likely to reflect progress on the nonhealth goals. Early child nutrition and health, for example, affect educational outcomes for school-age children.

- Rapid progress on the income poverty goal would speed progress on the health goals, as would rapid progress on the education and gender equality goals.

★ Throughout the report we interpret "health" broadly. For example, nutrition is both a key aspect of health in its own right and a key influence on other aspects of health.

What's the score at half time?

Tracking progress toward the health goals is not straightforward because of differences in how the indicators are defined, which measurement instruments are used, how frequently information is collected, and how much effort has been invested in developing measurement systems (see appendix B). And as with progress on anything, much depends on how it is measured. Are we talking about countries being on track to hit the Millennium Development Targets or about how close countries come to hitting the targets? Are we talking about the number of countries that are on track or the number of people living in on-track countries? Are we talking about progress at the global level, at the level of the World Bank region, or at the level of different income groupings of countries (low, middle, or high)? Are we talking about progress for populations as a whole or for specific sections of the population, such as the poor? Countries may, after all, hit the Millennium Development Target for the whole population and yet leave some groups (the poor, women, ethnic minorities) or regions behind.

Prospects for meeting the malnutrition target are reasonably good

Goal 1 calls for halving the proportion of people suffering from hunger between 1990 and 2015, an average annual reduction of 2.7 percent. One of the two indicators tracking progress toward this goal is the prevalence of underweight children among children under five.

Five of the six Bank regions achieved population-weighted average annual reductions in underweight children of 2.7 percent or more in the 1990s (figure 2.1).[†] Upper middle-income countries and particularly lower middle-income countries exceeded the target (see figure 2.1). Not surprisingly, then, the developing world as a whole is on track to reach the malnutrition target, having achieved a population-weighted average annual decline of 5 percent in the 1990s. More than 50 percent of the developing world's population lives in an on-track country for the malnutrition goal (figure 2.2). In East Asia and South Asia, the figure is more than 85 percent, and in low-income countries, the figure is 64 percent.

Against this good news is some inevitable bad news. Sub-Saharan Africa saw barely any change in child malnutrition in the 1990s. Only 17 percent of countries there are on track to meet the malnutrition goal (figure 2.3), and only 12 percent of people there live in an on-track country. Malnutrition has been falling more slowly in low-income countries than in middle-income countries. In the

---

† See appendix A for a full explanation of data sources and methods used.

Table 2.1 Goals, targets, and indicators—many of them for health

Millennium Development Goal	Targets	Indicators	Additional monitoring indicators
Goal 1: Eradicate extreme poverty and hunger	Halve, between 1990 and 2015, the proportion of people whose income is less than $1 a day.		
	Halve, between 1990 and 2015, the proportion of people who suffer from hunger.	Prevalence of underweight children under five years of age Proportion of population below minimum level of dietary energy consumption	*Core intermediate indicators* Percentage of children 6–59 months who received one dose of vitamin A in the past six months; proportion of infants under six months who are exclusively breastfed *Optional indicators* Low birth weight incidence rate; proportion of mothers receiving vitamin A supplementation by eight weeks postpartum *Indicators requiring further research* Timely complementary feeding; recuperative feeding
Goal 4: Reduce child mortality	Reduce by two-thirds, between 1990 and 2015, the under-five mortality rate.	Under-five mortality rate Infant mortality rate Measles immunization among children under one	*Core intermediate indicators* Proportion of infants under six months who are exclusively breastfed; proportion of surviving infants who have received a dose of measles vaccine by their first birthday; proportion of children with fast or difficult breathing in the past two weeks who received an appropriate antibiotic; proportion of children with diarrhea in the past two weeks who received oral rehydration therapy; proportion of children under five who slept under an insecticide-treated net the previous night (in malarious areas); proportion of children with fever in the past two weeks who received an appropriate antimalarial (in malarious areas) *Optional indicators* Vitamin A supplementation; proportion of infants six- to nine-months-old receiving breast milk and complementary food; piped water and sanitation; female education; effects of income on mortality (such as access to water and sanitation, access to and use of cars); birth spacing *Indicators requiring further research* Perinatal and neonatal indicators (for example, deliveries attended by skilled personnel); indicators to capture determinants of death in the first days of life (such as identification and treatment of asphyxia, prevention and treatment of sepsis at birth)
Goal 5: Improve maternal health	Reduce by three-quarters, between 1990 and 2015, the maternal mortality ratio.	Maternal mortality ratio Proportion of births attended by skilled health personnel	*Core intermediate indicators* Contraceptive prevalence rate; percentage of women receiving any antenatal care; provision of emergency obstetric care; prevalence of syphilis in pregnant women and proportion properly treated; percentage of women receiving antenatal care who receive at least two intermittent preventive malaria treatments during pregnancy (in malarious areas) *Optional indicators* Prevention of mother-to-child transmission of HIV/AIDS; perinatal mortality rate; total fertility rate; female genital mutilation *Indicators requiring further research* Adolescent reproductive health; caesarean section rate

Millennium Development Goal	Targets	Indicators	Additional monitoring indicators
Goal 6: Combat HIV/AIDS, malaria, and other diseases	Halt by 2015 and begin to reverse the spread of HIV/AIDS.	HIV prevalence among 15- to 24-year-old pregnant women Condom use rate of the contraceptive prevalence rate Number of children orphaned by HIV/AIDS	*Core intermediate indicators* Percentage of people using a condom during most recent higher-risk sexual encounter; percentage of sexually transmitted infection clients who are appropriately diagnosed and treated according to guidelines; percentage of HIV-positive women receiving antiretroviral treatment during pregnancy to prevent mother-to-child transmission of HIV
	Halt by 2015 and begin to reverse the incidence of malaria and other major diseases.	Prevalence and death rate associated with malaria Proportion of population in malaria risk areas using effective malaria prevention and treatment measures	*Core intermediate indicators* Percentage of patients with uncomplicated malaria who received treatment within 24 hours of onset of symptoms; percentage of children under age five sleeping under insecticide-treated nets; percentage of pregnant women sleeping under insecticide-treated nets; percentage of pregnant women who have taken chemoprophylaxis or drug treatment for malaria
		Prevalence and death rates associated with tuberculosis Proportion of tuberculosis cases detected and cured under DOTS	*Core intermediate indicators* Percentage of estimated new smear-positive tuberculosis cases registered under the DOTS approach
Goal 7: Ensure environmental sustainability	Integrate the principles of sustainable development into country policies and reverse loss of environmental resources.		
	Halve by 2015 the proportion of people without sustainable access to safe drinking water.	Proportion of population with sustainable access to an improved water source, urban and rural	
	By 2020 achieve a significant improvement in the lives of at least 100 million slum dwellers.	Proportion of urban population with access to improved sanitation Proportion of households with access to secure tenure	
Goal 8: Develop a global partnership for development	Develop further an open, rule-based, predictable, nondiscriminatory trading and financial system.		
	Address the special needs of the least developed, land-locked, and small island developing countries.		
	Deal comprehensively with the debt problems of developing countries.		
	Develop and implement strategies for decent and productive work for youth.		
	In cooperation with pharmaceutical companies, provide access to affordable essential drugs in developing countries.	Proportion of population with access to affordable essential drugs on a sustainable basis	
	In cooperation with the private sector, make available the benefits of new technologies, especially information and communications.		

Source: Reference 18.

Figure 2.1 Progress on malnutrition, under-five mortality, and maternal mortality, by region and income

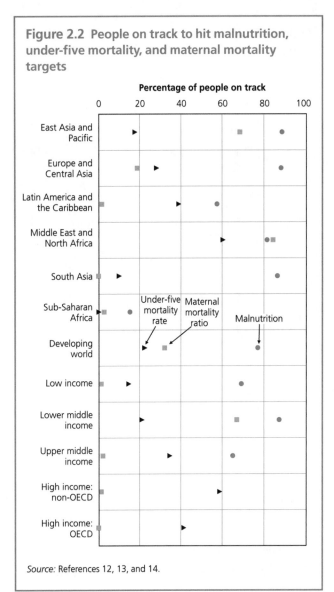

Average annual percentage change

East Asia and Pacific
Europe and Central Asia
Latin America and the Caribbean
Middle East and North Africa
South Asia
Sub-Saharan Africa
Developing world
Low income
Lower middle income
Upper middle income
High income: non-OECD
High income: OECD

Maternal mortality ratio
Under-five mortality rate
Malnutrition

Source: References 12, 13, and 14.

Figure 2.2 People on track to hit malnutrition, under-five mortality, and maternal mortality targets

Percentage of people on track

East Asia and Pacific
Europe and Central Asia
Latin America and the Caribbean
Middle East and North Africa
South Asia
Sub-Saharan Africa
Developing world
Low income
Lower middle income
Upper middle income
High income: non-OECD
High income: OECD

Under-five mortality rate
Maternal mortality ratio
Malnutrition

Source: References 12, 13, and 14.

low-income countries, malnutrition has declined only 2.6 percent a year—just short of the target rate. Even in the regions experiencing high average annual declines in malnutrition, several countries have fallen short of the target rate of 2.7 percent (figure 2.4). The East Asia and the Pacific region is well on target, for example, but nearly half the countries there are currently off target. But things could have been worse. That 17 percent of Sub-Saharan countries and 20 percent of low-income countries are on track provides some hope for other Sub-Saharan and low-income countries.

How have the poor fared in reducing malnutrition? For the 17 countries with disaggregated trend data, the average rate of reduction of malnutrition in the 1990s was broadly similar for the poorest 20 percent of the population and for the population as a whole (figure 2.5). In two coun-

tries—Colombia and Tanzania—progress was substantially faster among the very poor than among the whole population. But in several countries—including Bangladesh and Bolivia, often held up as examples of countries that have implemented propoor policies—child malnutrition has been falling more slowly among the very poor.

Child mortality: Poor progress

The targets call for a two-thirds reduction in infant and under-five mortality rates between 1990 and 2015, an average reduction of 4.3 percent a year. But no Bank region achieved a population-weighted annual average reduction in excess of 4.3 percent in the 1990s (see figure 2.1). The only countries on target are the high-income countries—indicating that, contrary to what is often claimed, large percentage reductions in child mortality are

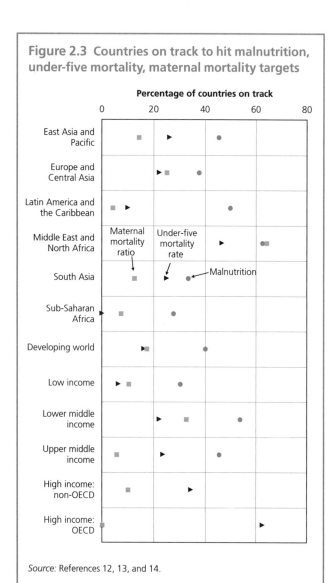

Figure 2.3 Countries on track to hit malnutrition, under-five mortality, maternal mortality targets

Percentage of countries on track

Source: References 12, 13, and 14.

Figure 2.4 Some countries are reducing malnutrition quickly. In others malnutrition has fallen less slowly, and in some it has increased.

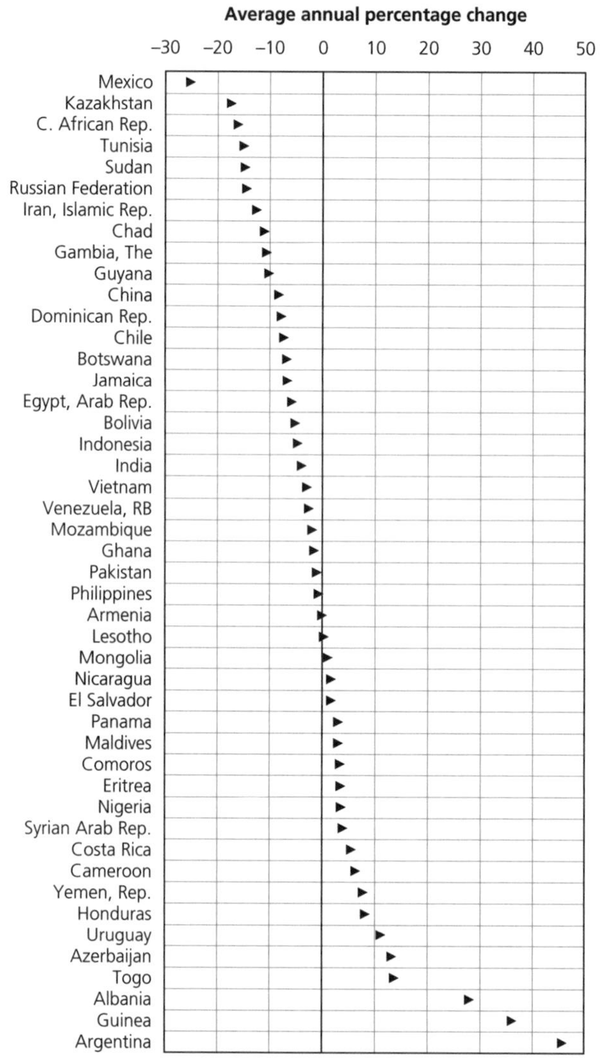

Average annual percentage change

Source: Reference 13.

possible even at low levels of mortality. The goals, which are defined in terms of percentage reductions rather than absolute levels, are as relevant to middle-income and high-income countries as they are to low-income countries. As a group, the middle-income countries experienced slower annual reductions in child mortality than the high-income countries, and they are off track for the child mortality target. The upper middle-income countries have fared better and are just on track, while the lower middle-income countries are badly off track.

The widening gap between poor and better-off countries is mirrored at the country level. And gaps in child mortality between the poor and the better off are widening within countries, too. On average, the child mortality rate among the poorest 20 percent of the population fell just half as fast as for the whole population (figure 2.6 and appendix B). And there is more bad news. Only 16 percent of coun-

tries are on track for the under-five mortality target, and only 22 percent of the developing world's population lives in an on-track country (see figures 2.2 and 2.3). Not a single Sub-Saharan country is on track for the child mortality target. And in all regions—especially Latin America and the Caribbean, the Middle East and North Africa, and Sub-Saharan Africa—the rate of decline of under-five mortality was greater in the 1980s than in the 1990s (figure 2.7).

The news on child mortality is not all bad, however. Although mortality rates fell more rapidly, on average, in the 1980s than in the 1990s, 38 percent of countries saw a faster decline in the 1990s than in the 1980s (figure 2.8). For Sub-Saharan Africa the figure was 41 percent, and half the region's

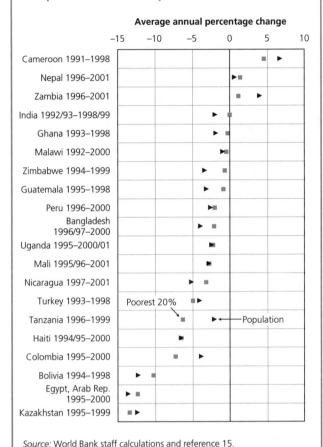

Figure 2.5 How the poor have fared on malnutrition reductions—absolutely and compared with the less poor

Average annual percentage change

Cameroon 1991–1998
Nepal 1996–2001
Zambia 1996–2001
India 1992/93–1998/99
Ghana 1993–1998
Malawi 1992–2000
Zimbabwe 1994–1999
Guatemala 1995–1998
Peru 1996–2000
Bangladesh 1996/97–2000
Uganda 1995–2000/01
Mali 1995/96–2001
Nicaragua 1997–2001
Turkey 1993–1998
Tanzania 1996–1999
Haiti 1994/95–2000
Colombia 1995–2000
Bolivia 1994–1998
Egypt, Arab Rep. 1995–2000
Kazakhstan 1995–1999

Poorest 20%

Population

Source: World Bank staff calculations and reference 15.

Figure 2.6 How the poor have fared on under-five mortality reductions—absolutely and compared with the less poor

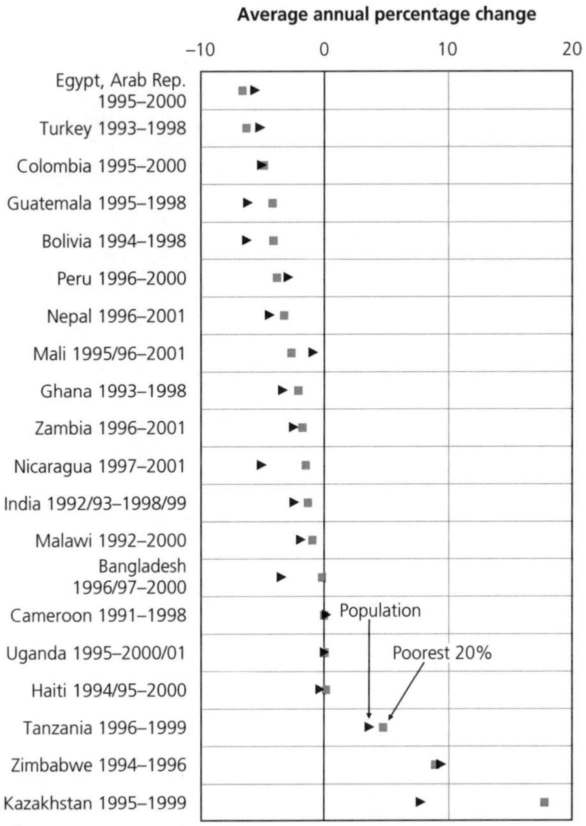

Average annual percentage change

Egypt, Arab Rep. 1995–2000
Turkey 1993–1998
Colombia 1995–2000
Guatemala 1995–1998
Bolivia 1994–1998
Peru 1996–2000
Nepal 1996–2001
Mali 1995/96–2001
Ghana 1993–1998
Zambia 1996–2001
Nicaragua 1997–2001
India 1992/93–1998/99
Malawi 1992–2000
Bangladesh 1996/97–2000
Cameroon 1991–1998
Uganda 1995–2000/01
Haiti 1994/95–2000
Tanzania 1996–1999
Zimbabwe 1994–1996
Kazakhstan 1995–1999

Population

Poorest 20%

Source: World Bank staff calculations and reference 15.

people live in a country that accelerated its rate of decline of child mortality in the 1990s. This partly reflects the fact that Ethiopia and Uganda improved their performance in the 1990s. This is also a cause for hope: despite HIV/AIDS, many Sub-Saharan countries have shown themselves able to accelerate the rate of decline of under-five mortality.

Maternal mortality: Insufficient progress

The Millennium Development Goals call for a three-quarters reduction in the maternal mortality ratio between 1990 and 2015, an average annual reduction of 5.4 percent.

The developing world as a whole is off target, having registered an average population-weighted decline of just 3.2 percent in the 1990s (see figure 2.1).‡ Indeed, only one region—the Middle East and North Africa—is on target, though East Asia and the Pacific comes fairly close, with an

estimated annual reduction of 4.5 percent. Across the developing world, 17 percent of countries are on track to achieve the maternal mortality target, but there are large variations across regions, ranging from 4 percent in Latin America and the Caribbean to 64 percent in the Middle East and North Africa. For the developing world as a whole, 32 percent of the population lives in an on-track country. But the 12 percent of countries on track in South Asia have a negligible share of that region's population.

Communicable diseases: Too little progress

The goals call for a reversal in the spread of HIV/AIDS and other communicable diseases and the beginning of a decline in incidence. According to UNAIDS, the AIDS epidemic led to the deaths of an estimated 3.1 million people in 2002, and an estimated 5 million people were living with HIV infection in 2002. Some countries have been devastated by HIV/AIDS. In Botswana the rate of increase in the number of new cases appears to have peaked in the

‡ More accurately, a country's estimated rate of reduction is weighted by the number of births.

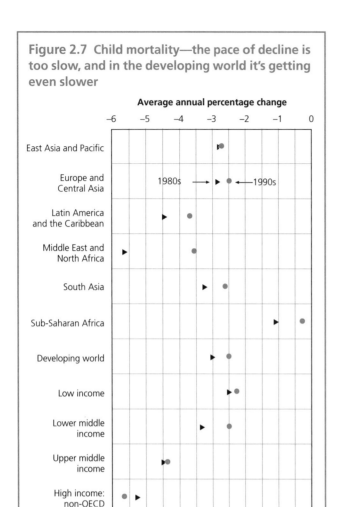

Figure 2.7 Child mortality—the pace of decline is too slow, and in the developing world it's getting even slower

Average annual percentage change

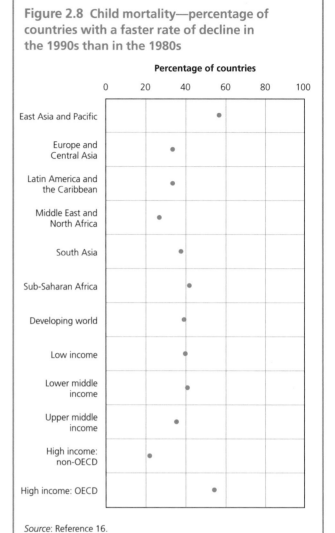

Figure 2.8 Child mortality—percentage of countries with a faster rate of decline in the 1990s than in the 1980s

Percentage of countries

late 1990s—but not until the prevalence of HIV reached a staggering 44 percent in urban areas. Yet there are some hopeful signs. In Uganda HIV prevalence in Kampala has been declining steadily—from a high of 30 percent in 1990 to 11 percent in 2000—and similar rates of decline have been observed in other areas of the country (figure 2.9). In Côte d'Ivoire HIV prevalence in major urban areas has declined for the last three years for which data are available.

The number of countries implementing directly observed treatment, short-course (DOTS) regimens for tuberculosis has increased to 155 (of 210). More than 10 million patients have been diagnosed and treated in DOTS programs since 1995. While some countries have made rapid progress in DOTS detection rates, those with high tuberculosis burdens are not increasing case detection rates toward the 70 percent target in DOTS areas. Treatment success under DOTS for 2000 was 82 percent on average but substantially below average in Africa (72 percent).

Figures 2.10 and 2.11 show DOTS detection and cure rates for selected countries in Sub-Saharan Africa.

Will the second half go better?

As the well-known stock market dictum warns—and as figure 2.12 shows for under-five mortality—past performance is not necessarily a good predictor of future performance. The fact that a country is on track on the basis of its performance in the 1990s does not guarantee that it will maintain the required annual rate of reduction of malnutrition or mortality in 2000–15. It is also possible, of course, that countries that are currently off track may get on track during the second half. What are the likely future trends in the various country-level determinants of malnutrition and mortality? Will countries grow more rapidly in the new millennium than in the 1990s? If so, how much extra mortality reduction will this faster growth buy?

Figure 2.9 Trends in HIV prevalence among pregnant women in Uganda, 1990–2001

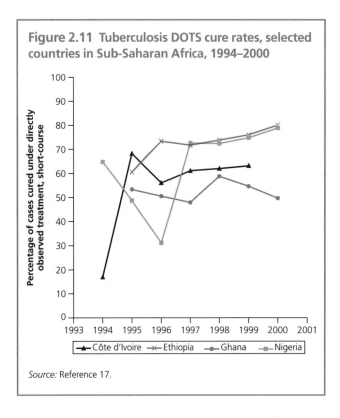

Figure 2.11 Tuberculosis DOTS cure rates, selected countries in Sub-Saharan Africa, 1994–2000

Source: Reference 12.

Source: Reference 17.

Figure 2.10 Tuberculosis DOTS detection rates, selected countries in Sub-Saharan Africa, 1995–2001

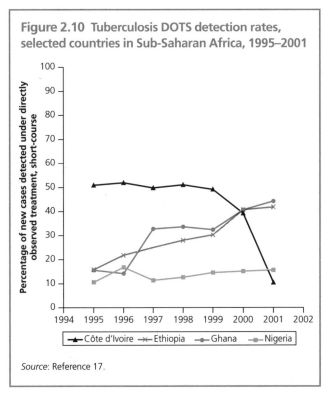

Source: Reference 17.

Economic growth will increase in the new millennium, except in East Asia

The World Bank[3] estimates that growth will fall somewhat in East Asia, turn from negative to positive growth in Europe and Central Asia and Sub-Saharan Africa, and increase somewhat in Latin America and the Caribbean,

the Middle East and North Africa, and South America (figure 2.13). Given mortality's and malnutrition's close links with per capita income,[4,5] the increase in growth will help push countries toward the goals, especially in Europe and Central Asia, where the change in growth is appreciable. But even with faster growth, per capita incomes will rise at more than 2 percent a year in only two regions—East Asia and the Pacific and South Asia.

Primary education completion will probably increase more rapidly in the new millennium

The Millennium Development Goals call for 100 percent completion rates at primary level, and it is likely that *Education for All* and the *Fast Track Initiative* will accelerate progress toward universal primary completion. The health payoffs to this in the second half are unclear. An increase in the primary completion rate in 2000 will not filter through into higher levels of educational attainment among women of childbearing age until 2005 or so. And the first full round of effects on under-five mortality will not be felt until 2010. Since only a small percentage of births are to 15-year-olds, the bulk of any child survival payoffs associated with an increased primary completion rate in 2000 will come after 2010—mostly well after 2015.

Even beyond 2015 it is unlikely that increases in primary school completion rates will yield appreciable payoffs in better health outcomes. A recent multicountry study[6] using Demographic and Health Surveys data found that

Figure 2.12 Past performance is not necessarily a good predictor of future performance: under-five mortality

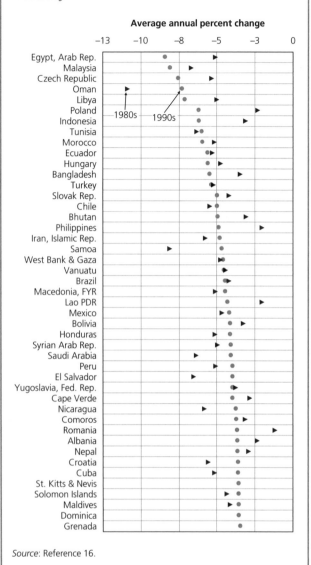

Average annual percent change

| | −13 | −10 | −8 | −5 | −3 | 0 |

Egypt, Arab Rep.
Malaysia
Czech Republic
Oman
Libya
Poland
Indonesia
Tunisia
Morocco
Ecuador
Hungary
Bangladesh
Turkey
Slovak Rep.
Chile
Bhutan
Philippines
Iran, Islamic Rep.
Samoa
West Bank & Gaza
Vanuatu
Brazil
Macedonia, FYR
Lao PDR
Mexico
Bolivia
Honduras
Syrian Arab Rep.
Saudi Arabia
Peru
El Salvador
Yugoslavia, Fed. Rep.
Cape Verde
Nicaragua
Comoros
Romania
Albania
Nepal
Croatia
Cuba
St. Kitts & Nevis
Solomon Islands
Maldives
Dominica
Grenada

1980s   1990s

Source: Reference 16.

Figure 2.13 Growth rates of per capita income: actual 1990–2000 and forecasts for 2001–15

Legend: ■ 1990–2000 □ 2001–15

Y-axis: 7%, 6%, 5%, 4%, 3%, 2%, 1%, 0%, −1%, −2%, −3%

X-axis categories: East Asia and Pacific; Europe and Central Asia; Latin America and the Caribbean; Middle East and North Africa; South Asia; Sub-Saharan Africa

Source: Reference 3.

while secondary education can exert a significant effect on infant mortality, primary education does so in only a few countries.[§] This is consistent with the finding[7] that better-educated women achieve better health outcomes not by using health-specific knowledge acquired at school but by using the general numeracy and literacy skills they are taught at school to acquire health-specific knowledge later on in life. The implication is not that primary schooling necessarily has limited and possibly negligible payoffs for child and maternal health. It is that current average levels

of quality are probably too low for girls to acquire the literacy and numeracy skills needed to develop enough health-specific knowledge later in life.

Gender gaps in secondary education may well narrow in the new millennium

One of the Millennium Development Goals is to promote gender equality and empower women. If the elimination of gender disparities at all levels of education entails faster growth in secondary school completion rates among girls, it could have significant consequences for maternal and child health outcomes. To achieve parity with boys by 2015 in the proportion of the population 15 and older that completes secondary education, girls' completion rates will have to grow faster in the new millennium than in the 1990s in most regions, especially in East and South Asia (figure 2.14).★★

Attaining the drinking water and sanitation goals would entail faster growth in access in the new millennium

The Millennium Development Goals (and the Johannesburg goals) call for halving the proportion of the world's popula-

[§] This is consistent with cross-country econometric work undertaken for this report that finds that while female *secondary* education significantly reduces maternal mortality, female *primary* education has no significant effect on any Millennium Development Goal outcome (see appendix A).

★★ In this simulation it is assumed that the proportion of males in each World Bank region who complete secondary education continues to grow in 2001–15 at the same rate it grew during the second half of the 1990s. The figure for females is then brought up to the level that males would reach in 2015, on the assumption that the figures for both males and females grow linearly.

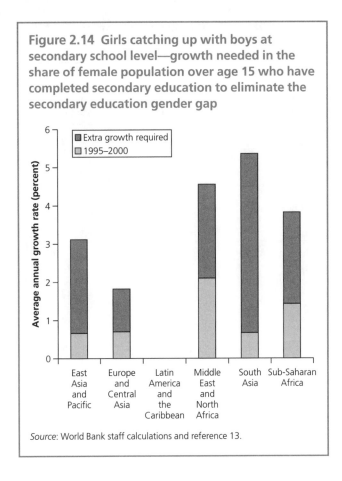

Figure 2.14 Girls catching up with boys at secondary school level—growth needed in the share of female population over age 15 who have completed secondary education to eliminate the secondary education gender gap

Average annual growth rate (percent)

■ Extra growth required
□ 1995–2000

East Asia and Pacific | Europe and Central Asia | Latin America and the Caribbean | Middle East and North Africa | South Asia | Sub-Saharan Africa

Source: World Bank staff calculations and reference 13.

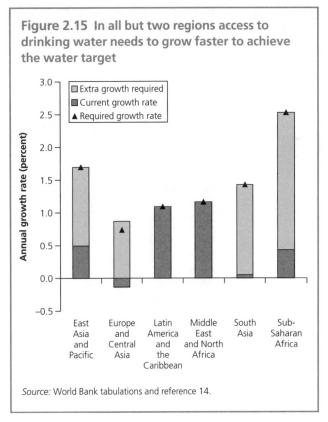

Figure 2.15 In all but two regions access to drinking water needs to grow faster to achieve the water target

Annual growth rate (percent)

□ Extra growth required
■ Current growth rate
▲ Required growth rate

East Asia and Pacific | Europe and Central Asia | Latin America and the Caribbean | Middle East and North Africa | South Asia | Sub-Saharan Africa

Source: World Bank tabulations and reference 14.

tion without access to safe drinking water and sanitation between 1990 and 2015. If drinking water access rates grow linearly at the trend rates of the 1990s, only Latin America and the Caribbean and the Middle East and North Africa will achieve the Millennium Development Target. To achieve the water target, access rates would need to grow much more rapidly, especially in Sub-Saharan Africa, where access is currently growing by 0.43 percent a year but would need to grow by 2.53 percent a year to meet the goal (figure 2.15). If access rates were to grow rapidly enough to achieve the water target, the under-five and maternal mortality rates could fall appreciably.

Even with economic growth and faster progress on the nonhealth goals, many regions will still miss many of the health targets

Faster economic growth and achievement of the gender and water goals will lead to appreciable declines in mortality and malnutrition (see appendix A for methods). In Europe and Central Asia progress on these three fronts might add as much as 1.4 percentage points to the rate of decline of under-five mortality, 1.1 percentage points to the rate of decline of maternal mortality, and just under 1 percentage point to the annual rate of reduction of underweight (table 2.2). In South Asia it might add as much as 2.6 percentage

points to the annual rate of reduction of maternal mortality, taking the annual rate of decline from 2.9 percent to 5.5 percent. These contributions will push countries and regions firmly toward the Millennium Development Targets, but for the most part they will not get them there. (An exception is maternal mortality in East Asia.) In Europe and Central Asia and South Asia the impetus is also large— but for the relatively slow progress in the 1990s, the antici- pated faster economic growth and faster progress on girls' education might have allowed both regions to hit the maternal mortality targets. The picture is bleakest for under- five mortality and for Sub-Saharan Africa. Even with the one extra percentage point annual reduction in under-five mortality driven by economic growth and achievement of the gender and water targets, the projected reduction of under-five mortality for 2000–15 is still only 1.6 percent a year in Sub-Saharan Africa.

Why the picture may be bleaker

The assumptions about future trends in the determinants of the Millennium Development Goals used for the simu- lations conducted here are probably overly optimistic. It is assumed that progress on eliminating gender gaps in sec- ondary education and expanding access to drinking water is fast enough to achieve the relevant target. It is also assumed that in the absence of faster economic growth and accelerated progress toward the gender and water

Table 2.2 Economic growth and attainment of the gender and water targets will push countries toward the health targets but leave many a long way from them

Millennium Development Goal	Region	Target growth rate 1990–2015 (percent)	Current growth rate 1990–2000 (percent)	Contributions from faster economic growth and progress toward gender and water targets (percent)	Revised growth rate (percent)
Under-five mortality rate	East Asia and the Pacific	–4.3	–2.7	–0.2	–2.9
	Europe and Central Asia	–4.3	–2.5	–1.4	–3.9
	Latin America and the Caribbean	–4.3	–3.7	0.0	–3.7
	Middle East and North Africa	–4.3	–3.6	–0.1	–3.7
	South Asia	–4.3	–2.6	–0.6	–3.2
	Sub-Saharan Africa	–4.3	–0.3	–1.0	–1.3
Maternal mortality ratio	East Asia and the Pacific	–5.4	–4.5	–1.7	–6.3
	Europe and Central Asia	–5.4	–4.3	–1.0	–5.3
	Latin America and the Caribbean	–5.4	–1.5	0.0	–1.5
	Middle East and North Africa	–5.4	–6.9	–0.8	–7.8
	South Asia	–5.4	–2.9	–2.6	–5.5
	Sub-Saharan Africa	–5.4	–1.6	–2.4	–4.1
Underweight	East Asia and the Pacific	–2.7	–6.7	0.2	–6.6
	Europe and Central Asia	–2.7	–9.6	–0.9	–10.5
	Latin America and the Caribbean	–2.7	–4.1	0.0	–4.1
	Middle East and North Africa	–2.7	–6.3	–0.1	–6.4
	South Asia	–2.7	–3.5	–0.1	–3.6
	Sub-Saharan Africa	–2.7	–0.2	–0.3	–0.5
Tuberculosis mortality	East Asia and the Pacific	n.a.	n.a.	0.2	0.2
	Europe and Central Asia	n.a.	n.a.	–1.1	–1.1
	Latin America and the Caribbean	n.a.	n.a.	0.0	0.0
	Middle East and North Africa	n.a.	n.a.	–0.1	–0.1
	South Asia	n.a.	n.a.	–0.1	–0.1
	Sub-Saharan Africa	n.a.	n.a.	–0.3	–0.3

n.a. Not applicable (no targets for tuberculosis mortality).

Source: World Bank staff calculations.

goals, the pace of decline would continue at the rate of the 1990s. Both assumptions are probably overly optimistic. Changes in three variables found to be good predictors of maternal mortality are likely to be less conducive to reductions in maternal mortality in the new millennium than they were in the 1990s (box 2.1). In the absence of faster economic growth and accelerated progress on the nonhealth goals, maternal mortality will probably decline less quickly in the new millennium than in the 1990s.

So why do the Millennium Development Goals matter?

The upshot of all this: even if economic growth accelerates as *Global Economic Prospects* predicts, and even if progress toward

the gender and water goals is substantially accelerated, the developing world is likely to wake up on the morning of January 1, 2016, some way from the health targets; in Sub-Saharan Africa, it may be a long way. So why should the Millennium Development Goals be taken seriously?

Progress can be quickened, irrespective of the targets

Accelerating progress on the various health goals is critical—even if the targets will not be reached. Reversing negative trends in Sub-Saharan Africa and accelerating slow progress in other regions are vital. A key message of this report is that progress can be accelerated through a judicious mix of spending and reform of both policies and institutions. Countries can set—and are setting—their own development targets, based on the Millennium Development Goals, but

Box 2.1 Why the decline in maternal mortality is slowing

The Millennium Development Goal for maternal health is to reduce the maternal mortality ratio by three-quarters between 1990 and 2015. In addition to the challenge of accomplishing such a large reduction, it will be difficult in many countries to measure whether the goal has been achieved or whether countries have recently been making enough progress to be on track to reach the goal. Trends in maternal mortality ratios are difficult to establish for several reasons:

- Measurement of maternal mortality is complex, partly because of the concept itself (a cause-specific mortality rate) and because of the rarity of maternal mortality. Estimates based on hospital studies suffer from a lack of representativeness. Vital registration systems exist in many countries, but the incompleteness of the systems is a major obstacle to their use in epidemiology. Household surveys using respondents' reports on the mortality of sisters have provided most of the measured estimates of maternal mortality in developing countries. But estimates based on this approach usually lack precision and are typically for several years in the past.

- Maternal deaths are frequently misclassified. Even in countries with complete coverage of deaths in vital registration, maternal deaths may be misclassified in 50 percent of cases.[8]

- Baseline estimates have not been collected in many countries, and too few additional estimates are likely to be forthcoming. This is the most serious obstacle to monitoring trends in maternal mortality.

To overcome the paucity of the data, UNICEF and the World Health Organization (WHO) have developed models to predict the maternal mortality ratio from a set of variables that are known to be related to maternal mortality. Such model-derived estimates have been issued for 1990 and 1995, and a set of estimates for 2000 was released as this report was being completed. Because the models use different variables, the results of the three exercises are not comparable, and the data cannot be used to analyze trends over time.

New analysis

Analysis for this report uses the model developed by WHO-UNICEF for countries without vital registration data or reliable survey estimates to generate the 1995 estimates and extends the period back to 1990 and forward to 2015.[8] Estimates of progress from 1990 to 2001 are made by calculating the rate of change in the maternal mortality ratio for this period, which is then compared with the rate of change needed to achieve the Millennium Development Goal by 2015.

The model estimates the proportion of deaths of women of reproductive age due to maternal causes from the following variables: the proportion of births with a skilled health care worker; the general fertility rate; whether a country is in formerly socialist Europe; whether a country is in Latin America, South or West

Asia, or Africa; whether death registration is complete; and the prevalence of HIV among adults.

Skilled attendance at delivery has a negative correlation with maternal mortality (and is an indicator used to measure the Millennium Development Goals for maternal health by itself). HIV prevalence and the resulting mortality from AIDS reduces the exposure to death from other causes, including maternal mortality. Higher fertility rates tend to lead to higher maternal mortality ratios, because more high-risk pregnancies occur.

Data for these variables for 1990, 1995, and 2001 are estimated from World Bank and UN databases. Projections for 2015 are based on extrapolated trends in the proportion of skilled attendants in the 1990s and on the assumption of gradually increasing or decreasing HIV prevalence, depending on trends in the 1990s. The general fertility rate is estimated from projections of the number of births and the number of females between 15 and 49 (see appendix B).

The estimated proportion of deaths of women of reproductive age is applied to the overall envelope of deaths to women 15–49 (estimated and projected) to obtain the number of deaths due to maternal causes for all countries. The maternal mortality ratio is then calculated by dividing this number by the estimated or projected number of births.

Results: 1990–2001

Skilled attendance at birth rose, fertility declined, and HIV/AIDS increased (see table) in all Bank regions in the 1990s. In each case the effect was to reduce the proportion of deaths of women of reproductive age (PMDF). In East Asia and the Pacific, Europe and Central Asia, and the Middle East and North Africa, the number of female deaths also fell, reinforcing the effect of the declining PMDF. However, the number of births fell in these three regions, putting upward pressure on the maternal mortality ratio. The maternal mortality ratio is estimated to have fallen in all three regions, though by a smaller percentage than the PMDF in East Asia and the Pacific and in Europe and Central Asia. In the Middle East and North Africa, the decline in the number of births was small, and the maternal mortality ratio fell by a larger percentage than the PMDF. In Latin America and the Caribbean, Southeast Asia, and Sub-Saharan Africa, the number of female deaths rose during the 1990s, partly offsetting the fall in the PMDF. In Latin America and the Caribbean, Southeast Asia, and Sub-Saharan Africa, the maternal mortality ratio is estimated to have fallen less than in the other three regions, in part because of relatively small percentage reductions in the PMDF, in part because of increases in female deaths.

Projections for 2001–15

The extrapolated trend in skilled attendance at birth will further reduce the PMDF. In some countries, however, skilled atten-

(continued)

Box 2.1 Why the decline in maternal mortality is slowing (continued)

dance has already reached high levels and has limited room for future increases; in only two regions (Latin America and the Caribbean and Southeast Asia) are attended deliveries expected to increase at a faster rate than in the 1990s. The general fertility rate is projected to continue to decline but at a slower rate than in the 1990s, except in Sub-Saharan Africa, where it is projected to decline more rapidly. HIV/AIDS prevalence will continue to increase or decline, depending on trends in the 1990s, but the rate of increase or decline will slow.

The result of these projected changes in the independent variables is that the PMDF will keep falling, but at a slower rate than in the 1990s, except in Southeast Asia. Beginning in 2001, female deaths are expected to rise in all regions except the Middle East and North Africa, partly offsetting the fall in the PMDF. The net effect is likely to be a reduction in the number of maternal deaths, but—partly because of changing numbers of births—the maternal mortality ratio is projected to decline more slowly than in the 1990s, except in Latin America and the Caribbean.

Maternal mortality ratio trends and forecasts

	East Asia and the Pacific	Europe and Central Asia	Latin America and the Caribbean	Middle East and North Africa	Southeast Asia	Sub-Saharan Africa
1990–2000 growth rates						
Attended deliveries	1.9%	1.1%	0.2%	3.7%	2.1%	1.8%
Gross fertility rate	–0.6%	–0.9%	–0.5%	–0.7%	–0.4%	–0.2%
HIV/AIDS	72.5%	74.7%	80.5%	61.6%	78.5%	101.4%
Proportion of deaths of women of reproductive age	–4.6%	–5.6%	–3.4%	–5.4%	–2.7%	–2.1%
Number of female deaths	–1.1%	–0.1%	2.1%	–0.7%	0.8%	3.2%
Number of births	–1.6%	–2.2%	–0.2%	–0.3%	–0.1%	1.9%
Maternal mortality ratio	–4.5%	–4.3%	–1.5%	–6.9%	–2.9%	–1.6%
2001–2015 growth rates						
Attended deliveries	1.6%	0.2%	0.5%	1.3%	2.8%	1.5%
Gross fertility rate	–0.2%	–0.2%	–0.4%	–0.3%	–0.4%	–0.3%
HIV/AIDS	1.4%	4.9%	1.2%	4.7%	–0.2%	0.8%
Proportion of deaths of women of reproductive age	–2.9%	–2.6%	–3.0%	–2.8%	–3.2%	–2.1%
Number of female deaths	2.1%	1.3%	0.3%	–1.0%	2.1%	3.0%
Number of births	–0.3%	–0.6%	–0.6%	0.9%	–0.2%	1.1%
Maternal mortality ratio	–1.5%	–1.1%	–1.9%	–4.8%	–2.5%	–1.3%

they are tailoring the targets to local circumstances. In some countries the targets may be more ambitious than the Millennium Development Targets. In others realism will require the setting of less ambitious targets. The important thing is that the goals be pursued and that realistic but challenging targets be aimed at.

Progress needs to be for everyone, not just the better off

Progress toward the Millennium Development Targets is uneven within countries (see figures 2.5 and 2.6). For under-

five mortality—less so for child malnutrition—the poor are progressing less quickly than the better off. There is an urgent need to ensure that countries do not progress toward the Millennium Development Goals by focusing on the low-hanging fruit, leaving the poor behind in the process. Countries and regions that are on track cannot be complacent. For example, the Middle East and North Africa region has better prospects than most for reaching the targets, but it has some of the largest inequalities across wealth groups in the Millennium Development Indicators. The challenge there is to ensure that progress for the whole population is accompanied by narrowing the gaps between the poor and the better off. In Egypt in the late 1990s under-five mortality fell more rapidly among the poor than among the whole population (see figure 2.6). That should inspire other countries to reach out to the poor in their efforts to hit the targets.

Goals help focus on outcomes

A major attraction of the Millennium Development Goals is that they provide an opportunity to refocus attention in the health sector on outcomes. Focusing on a specific set of outcomes requires choosing a limited set of corresponding interventions and devising strategies to ensure that everyone who could benefit from these interventions—whether affluent or poor—actually gets them. This approach forces us to think about why coverage levels are often so low and about the role of household factors, community factors, and health system factors.

The appropriate strategy will usually entail working at all levels. The role of households in initiating and delivering care cannot be ignored. The role of communities in shaping demand and delivering interventions is often crucial, especially in poorer communities. Also crucial is the health system—providers and their links to one another, the human and material inputs they have available to them, the incentives they face, the organizational and regulatory structure they work in.

These factors have long been considered important in the health sector. What is different about the Millennium Development Goals is that they force us to take stock of whether the general debates surrounding the health sector have done enough to generate strategies for raising the coverage levels of the very specific set of interventions of relevance to the goals.

Public policy debates in the health field too often focus on the delivery of services in health facilities. Indeed, analysis and debate often center on the delivery of care in public facilities. The Millennium Development Goals, with their focus on outcomes, provide a powerful reminder that such perspectives are unduly narrow. The preventive care and treatment that households themselves deliver are important to health outcomes. The care delivered outside the public sector is also important. The Millennium Development Goals provide a chance to refocus health policy on health outcomes and the major determinants, core interventions, and delivery strategies—and in the process to forge closer links between health ministries and other organizations that can help achieve these outcomes, including other government ministries.

The goals remind us of what is achievable

The value of the Millennium Development Goals goes beyond getting policymakers to focus more on outcomes.

True, the targets are ambitious. But if they had been set so low that developing countries could have achieved them by making progress at current rates, they would have been criticized for being unambitious. In the 1990s, 20 percent of developing countries achieved the target 4.3 percent annual reduction in under-five mortality. And several countries accelerated their annual reductions—Egypt from 5 percent to 8.5 percent, Indonesia from about 3 percent to 6.25 percent, and Bangladesh from about 3 percent in the 1980s to 5.5 percent in the 1990s.

What this suggests is that the world should not abandon hope for the countries off track on reaching the goals. Annual rates of under-five mortality reduction in excess of 4.3 percent are possible. Some developing countries with impressive rates of decline in the 1980s accelerated those rates in the 1990s. A final reason for hope: many countries not on track for the under-five mortality target achieved (or were close to achieving) the required annual percentage reduction in the 1980s (see figure 2.12). All this suggests that, while the targets are ambitious, they are not impossible for the majority of developing countries. Countries off track should be encouraged to ask how they can get on track—or back on track.

There is reason to hope that developing countries can make faster progress toward the other Millennium Development Goals as well.[9] Several countries have achieved significant reductions in maternal mortality rates. Sri Lanka, a poor country, reduced the maternal mortality ratio from 555 to 24 per 100,000 live births between 1950 and 1995.[10] Malaysia reduced its maternal mortality ratio from 500 to 21 over the same period. And China, Egypt, and Honduras greatly improved maternal health outcomes in the 1990s.[11]

There are encouraging examples for communicable disease, too. Tuberculosis case detection under the recommended DOTS approach increased steadily through the late 1990s—from 7.5 percent of tuberculosis cases in 1995 to 33 percent in 2001, although the scaling-up is still too slow. Even so, large countries such as China, India, Indonesia, Pakistan, the Philippines, and the Russian Federation are all moving to scale up more quickly, with some successes so far. The epidemiological impact of service interventions is measurable. In China the areas of 16 provinces where DOTS had been applied, with World Bank support, saw a 36 percent drop in tuberculosis prevalence between 1990 and 2000—a decline that was more than 10 times greater than in nonintervention areas. In Peru reaching cure and case detection targets was associated with a rapid decline in incidence.

Sustained reductions in HIV infection have been achieved in Thailand through government efforts to promote safer sex. The HIV prevalence rate has been reduced among 13–19 year-olds in Masaka, Uganda. The spread of

HIV has been contained in Senegal through a broad-based response to keep HIV prevalence low among pregnant women and steps to maintain a high level of condom use to prevent sexually transmitted infections among sex workers. In the effort to roll back malaria, free treatment and insecticide-treated nets have reduced malaria deaths in Vietnam and coastal Kenya, while insecticide spraying and effective case management have reduced malaria in Azerbaijan.

The rest of the report

That some countries—and indeed some regions—have achieved the target rates of improvement in the Millennium Development Indicators points to the need to understand what has been responsible for the successes and the failures. Chapter 3 reviews the interventions available for reducing child and maternal mortality, malnutrition, and communicable disease mortality. It argues that, together, they constitute a powerful arsenal of weapons to take on the Millennium Development Goals and that gaps in the arsenal have not, for the most part, held countries back. The report's second part argues that the causes of slow progress lie elsewhere—in low levels of government health spending and, even more, in poor policies and institutions across the entire health sector.

References

1. Claeson, M., and E. Bos. 2002. Health, Nutrition and Population Development Goals: *Measuring Progress Using the Poverty Reduction Strategy Framework*. Report of a World Bank Consultation, November 28–29. World Bank, Health, Nutrition and Population Department, Washington, DC.

2. Short, C. 1999. "Better Health for the Poor of the World." Speech to the King's Fund. London, Department for International Development.

3. World Bank. 2003. *Global Economic Prospects and the Developing Countries*. Washington, DC.

4. Pritchett, L., and L.H. Summers. 1996. "Wealthier Is Healthier." *Journal of Human Resources* 31 (4): 841–868.

5. Haddad, L. 2003. "What Can the Analysis of Food Security and Nutrition Add to Poverty Diagnosis?" World Bank, Washington, DC.

6. Desai, S., and S. Alva. 1998. "Maternal Education and Child Health: Is There a Strong Causal Relationship?" *Demography* 35 (1): 71–81.

7. Glewwe, P. 1993. "Why Does Mother's Schooling Raise Child Health in Developing Countries?" *Journal of Human Resources* 34 (1):124–159.

8. Hill, K., C. Abou Zhar, and T. Wardlaw. 2001. "Estimates of Maternal Mortality for 1995." *Bulletin of the World Health Organization* 79 (3):182–193.

9. World Health Organization. 2002. *Health: A Key to Prosperity: Success Stories in Developing Countries*. Geneva.

10. Pathmanathan, I., J. Liljestrand, J.M. Martins, L.C. Rajapaksa, C. Lissner, A. de Silva, S. Selvaraju, and P.J. Singh. 2003. *Investing in Maternal Health: Learning from Malaysia and Sri Lanka*. Washington, DC: World Bank.

11. Koblinsky, M.A., ed. 2003. *Reducing Maternal Mortality: Learning from Bolivia, China, Egypt, Honduras, Indonesia, Jamaica, and Zimbabwe*. Washington, DC: World Bank.

12. UNAIDS. 2002. *Report on the Global HIV/AIDS Epidemic*. Geneva.

13. Barro, R.J., and J.-W. Lee. 2000. "International Data on Educational Attainment Updates and Implications." NBER Working Paper 7911, National Bureau of Economic Research, New York.

14. UNICEF. 2003. Statistics: Water and sanitation. http://www.childinfo.org/eddb/water.htm.

15. ORC Macro. 2003. Demographic and Health Surveys. http://www.measuredhs.com/.

16. UNICEF. 2003. Statistics: Child mortality. http://www.childinfo.org/cmr/revis/db2.htm.

17. World Health Organization. 2003. *Global Tuberculosis Control*. Geneva.

18. United Nations. 2004. "Millennium Development Goals." New York.

CHAPTER 3

Effective Interventions Exist—They Need to Reach More People

Suneeta, a Bengali woman living in a rural village, falls ill with chronic cough, fever, weight loss, and other problems. Others around her may have previously been ill with similar symptoms. She may delay seeking care due to other duties or a lack of funds to pay for travel or consults. She may purchase medicines from a drug seller or visit a traditional healer or private physician. She may take drugs sporadically until her money runs out, her symptoms remain, and she becomes further incapacitated. Her family or neighbors may then bring her to a health center or hospital, where she sees a nurse auxiliary who may or may not refer her to a physician. The physician may charge her for an X-ray or treat her with general antibiotics and send her home or refer her for a free sputum smear exam if available.

Suneeta is found to have active infectious tuberculosis. The physician or nurse may tell her about tuberculosis—or due to a lack of interest or time, tell her only that she needs to take more medicines. They may give her a month's worth to take home or tell her to attend the health clinic every day, even though it is two hours to get there from her home. Worse yet, they may tell her to buy the medicines elsewhere, if no drugs are in stock. She might get only two of the four medicines she needs, and family members who may also have become infected or ill may not be seen by the health provider. The health provider may not be able to follow up to see whether Suneeta tolerated the medicines, took them regularly, was cured, remained ill, or died. No

functioning information system may be in place to register that a case was detected and treated. No supervisors visit the facility to provide training or feedback on performance.

It is not the lack of an effective intervention for tuberculosis that explains this sequence of events. It is the delays in seeking care, the insufficiently skilled or inadequately paid staff, the lack of patient and community health education, the poor supply chains, the failure to report the tuberculosis case, the lack of follow-up with the patient or her close contacts, and the poor supervision in the use of the medicines that explain the risk of failed treatment, chronic disease, or death for the patient. This situation can also contribute to the spread of infection in the community and to the emergence of drug-resistant organisms, which pass from community to community and across borders.

It is not a lack of interventions that is the main obstacle to faster progress toward the Millennium Development Goals—it is the low levels of use, especially among the poor, of existing effective interventions. Globally, the use of effective interventions for child health is typically below 50 percent, and in many poor countries the figure is much lower. Using all known interventions appropriately—achieving 99 percent coverage rates—could avert 63 percent of child deaths and 74 percent of maternal deaths.

Effective interventions exist—
for all the health targets

Interventions are being developed and tested for each of the Millennium Development Targets, with the potential to substantially reduce mortality and ill health. That is for the future—though in some cases the not-too-distant future.

What matters for the present is the impressive array of interventions now available to fight child malnutrition, child mortality, maternal mortality, and communicable disease mortality (table 3.1). Not all the evidence is equally strong, and not all interventions are equally effective. But overall the interventions listed in table 3.1 constitute a powerful arsenal for preventing and treating the main causes of death and malnutrition.

Take child mortality. Three causes of death—diarrhea, pneumonia, and malaria—account for 52 percent of deaths worldwide (figure 3.1). Neonatal causes account for another 33 percent, measles for 3 percent, and AIDS for 1 percent. Malnutrition is an underlying cause in

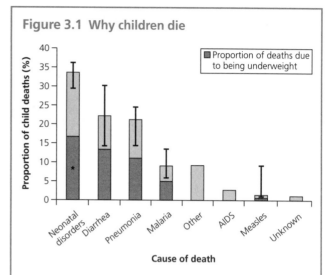

Figure 3.1 Why children die

Note: Bars indicate uncertainty bounds.

*Work in progress to establish cause-specific contribution of being underweight to neonatal deaths.

Source: Reference 2.

Reprinted with permission from Elsevier (*The Lancet,* 2003, vol. 361, page 6).

Table 3.1 Effective interventions for reducing illness, deaths, and malnutrition

Goal	Preventive interventions	Treatment interventions
Reduce child mortality	Breastfeeding; hand-washing; safe disposal of stool; use of latrine; safe preparation of weaning foods; use of insecticide-treated nets; complementary feeding; immunization; micronutrient supplementation (zinc and vitamin A); antenatal care, including steroids and tetanus toxoid; antimalarial intermittent preventive treatment in pregnancy; newborn temperature management; nevirapine and replacement feeding; antibiotics for premature rupture of membranes; clean delivery	Case management with oral rehydration therapy for diarrhea; antibiotics for dysentery, pneumonia, and sepsis; antimalarials for malaria; newborn resuscitation; breastfeeding; complementary feeding during illness; micronutrient supplementation (zinc and vitamin A)
Reduce maternal mortality	Family planning, intermittent malaria prophylaxis, use of insecticide-treated bednets, micronutrient supplementation (iron, folic acid, calcium for those who are deficient)	Antibiotics for preterm rupture of membranes, skilled attendance (especially active management of third stage of labor), basic and emergency obstetric care
Improve nutrition	Exclusive breastfeeding for six months, appropriate complementary child feeding for next 6–24 months, iron and folic acid supplementation for children, improved hygiene and sanitation, dietary intake of pregnant and lactating women, micronutrient supplementation for prevention of anemia and vitamin A deficiency for mothers and children, anthelminthic treatment in school-age children	Appropriate feeding of sick child and oral rehydration therapy, control and timely treatment of infectious and parasitic diseases, treatment and monitoring of severely malnourished children, high dose treatment of clinical signs of vitamin A deficiency
Prevent and combat HIV/AIDS	Safe sex, including condom use; use of unused needles by drug users; treatment of sexually transmitted infections; safe, screened blood supplies; use of antiretrovirals in pregnancy to prevent maternal to child transmission and after occupational exposure	Treatment of opportunistic infections, cotrimoxazole prophylaxis, highly active antiretroviral therapy, palliative care
Prevent and combat tuberculosis	Directly observed treatment of infectious cases to prevent transmission and emergence of drug resistant strains and treatment of contacts, BCG immunization.	Directly observed treatment to cure symptomatic cases, including early cases of tuberculosis
Prevent and combat malaria	Use of insecticide-treated nets, indoor residual spraying (in epidemic-prone areas), intermittent presumptive treatment of pregnant women	Rapid detection and early treatment of uncomplicated cases, treatment of complicated cases (such as cerebral malaria and severe anemia)

Note: "Intervention" refers to the direct action that leads to prevention or cure. The act of immunization, not the vaccine itself, is the intervention. Case management, not medicines or vitamins, is the intervention. Counseling for safer sex is not an intervention in this sense—safer sex is.

nearly half of under-five deaths. For each of these causes of death, there is at least one proven effective preventive intervention and at least one proven effective treatment intervention (figure 3.2). And each can be delivered in a low-income setting. In most cases, there are several proven effective interventions. For example, for diarrhea—the second-leading cause of child deaths—there are no fewer than five proven preventive interventions (breastfeeding, complementary feeding, hygiene and use of safe water, zinc, and vitamin A) and no fewer than three proven treatment interventions (oral rehydration therapy, antibiotics, and zinc). Many of these interventions can be—and are—delivered by households, but many are not.

Similar arguments can be made for the other goals. Some interventions for maternal mortality are delivered by the household (nutrition, family planning), but most are not (figure 3.3). And for those delivered by households, there is typically little—if any—scientific evidence available on impact.

Because of the multiple and interrelated causes of childhood and maternal deaths, integrated strategies, such as Integrated Management of Childhood Illness (IMCI) and Integrated Management of Pregnancy and Childbirth (IMPAC) have been introduced in many countries. Delivery of these bundled interventions has the potential to yield greater efficiency, synergy, and impact—if implemented on scale and not underused.

Effective interventions are underused—especially by the poor

The proximate cause of the high rates of death and malnutrition in the developing world is that, for one reason or another, people do not receive the interventions that could save their life or make them well nourished. In upper middle-income and high-income countries, 90 percent of children receive diphtheria, pertussis, and tetanus (DPT3) vaccinations; more than 90 percent of babies are delivered by a medically trained person; and more than 90 percent of pregnant women have at least one antenatal visit (figure 3.4). In low-income and lower middle-income countries, the figures are much lower—often dramatically so. In South Asia less than 50 percent of pregnant women receive antenatal checkups, and only 20 percent of babies are delivered by a medically trained person (figure 3.5). In some countries less than 20 percent of children with acute respiratory infections are seen by a medically trained person (figure 3.6)—despite the fact that pneumonia, the most severe respiratory infection, can be treated with an antibiotic. The story is similar for other childhood interventions and for interventions for other Millennium Development

Goals (box 3.1). In short, there is substantial underuse of effective interventions in the developing world.

Just as shortfalls in coverage vary across countries, they vary within countries. The poor and other deprived groups invariably lag behind the population in many preventive and curative health interventions. They are less likely to receive full basic immunization coverage (bacillus of Calmette and Guerin [BCG], measles, and DPT) (figure 3.7); to have their deliveries attended by a medically trained person; or to have at least one antenatal care visit to a medically trained person. The trends in use by wealth group are more encouraging. For the most part, the poor are making more rapid progress than the better off, who already have high coverage rates for many interventions (see tables in appendix D). Progress has been more propoor in professionally delivered interventions (skilled attendance, treatment of common childhood illnesses) than in home-delivered interventions (breastfeeding, timely complementary feeding, and vitamin A supplementation) (figure 3.8).

The underuse of effective interventions costs lives

The low use of effective interventions—in the developing world and among the poor—translates into rates of mortality, morbidity, and malnutrition that are far higher than they need be.

Take child mortality. If the use of all the proven effective childhood preventive and treatment interventions were to rise from its current level to 99 percent (95 percent for breastfeeding), the number of under-five deaths worldwide would fall dramatically (figure 3.9). Deaths from malaria and measles could be all but eliminated, and deaths from diarrhea, pneumonia, and HIV/AIDS could be dramatically reduced. Overall, a reduction in childhood deaths of 63 percent could be achieved by increasing coverage rates to 99 percent.

Of these 6 million averted deaths worldwide, perhaps half would result from increased coverage of home-delivered interventions.★ This fraction will vary according to the relative importance of different causes of death. In Brazil and China, just under half of child deaths are neonatal,[2] for which the relevant effective interventions are professionally delivered. In much of Sub-Saharan Africa, by contrast,

★ This is a preliminary estimate, based on the figures in table 2 of Jones and others.[1] It classifies breastfeeding, insecticide-treated materials, complementary feeding, hygiene and use of clean water, vitamin A supplementation, oral rehydration therapy, and antimalarials as home-delivered interventions. The figure is a tentative estimate because unlike table 3 in Jones and others, no account is taken in table 2 of competing risks (in principle, a child could be saved several times over in this calculation).

Figure 3.2 The arsenal of effective interventions against childhood killers

	Diarrhea	Pneumonia	Measles	Malaria	HIV/AIDS	Birth asphyxia	Preterm delivery	Neonatal tetanus	Neonatal sepsis
Preventive interventions									
Breastfeeding	1	1							1
Insecticide-treated materials				1			1		
Complementary feeding	1	1	1	1					
Water, sanitation, hygiene	1								
Hib vaccine		1							
Zinc	1	1		2					
Vitamin A	1		2	2					
Antenatal steroids							1		
Newborn temperature management							2		
Tetanus toxoid								1	
Nevirapine and replacement feeding					1				
Antibiotics for premature rapture							2		2
Clean delivery							1	1	1
Measles vaccine			1						
Antimalarial prev. treatment in pregnancy									
Treatment interventions									
Oral rehydration therapy	1								
Antibiotics for pneumonia		1							
Antimalarials				1					
Antibiotics for sepsis									1
Newborn resuscitation						2			
Antibiotics for dysentery	1								
Zinc	1								
Vitamin A			1						

Causes of under-five deaths

Legend:
- 1 Level 1 (sufficient evidence)
- 2 Level 2 (limited or indirect evidence)
- No impact or no evidence

Source: Adapted from reference 1.

Figure 3.3 Interventions for reducing maternal mortality

		Causes of maternal death								
Interventions	Interventions	Hemorrhage	Puerperal infection	Eclampsia	Obstructed labor	Abortion complications	Malaria	Anemia	Tetanus	Other
Preventive	Iron supplementation in pregnancy							2		
	Folate supplementation in pregnancy							2		
	Balanced protein and energy supplements in pregnancy									2
	Treatment for iron deficiency in pregnancy							2		
	Calcium supplementation during pregnancy for preventing hypertensive disorders and related problems			2						
	Vitamin A supplementation during pregnancy	2	2	2						
	Use of insecticide treated nets for prevention of malaria						2	2		
	Intermittent malaria prophylaxis						1	1		
	Family planning	1	1	1	1	1				
	Continuity of caregivers during pregnancy and child birth									2
Primary clinical care	Antibiotics for preterm (before 37 weeks) rupture of membranes		1							
	Antibiotics for prelabor (36 weeks or beyond) rupture of membranes		1							
	Antibiotics for treating bacterial vaginosis in pregnancy		2							
	Antihypertensive drug therapy for mild to moderate hypertension during pregnancy			2						
	Professional delivery servcies (skilled attendant)	2	2	2	2					
	Active versus expectant management in the third stage of labor	1								
Basic essential obstetric care	Management of primary postpartum hemorrhage with rectal Misoprostol administration	1								
	Treatment of secondary postpartum hemorrhage (between 24 hours and 12 weeks postnatal)	2								
Comprehensive essential obstetric care	Magnesium sulphate and other anticonvulsants for women with pre-eclampsia			2						
		1	1	1	1					

Interventions for reducing maternal mortality

Legend:
- 1 — Level 1 (sufficient evidence)
- 2 — Level 2 (limited or indirect evidence)
- No impact

Source: Reference 3.

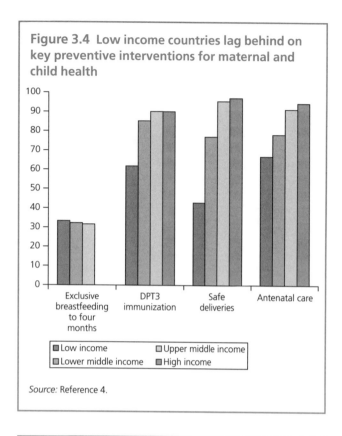

Figure 3.4 Low income countries lag behind on key preventive interventions for maternal and child health

Legend: Low income, Lower middle income, Upper middle income, High income

Source: Reference 4.

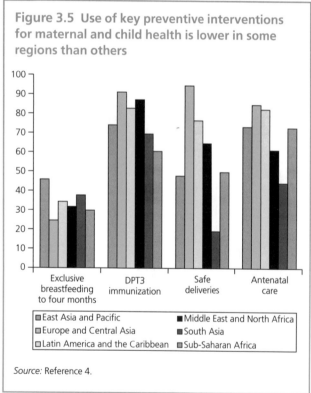

Figure 3.5 Use of key preventive interventions for maternal and child health is lower in some regions than others

Legend: East Asia and Pacific, Europe and Central Asia, Latin America and the Caribbean, Middle East and North Africa, South Asia, Sub-Saharan Africa

Source: Reference 4.

neonatal deaths account for about a quarter of child deaths, and malaria and diarrhea—two causes of death for which household-delivered interventions could be important—together account for more than half of child deaths.[2]

Figure 3.6 Some children with acute respiratory infections receive treatment—others don't

Level (%)

Tanzania 1999
Jordan 1997
South Africa 1998
Zambia 2001
Vietnam 1997
Indonesia 1997
Namibia 1992
India 1999
Uganda 2000
Pakistan 1990
Egypt, Arab Rep. 2000
Peru 2000
Philippines 1998
Nicaragua 2001
Kenya 1998
Comoros 1996
Zimbabwe 1999
Gabon 2000
Brazil 1996
Bolivia 1998
C. African Rep. 1994–95
Mauritania 2000
Guinea 1999
Côte d'Ivoire 1994
Mozambique 1997
Haiti 2000
Guatemala 1998
Nigeria 1990
Eritrea 1995
Madagascar 1997
Cambodia 2000
Mali 2001
Cameroon 2000
Yemen, Rep. 1997
Bangladesh 2000
Malawi 2000
Ghana 1998
Togo 1998
Nepal 2001
Niger 1998
Chad 1996–97
Morocco 1992
Ethiopia 2000
Rwanda 2000

Proportion of children with acute respiratory infections seen medically

Source: World Bank staff calculations and reference 5.

Spectacular reductions in mortality could also be achieved if coverage rates of the key maternal mortality interventions in figure 3.3 were increased from current levels to 99 percent. It is estimated that perhaps as many as 1391,000 deaths worldwide—74 percent of current maternal deaths—could be averted,[†] all from increased coverage of professionally delivered interventions. Four stand out as especially important (figure 3.10): access to essential obstetric care (52 percent of deaths averted), access to safe abortion services (16 percent), active rather than expectant management in the third stage of labor (10 percent), and the use of magnesium sulphate and other anticonvulsants for women with pre-eclampsia (8 percent).

[†] These are preliminary estimates. The details will be spelled out in a separate technical note.

Box 3.1 Low coverage of HIV/AIDS interventions

Most countries have developed strategic frameworks for HIV prevention, but only a fraction of people at risk have meaningful access to basic prevention and treatment.

Risk reduction behavior among young people

Survey results indicate that condom use with nonregular partners is higher in urban than in rural areas and higher among young men than among young women. Data also suggest that condom use varies considerably across countries, ranging from 2 percent to 88 percent in Sub-Saharan Africa. In this region, 15–20 percent of young people report having had sexual intercourse before the age of 15, with young women reporting an earlier median age of first sex than males.

Management of sexually transmitted infections

Because untreated sexually transmitted infections increase the risk of HIV transmission by several orders of magnitude, control of sexually transmitted infection is a fundamental element of effective HIV prevention. Yet from limited information received, only one in four countries in Sub-Saharan Africa reports that at least 50 percent of sexually transmitted infection patients are appropriately diagnosed, counseled, and treated.

Prevention of mother-to-child transmission

Four years after research indicated that a relatively inexpensive single dose of nevirapine to mother and newborn significantly reduced the odds of HIV transmission to the infant, prevention of mother-to-child transmission (PMTCT) coverage remains virtually nonexistent in many heavily affected countries. Apart from Botswana, where coverage reached 34 percent by the end of 2002, PMTCT remains extremely low in countries hardest hit by HIV/AIDS.

Antiretroviral therapy

While an estimated 6 million people in low- and middle-income countries currently need antiretroviral therapy, only 300,000 were obtaining such therapy by the end of 2002. Although coverage remains low in Sub-Saharan Africa, Botswana, Cameroon, Nigeria, and Uganda have made serious efforts to increase antiretroviral therapy coverage through the public and private sectors. Caribbean countries report coverage of less than 1 percent. In Asia, where more than 7 million people are living with HIV/AIDS, no country has exceeded 5 percent coverage.

Source: World Bank.

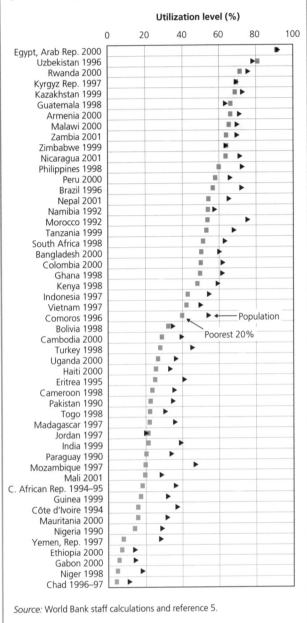

Figure 3.7 Proportion of children age 12–23 mos who received full basic immunization coverage— poorest 20 percent vs. population as a whole

Source: World Bank staff calculations and reference 5.

The challenge

If the lack of interventions is not holding countries back from achieving the goals, what is? Part II of the report investigates this question. Chapter 4 argues that a lack of government health spending is only part of the story of low coverage rates. It makes the case that governments need to improve their targeting of health spending, but even more they need to improve their policies and the institutions of the health sector—very broadly defined. The rest of part II shows how.

Figure 3.8 Use trends for household-delivered and professionally delivered interventions

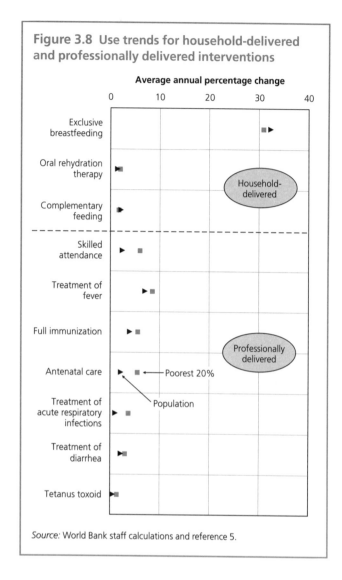

Source: World Bank staff calculations and reference 5.

Figure 3.9 Full use of existing interventions would dramatically cut child deaths

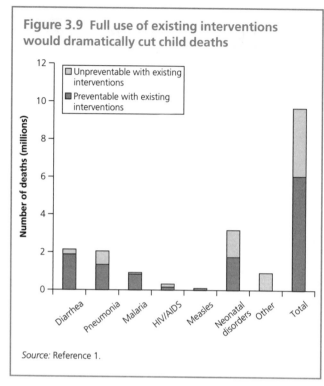

Source: Reference 1.

Figure 3.10 Full use of existing interventions would dramatically cut maternal deaths

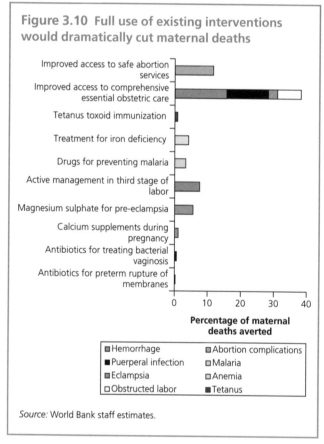

Source: World Bank staff estimates.

References

1. Jones, G., R.W. Steketee, R.E. Black, Z.A. Bhutta, and S.S. Morris. 2003. "How Many Child Deaths Can We Prevent This Year?" *Lancet* 362 (9377): 65–71.

2. Black, R.E., S.S. Morris, and J. Bryce. 2003. "Where and Why Are 10 Million Children Dying Every Year?" *Lancet* 361 (9376): 2226–2234.

3. Ramana, G. 2003. Personal communication. Senior Public Health Specialist, Health, Nutrition and Population Department, World Bank, Washington, DC.

4. World Bank. 2003. *World Development Indicators 2003*. Washington, DC: World Bank.

5. ORC Macro. 2003. Demographic and Health Surveys. http://www.measuredhs.com/.

CHAPTER 4

Extra Government Health Spending Is Necessary but Not Sufficient— Health Sector Strengthening Is Also Required, and Spending Needs to Be Better Targeted

Views diverge widely on government health spending. One view holds that low government health spending in the developing world is the cause of poor health indicators. According to this view, government health spending needs to be increased substantially and financed largely through development assistance.[1] At the other extreme is the view that government health spending has little impact on health outcomes at the margin, reflecting the multitude of weak links in the chain running from government spending to health outcomes.[2-4] According to this view, more government health spending would be unproductive; the focus should instead be on strengthening the weak links.

This chapter argues for a more nuanced view. Adding to government health budgets and scaling up proportionally all government health programs has an impact on Millennium Development Goal outcomes in well-governed countries. But the impact of such across-the-board increases on health outcomes would be modest, so substantial increases in spending would be needed. Carefully targeted spending can improve Millennium Development Goal outcomes even in poorly governed countries. But policies and institutions need to be strengthened if across-the-board increases in spending are to be productive.

Shaping strong policies and institutions for achieving the goals requires broad thinking, across a wide variety of policy instruments and areas. They include those not normally considered integral parts of the health sector, such as households and communities, and those outside the health sector, such as water, sanitation, transport, and education.

The limits and returns to government health spending

The impact of government spending on mortality depends in part on its impact on coverage rates—and in part on the impact of coverage rates on mortality. The case for substantial increases in government health spending has been weakened by the absence of firm evidence on the first of these links. It is also weakened by the failure to factor in the contributions and resource requirements associated with changes in other sectors (water, sanitation, roads, female education).[5]

The case against extra government health spending is built on empirical evidence that shows that additional government health spending has no perceptible impact on infant and under-five mortality, once other influences are held constant.[2] But this analysis has limitations. It refers simply to child mortality, not to health outcomes in general. Child mortality differs from, say, maternal mortality in that several of the interventions aimed at children are delivered by the household, while almost all interventions aimed at mothers are delivered by professional providers. It is unlikely that, say, maternal mortality is as unresponsive (or inelastic) to government health spending as child mortality is. The results are also very general: they indicate what happens to child mortality among the population as a whole, in an average country. As a result, they hide significant spending effects among specific subpopulations and specific types of countries. Finally, the results indicate what would happen to child mortality if additional government spending were to take the form of a proportional scaling-up of all government health programs. They do not show what would happen if extra spending focused on specific subpopulations or specific programs.

The importance of good policies and institutions

For the developing world as a whole, then, and for populations as a whole, proportional scaling-up of government health programs has no perceptible impact on child mortality, once other influences are held constant.[2] But recent evidence suggests that scaling up does make a difference for specific subpopulations and specific types of countries.

Child mortality among the poor—whether the poorest 20 percent of the population or those living under $1 (or $2) a day—does improve with additional government health spending.[6-8] And among countries with good governance (measured by the quality of the bureaucracy), additional government health spending reduces child mortality (see the first panel of table 4.1).[9] This finding is

consistent with recent World Bank studies on aid effectiveness.[10,11] In countries with "good" policies and institutions (strong property rights, absence of corruption, a good bureaucracy), an extra 1 percent of GDP in aid has been estimated to lead to a decline in infant mortality of 0.9 percent. By contrast, in countries in which policies are only average, the impact is just 0.4 percent. Where policies are "bad," aid has no statistically significant effect on infant mortality.

These findings are also borne out in the results of a study undertaken for this report (see table 4.1 and appendix A), in which the quality of policies and institutions was measured by the World Bank's Country Policy and Institutional Assessment (CPIA) Index. As policies and institutions improve, this index increases from 1 to a maximum of 5 (figure 4.1). As the second panel of table 4.1 shows, the elasticity also increases in absolute size—government spending has a larger impact on health outcomes at the margin in better-governed countries. For example, at a CPIA score of 4 (one standard deviation above the mean), a 10 percent increase in the share of GDP devoted to government health spending results in a 7.2 percent decline in the maternal mortality ratio.

The elasticities in the second panel of table 4.1 reinforce the finding that across-the-board increases in government health spending have no perceptible impact on under-five mortality in poorly governed countries. But they also show something new: the same is true of other Millennium Development Goal outcomes. Whether the outcome is underweight, maternal mortality, or tuberculosis mortality, in countries one standard deviation below the mean CPIA score, across-the-board additions to government health spending have no significant effect. Indeed, for malnutrition and tuberculosis mortality, the CPIA score has to get above the population-weighted average of 3.5 for additional government health spending to have any bite.

The message, then, is clear. In countries with poor governance—and weak policies and institutions—improvements need to occur in these areas if additions to government health budgets are to have any impact. These improvements may require reforms that entail transition costs, which may need to be covered by government spending. And it may be possible to phase in the additional government health spending as these reforms are being implemented. But the fact remains: in these countries, extra government health spending by itself will do little, if anything, to accelerate movement toward the Millennium Development Targets. This is why the rest of part II—the bulk of the report—is devoted to the difficult but often overlooked question of how to shape effective policies and institutions in the health sector.

Table 4.1 Elasticities of Millennium Development Goal outcomes to government health spending, as a percent of GDP, by quality of policies and institutions

Governance score	Under-five mortality	Maternal mortality ratio	Underweight among children under five	Tuberculosis mortality
Quality of bureaucracy index				
2.2	−0.350	—	—	—
3.7	−0.450*	—	—	—
5.2	−0.560*	—	—	—
CPIA index				
1.0	0.799	−0.622	0.130	0.651
2.0	0.507	−0.654	−0.087	0.276
3.0	0.215	−0.687	−0.305	−0.098
3.25	0.142	−0.695*	−0.360	−0.192
3.5	0.069	−0.703*	−0.414	−0.285
4.0	−0.077	−0.720*	−0.523*	−0.472
4.5	−0.223	−0.736*	−0.632*	−0.659*
5.0	−0.369	−0.752*	−0.740*	−0.847*

— Not available.

Note: An elasticity of −0.622 means that a 10 percent increase in spending reduces mortality by 6.22 percent. The values 2.2, 3.7, and 5.2 are, respectively, one standard deviation below the mean, the mean, and one standard deviation above the mean. The means are based on a sample that includes industrial and developing countries. The population-weighted mean CPIA score is 3.5, with a standard deviation of 0.4. These figures are based on developing countries only, though industrial countries were also included in the regression (with CPIA values set at 5).

*Significantly different from zero at the 90 percent confidence level or above.

Source: Elasticities for the quality of bureaucracy index are from reference 9. Elasticities for the CPIA Index are based on a study undertaken for this report (see appendix A for details).

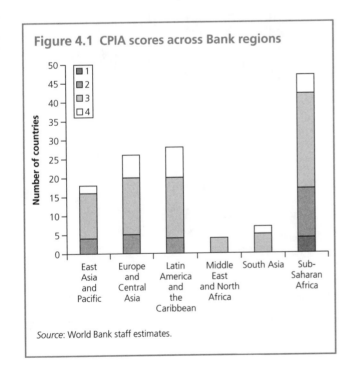

Figure 4.1 CPIA scores across Bank regions

Source: World Bank staff estimates.

More government spending in well-governed countries—how large are the returns relative to the Millennium Development Goal challenge?

In well-governed countries, and ones with good policies and institutions, there is scope for improving health outcomes through a proportional scaling-up of government health programs. According to the upper panel of table 4.1, extra government health spending would reduce child mortality in countries with above-average governance conditions. According to the lower panel, it would reduce maternal mortality ratio in countries with above-average CPIA scores and reduce malnutrition and tuberculosis mortality in countries with CPIA scores that are respectively 1.00 and 1.75 standard deviations above the mean. So well-governed countries in the developing world could, in principle, accelerate progress toward the health goals simply by adding to government health budgets. But how much extra momentum could they achieve by doing so? Or to put the question the other way around, how much extra would they need to spend to hit the Millennium Development Targets?

What would extra government health spending in well-governed countries actually achieve?

Figure 4.2 shows how much faster child malnutrition, under-five mortality, and maternal mortality would fall per year if an additional 2.5 percentage points were added to the annual growth rate of government health spending as a share of GDP, assuming the country in question has a CPIA score of 4 (one standard deviation above the mean). Also shown are the current rate of reduction of the Millennium Development Indicator, the estimated contributions from faster economic growth and quicker growth in girls' secondary school completion and access to drink-

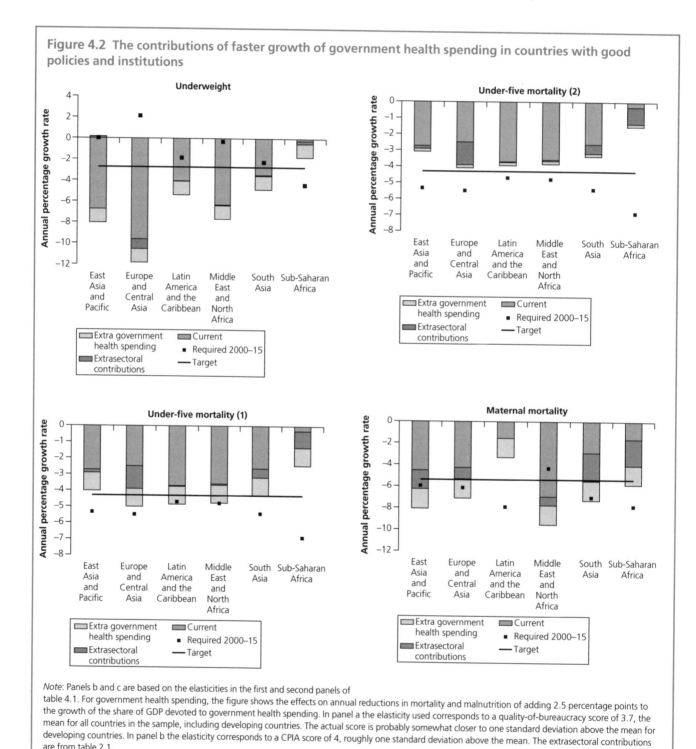

Figure 4.2 The contributions of faster growth of government health spending in countries with good policies and institutions

Note: Panels b and c are based on the elasticities in the first and second panels of table 4.1. For government health spending, the figure shows the effects on annual reductions in mortality and malnutrition of adding 2.5 percentage points to the growth of the share of GDP devoted to government health spending. In panel a the elasticity used corresponds to a quality-of-bureaucracy score of 3.7, the mean for all countries in the sample, including developing countries. The actual score is probably somewhat closer to one standard deviation above the mean for developing countries. In panel b the elasticity corresponds to a CPIA score of 4, roughly one standard deviation above the mean. The extrasectoral contributions are from table 2.1.

Source: World Bank staff estimates.

ing water, the target rate of reduction, and the required rate of reduction for the period 2000–15 given progress in the 1990s. For example, in East Asia and the Pacific under-five mortality fell by only 2.7 percent a year in the 1990s, so it would need to fall by 5.3 percent a year in 2000–15 for the region to achieve the targeted two-thirds reduction between 1990 and 2015.

For the maternal mortality ratio, the contribution from an additional 2.5 percentage points of growth in government health spending as a share of GDP would be substantial, pushing two regions (Europe and Central Asia and South Asia) up to their required rates of reduction for 2000–15. For malnutrition the contribution would also be appreciable but unnecessary given trends to date, except in Sub-Saharan Africa, where it would be insufficient to get the region to the target. For under-five mortality the estimated contribution of extra health spending depends on the set of elasticity estimates used. If the first set is used, Latin America and the Caribbean and the Middle East and North Africa would hit the under-five mortality targets if

an additional 2.5 percentage points were added to the rate of growth of government health spending as a share of GDP. If the second set is used, the extra government health spending would have little—if any—impact.

How much would reaching the Millennium Development Goals cost in well-governed countries?

Another way of looking at the spending question is to ask how much faster government health spending as a share of GDP would need to grow to hit the Millennium Development Targets in well-governed countries. Would such extra growth be reasonable? Table 4.2 presents estimates for two scenarios—one in which the expected economic growth materializes and the other relevant Millennium Development Goals are met, another in which growth fails to materialize and there is no acceleration in the rate of progress toward these other goals. Obviously in the second case, the costs of reaching the health goals will be higher, because the health sector cannot ride as much on the coattails of other sectors.

Table 4.2 How far would the share of GDP devoted to government health spending need to rise in well-governed countries to meet the Millennium Development Goals?

| Region | 2000 values | Annual percentage change in 1990s | Assumes that 1990s trend continues[a] | Assumes that economic growth accelerates and other Millennium Development Goals are met | | | Assumes that economic growth continues at current rate and no acceleration occurs in progress toward other Millennium Development Goals | | |
				Under-weight	Under-five mortality	Maternal mortality	Under-weight	Under-five mortality	Maternal mortality
East Asia and the Pacific	1.7	−0.2	1.7	1.7	3.7	1.7	1.7	3.9	2.2
Europe and Central Asia	3.5	0.5	3.8	3.8	6.3	4.5	3.8	9.9	5.5
Latin America and the Caribbean	3.4	4.6	6.6	6.6	9.0	22.3	6.6	9.1	22.3
Middle East and North Africa	2.3	6.2	5.7	5.7	8.1	5.7	5.7	8.3	5.7
South Asia	0.9	0.7	1.0	1.0	2.1	1.4	1.0	2.6	2.4
Sub-Saharan Africa	1.8	1.2	2.2	6.4	12.2	4.6	6.8	16.5	7.4
Developing countries	1.6	1.0	2.1	2.6	4.6	3.8	2.6	5.5	4.6

Note: Averages are population weighted. Under-five mortality estimates based on elasticity in first panel of table 4.1 corresponding to a quality-of-bureaucracy score of 3.7. This is the mean for all countries in the sample, including developing countries. The figure for developing countries is probably closer to one standard deviation above the mean. For underweight and maternal mortality, elasticities correspond to a CPIA score of 4, roughly one standard deviation above the mean. Developing world averages are weighted by regional populations.

[a]Assumes compound growth.

Source: Baseline data are from reference 30. Estimated 2015 values are derived using regressions in appendix A. Extrasectoral contributions from table 2.1.

In East Asia and the Pacific the share of GDP devoted to government health spending was a little over 1.7 percent in 2000, and the share shrank at –0.2 percent a year in the 1990s. If this trend were maintained, the share would be about 1.67 percent in 2015. If economic growth is as expected in the new millennium (a slight reduction is anticipated for East Asia and the Pacific), and the other relevant goals are reached, East Asia and the Pacific would hit the underweight and maternal mortality ratio targets even without additional health spending. It would, however, miss the under-five mortality target—an additional five percentage points would need to be added to the rate of growth of the government health share of GDP to hit the target, taking it to 3.7 percent in 2015. If there were no change in economic growth in the new millennium and no acceleration in progress toward the other goals, the rate of growth of the government health share of GDP would have to rise to 3.9 percent, more than twice the projected 2015 value based on 1990s trends.

For all regions except Latin America and the Caribbean the binding constraint is under-five mortality—government spending has to rise faster to hit this target than it does to hit the others. And the results for under-five mortality may be overly optimistic, based on the elasticities in the first panel rather than the second. Since the second set of estimated elasticities is not statistically significant, the extra spending required could be infinite. Looking across the developing world, well-governed countries could achieve the goals if they raised the share of GDP devoted to government health spending to 4.6–5.5 percent in 2015, depending on whether anticipated economic growth materializes and the other relevant targets are hit. This is two to three times the GDP share projected for 2015 on the basis of 1990s trends.

In Sub-Saharan Africa the implied increases in the GDP share going to government health programs are even less palatable. Even in the optimistic first scenario, the share would need to rise to 12.2 percent by 2015. In the second scenario, the required share in 2015 would be even more unrealistic—16.5 percent. And this applies only to countries whose quality of policies and institutions is above average. Sub-Saharan Africa has few of them: only five of 47 Sub-Saharan countries had a CPIA in 2000 of at least 4. For the other Sub-Saharan countries, accelerated progress toward the goals will not happen through extra spending alone, however large the increases.

The bottom line

So, yes, in well-governed countries, additions to government health budgets will by themselves lead to reductions in malnutrition and mortality. But the implied increases in

the share of GDP to be devoted to government health spending are impressively large. In the few well-governed countries in Sub-Saharan Africa, the share might need to be nearly eight times what it is predicted to be in 2015 based on current trends. In poorly governed countries, then, extra spending alone will not result in faster progress toward the goals. In well-governed countries it will, but the implied resource increases are unrealistically high. This second group of countries faces two options: raising the productivity of existing spending and targeting additional spending carefully.

Improving expenditure allocation and targeting

It is important to be clear about what the elasticities in table 4.1 show. They are estimates of the effects at the margin of adding to the government's health budget on the assumption that the additional spending will be allocated across programs and institutions in proportion to current allocations. From the viewpoint of expanding health budgets—through, say, budgetary support by external donors—these calculations are clearly highly relevant. But even here they may be misleading if budget support is linked to policy changes that entail shifts in spending patterns or a different spending pattern for the extra spending. The elasticities in table 4.1 do not tell us what health impacts will be achieved if, rather than making additions to a ministry of health budget without changing the composition of government health spending, additional resources were instead spent in very specific and targeted ways.

Geographic targeting

The poorest district in Lesotho receives only 20 percent of the amount the capital city receives in per capita allocations of public expenditures on health—inequality that is not resolved when accounting for nongovernmental services. In Peru per capita spending allocated through the regional budget (which excludes teaching hospital allocations) is 66 percent higher in the Lima region than in the very poor regions.[12] In Bangladesh more developed districts receive more per capita than less developed districts.[13]

Resource-allocation formulas can reduce government spending gaps across regions and ensure that the poor also benefit from government spending. But they have an efficiency angle too—resources can be diverted from areas where the marginal benefit is probably fairly low (high-tech hospitals in the capital city) to those where the marginal benefit is likely to be high (immunization in rural areas).

Such formulas have narrowed regional gaps in industrial countries.[14] In developing countries, too, they have begun to be used. Bolivia has used these formulas since 1994 as part of its decentralization efforts—and in its allocation of newly available Heavily Indebted Poor Country (HIPC) Initiative resources. Funds went to municipalities on a per capita basis based on poverty indicators (the poorer the indicator, the larger the per capita amount allocated), with the mandate that municipalities spend such resources on prespecified health, education, and other social programs. The program has been associated with some fairly large—and propoor—improvements in maternal and child health indicators (chapter 5).

Changing the allocation of spending across levels of care

Spending on health in developing countries is characterized by a surprisingly high concentration of spending on secondary and tertiary infrastructure and on personnel, despite low bed-occupancy rates. Armenian hospitals, for example, receive more than 50 percent of the government budget for health. Health clinics and ambulatory facilities—according to household surveys, the preferred service providers for sick people in the poorest quintile—received just over 20 percent of expenditures.[15] This pattern is also seen in lower-income countries. In Tanzania government spending in hospitals accounted for about 60 percent of the budget in 2000, compared with only 34 percent of spending on preventive and primary care facilities. Recent government efforts to change this brought the respective proportions to 43 percent and 48 percent in 2002.

Simply reallocating the budget toward primary care need not result in higher payoffs to government health spending in lowering child and maternal mortality and malnutrition.[3,4] In many instances service providers have failed to deliver quality care or to use resources efficiently (chapter 6). So even though many key Millennium Development Goal interventions can be and are delivered at lower levels of care, simply redirecting money toward these facilities will not necessarily yield higher returns. The trick is to couple expenditure reallocations with measures to improve the performance of primary care facilities and district hospitals (chapter 6) and measures to ensure that households actually demand the relevant interventions (chapter 5).

Targeting specific programs

Programs such as Integrated Management for Childhood Illness and directly observed treatment, short-course (DOTS) therapy for tuberculosis are good examples of programs that may yield high returns to government spending. Both are the subject of ongoing evaluation, and

early results are encouraging.[16,17] A recent World Bank study[18] of the Millennium Development Goals in India provides further support for the idea that the way government spending is allocated across programs affects its impact on Millennium Development Indicators. The report finds that a one percentage point increase in the share of total government health spending devoted to public health and family welfare activities (prevention and control of diseases, population and family planning services, and maternal and child health programs, including immunization) leads to a reduction of about 0.8 infant deaths per 1,000 live births.

This effect—estimated holding constant the amount spent per capita on all medical, public health, and family welfare activities—is more pronounced for poor states and not statistically significant for nonpoor states. For the poor states, a one percentage point increase in the share of total government health expenditure on public health and family welfare is associated with a decrease of 1 infant death per 1,000 live births.

Targeting specific population groups

Many countries subsidize all government health services for everyone. These blanket schemes fail to target interventions that give rise to externalities, but they also fail to benefit the poor disproportionately (box 5.8 in chapter 5). This is so despite the stronger equity case for subsidizing care for the poor—and the fact that the poor tend to bear a disproportionate burden of child and maternal mortality and malnutrition. (Chapter 5 provides a variety of examples of programs that have successfully targeted government spending on poor and vulnerable groups, some of which have been evaluated and found to have had an impact.)

Using social investment funds to reach the poor

Targeting resources to poor regions and provinces may require nontraditional mechanisms for setting priorities and implementing programs. Social investment funds, which have achieved important impacts on such health outcomes as infant mortality rates (box 4.1), may fulfill such a role.

The returns to targeted spending from removing bottlenecks

Another approach is to assess—at the country level—health sector impediments to faster progress, identify ways to remove them, and estimate both the costs of removing them and the likely impacts of their removal on Millennium Development Goal outcomes (box 4.2).[22] Work along these lines has begun in several African countries and in India.

Box 4.1 Coupling targeting with institutional innovation through social investment funds

Social funds can be defined as "agencies that finance small projects in several sectors targeted to benefit a country's poor and vulnerable groups based on...demand generated by local groups and screened against a set of eligibility criteria."[19] Bolivia introduced the first such fund in 1986, when it established the Emergency Social Fund. International donors soon recognized the potential of the social fund as a channel for social investments in rural Bolivia and as an international model for community-led development.

In 1991 the Bolivian social fund began concentrating on delivering social infrastructure to historically underserved areas, moving away from emergency-driven employment generation projects. It proved that this type of institution could operate to scale, bringing small infrastructure investments to vast areas of rural Bolivia that line ministries had been unable to reach because of their weak capacity to execute projects. Providing financing to communities rather than implementing projects itself, the social fund rapidly absorbed a large share of public investment.

The concept spread quickly, as other countries sought to ease the social impact of economic crises and increase investment in underserved areas. Now established in most countries in Latin America, social funds have spread to Africa, the Middle East, Eastern Europe, and Asia. By May 2001 the World Bank had invested about $3.5 billion in social funds through more than 98 investment operations in 58 countries. These funds had also attracted more than $4.5 billion from other international agencies as well as from domestic financing from governments. Despite the sizable investments, however, the funds remain a small part of poverty and social protection activities in most countries, with total expenditures typically equal to less than 1 percent of GDP.

Social funds have the following common characteristics:

- *Second-tier agencies.* Social funds do not execute projects directly. Instead, they appraise, finance, and supervise investments carried out by other agencies, such as local representatives of line ministries, local governments, and nongovernmental organizations.

- *Multisectoral choice of investments.* Social funds typically offer implementing agencies a wide range of choices of investments to be financed in different sectors.

- *Demand-driven investments.* Social funds rely on project proposals submitted by a variety of local actors, including local governments, nongovernmental organizations, community groups, and others.

- *Operational autonomy and modern management practices.* Social funds reside in the public sector but operate like private firms. They are usually granted exceptional status, either as autonomous institutions or with operational autonomy under existing ministries.

A recent evaluation[20] of social funds was carried out in six countries: Armenia, Bolivia, Honduras, Nicaragua, Peru, and Zambia. Among other specific objectives, the study evaluated the degree to which social fund interventions reach poor areas and poor households and affect living standards (as measured by education and health outcomes). The study used panel data on project beneficiaries and comparison groups, applying several evaluation methodologies.

The results of the study are interesting because they reveal better targeting (especially in Peru) and positive health impacts (especially in Bolivia). The geographic distribution of social fund expenditures was propoor in all countries studied, with poor districts receiving more per capita than wealthier districts and the very poorest districts receiving shares exceeding their shares of the population. The high levels of investment in some of the poorest areas refute the idea that such areas are systematically incapable of accessing resources from demand-driven programs. But in most cases the overall distribution of resources at the household level was only mildly progressive. Positive discrimination toward poor households was best reached by latrine and health projects, with sewage projects benefiting the better off.

For health the research found that social fund health interventions had a positive impact on infrastructure quality and the availability of medical equipment and furniture. Essential drugs and replaceable medical supplies were generally more available in social fund facilities, though all facilities had difficulties securing adequate supply of essential drugs. Social fund facilities were also as well or better staffed than comparators. In Bolivia, perhaps because they went beyond simply improving infrastructure, interventions in health clinics raised utilization rates and were associated with substantial declines in under-five mortality rates.[20]

The results in under-five mortality rates in Bolivia are robust, based on three alternative methodologies: propensity score matching; changes in mortality using household surveys between treatment and comparison groups at two different dates (1993 and 1997), also known as double differences or difference in differences methodology; and econometric analysis estimation (Cox proportional hazard function). The changes in mortality using double differences show a statistically significant decline in the percentage of children dying, from 10.3 percent in 1993 to 6 percent in 1997 in the treatment group relative to an increase from 10.3 percent to 10.7 percent in the comparison group. The econometric estimates show a statistically significant decline in under-five mortality, from 88.5 to 65.6 deaths per 1,000 among children living in the service area of a health center that received social fund investment.

Source: Reference 21.

Box 4.2 Marginal budgeting for bottlenecks

Despite extensive sector reforms, the health systems in many developing countries still fail to reach large numbers of women and children—particularly the poor and most vulnerable of these populations—with interventions that could significantly reduce morbidity and mortality. Marginal budgeting for bottlenecks, recently developed by the United Nations Children's Fund, the World Bank, and the World Health Organization, has been tested in several countries. The tool helps policymakers and program managers improve the delivery of health services and interventions. It can help formulate medium-term national or provincial expenditure plans as well as Poverty Reduction Strategy Credits that explicitly link expenditure to health Millennium Development Goals and optimally allocate newly available resources to achieve such health outcome targets. It also allows the likely impact of alternative options on health outcomes to be assessed to improve the allocative efficiency of government health budgets. This distinguishes it from traditional approaches of programming and budgeting of health interventions.

Marginal budgeting for bottlenecks helps answer the following questions:

- What are the major health systems bottlenecks—"the weakest links in the chain"—that hamper the delivery of health services, and what can be done to address them?

- How much money is needed to achieve the expected results?

- How much can health outcomes be improved by removing the bottlenecks?

Marginal budgeting for bottlenecks consists of three modules: bottleneck identification, costing and budgeting, and expected impact.

Module 1: Bottleneck identification

The first module defines intervention packages according to service delivery mode: family and community-based care, population-oriented services, and individual-oriented clinical care. Current levels of coverage of these packages are estimated based on available country data. The module then uses proxy indicators from data sources such as Demographic and Health Surveys or Multiple Indicator Cluster Surveys to identify bottlenecks that hamper expansion of coverage levels. The identification of bottlenecks is performed in the following five broad categories: gaps in physical accessibility, human resources, supplies and logistics, demand and use, and technical and organizational quality.

Proxy indicators are used so that each intervention package can be adequately represented by a proxy intervention, which in turn has a proxy indicator for each corresponding constraint (or bottleneck). Mali used the proportion of deliveries attended by trained staff as a proxy for use of institutional professional deliveries (ideally measured by proportion of deliveries attended by a professional in a health center or hospital). The average of the values of the proxy indicators for a bottleneck—across an intervention package—represents the extent of the bottleneck at a particular level of service delivery. Based on an analysis of the realistic possibility that the bottleneck can be reduced in a certain time period, marginal budgeting for bottlenecks then sets a new target for the proxy indicator corresponding to the bottleneck—the "new performance frontier."

Module 2: Costing and budgeting

The costing and budgeting module estimates the volume of additional resources (the incremental cost) required to overcome the bottlenecks and achieving the new performance frontiers set in Module 1. It does so by costing a set of strategies or programs to address the bottlenecks in each intervention package. The costing module has six components, five corresponding to the categories of bottlenecks defined above. The sixth component adds the expected costs of needed stewardship to steer the increase in coverage levels. It includes costs for capacity strengthening, central supervision, research, and assistance with planning. The module can be applied to different regions (urban or rural, poor or rich, low or high morbidity and mortality). Such estimates can be used to assess resource allocation among regions. Once the marginal costs of addressing the bottlenecks within a certain time period have been identified, they can be spread over the time period using different budget formats.

Module 3: Expected impact

The expected impact module uses an epidemiometric model to calculate the potential impact on the Millennium Development Goals if the new performance frontiers for coverage levels of intervention packages are achieved. Providing policymakers with an idea of the consequences of their choices, it can serve as a basis for policy dialogue.

Source: Reference 22.

In Mali key bottlenecks to supporting home-based practices and delivering both periodic and continual professional care were identified. These included poor access to affordable commodities; the need for community-based support for home-based care; poor geographical access to preventive professional care (immunization, vitamin A supplementation, and antenatal care); shortages of qualified nurses and midwives; and the lack of effective third-party payment mechanisms for the poor for continual professional care. Removing these impediments at a cost of $12 per capita between 2002 and 2007 could reduce under-five mortality by 20–40 percent and maternal mortality by

Table 4.3 Marginal budgeting for bottlenecks—how targeting can raise government health spending elasticities

Country or state	Baseline under-five mortality rate	Under-five mortality reduction (percent)	Current government spending (U.S. dollars per capita)	Extra spending (U.S. dollars per capita)	Change in government spending per capita (percent)	Implied elasticity of under-five mortality rate to government health spending
Benin	158	59	12.00	7.32	61	−0.967
Ethiopia	185	31	4.00	3.77	94	−0.329
Madagascar	142	42	5.00	3.15	63	−0.667
Mali	231	57	10.00	8.13	81	−0.701
Gujarat (India)	85	16	4.69	1.53	33	−0.490
Orissa (India)	104	29	3.15	1.80	57	−0.508
Rajasthan (India)	115	29	4.61	1.77	38	−0.755

Source: Reference 31.

40–80 percent, depending on the poverty level of the region.

Cost and mortality estimates from studies such as this can be used to compute an implied elasticity of government health spending—the percentage change in mortality divided by the percentage change in spending. The implied elasticities (table 4.3) from several recent and ongoing exercises in marginal budgeting for bottlenecks are considerably larger than those in table 4.1, particularly because the poor quality of policies and institutions in these countries would mean elasticities in table 4.1 in the low and possibly insignificant range. The results suggest that in Ethiopia, spending an additional $7.32 per capita on removing the bottlenecks identified in the marginal budgeting for bottlenecks exercise would yield a return in lower child mortality considerably larger than what would be achieved if the extra money were simply added to the government's health budget. Only time—and careful monitoring and evaluation—will tell whether these estimates turn out to be accurate.

Improving policies and institutions— and the rest of the report

Without better policies and institutions, countries with low CPIA scores will not progress faster toward the Millennium Development Goals through extra government health spending. What do better policies and institutions entail in the health sector? Health systems are very broad—far broader than many people think. Weak policies and institutions can arise at several different points along the path from government health spending to health outcomes (figure 4.3). Part II of the report uses this framework to tackle the difficult question of how to build stronger policies and institutions.

Households are pivotal but often overlooked

Households play two roles in the health system (chapter 5). They are demanders of community-based and facility-based interventions, and they are deliverers of home-based interventions. For interventions that are—or ought to be—delivered by a professional (antenatal care, the safe delivery of a newborn, immunization), the patient (or the caregiver for a child) is crucial. He or she makes the initial contact and plays a key part in what follows, in compliance, follow-up, referral, and so on. If a mother fails to recognize the signs of a sick child and does not take the child to a provider, the consequences can be fatal. A recent study in Bolivia found that 60 percent of children who died during the period covered by the study had never been taken to a formal health care provider in the sickness episode culminating in their deaths.[23]

The household's role as a deliverer of care is also crucial. It is mothers who breastfeed their children, and it is they and other household members who purchase, treat, and use bednets. It is in the household that timely and appropriate complementary feeding gets provided to the growing child. It is the caregiver who administers oral rehydration therapy to a child with diarrhea and antimalarials to a child with fever. Much of a child's health is—or at least can be—"produced" in the household.

Policymakers can influence households through the resources households have at their disposal, including their knowledge of health matters, and through their influence on community factors, by affecting both social norms and infrastructure. All too often, however, health policy toward households is piecemeal and half-hearted, even failing to acknowledge that households are deliverers of health interventions.

Figure 4.3 Paths to better health, nutrition, and population outcomes

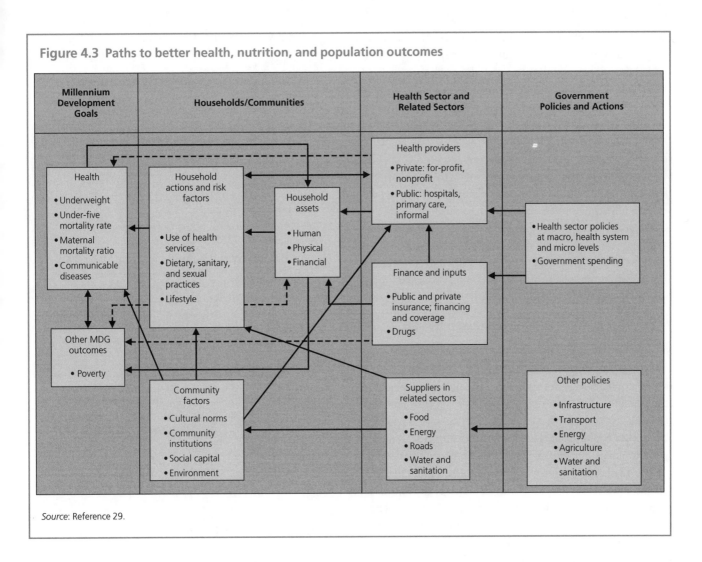

Source: Reference 29.

Improving provider accountability

Health providers in the public and private sectors play a key role in delivering interventions of relevance to the Millennium Development Goals. Yet they are often highly inefficient, deliver poor-quality care, and are unresponsive to patients, reflecting in part poor management and a lack of accountability to the public (chapter 6). Management often lacks an outcome focus, a clear delineation of responsibilities and accountabilities within provider organizations, and a proper link between performance, compensation, and promotion prospects. Citizens, in their capacities as patients, often exert less influence over providers than they could. In their capacities as voters, they often exert too little influence over policymakers, who in turn exert too limited influence over providers. The short route of accountability—from client to provider—can be strengthened through such schemes as vouchers, report cards, and citizen management groups. The long route—from citizen to policymaker to provider organization to frontline provider—can be strengthened through such schemes as contracting and public-private partnerships.

Strengthening input markets

Provider organizations do not operate in a vacuum—they rely on human resources and drugs to deliver services (chapter 7). In both "input markets," problems arise. Human resource stocks are often inadequate, and drugs are often unavailable. But there are other issues, too. Providers often are not as competent as they need to be. In Burundi in 1992 only 2 percent of children with diarrhea taken to health facilities were correctly diagnosed.[24] In the same facilities only 13 percent of children correctly diagnosed as having diarrheal disease were correctly rehydrated.[24] Even if patients are initiated in correct treatment, there is no assurance that it will be administered successfully: in India's public sector in the early 1990s less than 45 percent of patients diagnosed with tuberculosis were successfully treated.[25]

Mistakes and poor quality care are not inevitable. One strategy for preventing such problems is training (chapter 7). Another is improving program design—one of the issues of core public health functions (chapter 8). Both have proved effective. In Tanzania providers trained in the Integrated Management of Childhood Illness were twice as likely as other providers to prescribe antibiotics appropriately; in Bolivia they were 10 times more likely to recognize the danger signs of a sick child.[26,27] In India in 2002 the tuberculosis treatment success rate had risen to 84 percent where DOTS was implemented.[25] In Thailand the HIV infection rate among 21-year-old military conscripts dropped from 4 percent in 1993 to less than 1.5 percent in 1997 through active, effective, and open prevention efforts launched in 1991.[28]

For drugs it is not just that providers lack them in their facilities—often they prescribe inappropriate ones, often knowingly. Even if drugs are available and prescribed appropriately, poor households and poor countries may not be able to afford them (chapter 7).

Strengthening core public health functions

Strengthening core public health functions—monitoring, evaluation, surveillance, regulation, social mobilization, and intersectoral action—are also vital elements of a strategy for strengthening the health sector (chapter 8). Governments have the responsibility for achieving and measuring progress toward the health goals. They have to formulate the strategies and norms for disease prevention and control; establish the mechanisms for monitoring and evaluation; build institutions and the capacity to monitor, educate, and mobilize communities; and regulate and steer other sectors toward the health goals. The recent SARS epidemic drew attention to well-performing public health functions in preventing, controlling, and responding to new health challenges.

References

1. World Health Organization. 2001. *Macroeconomics and Health: Investing in Health for Economic Development.* Report of the Commission on Macroeconomics and Health. Geneva: WHO.

2. Filmer, D., and L. Pritchett. 1999. "The Impact of Public Spending on Health: Does Money Matter?" *Social Science and Medicine* 49 (10): 1309–1323.

3. Filmer, D., J. Hammer, and L. Pritchett. 2000. "Weak Links in the Chain: A Diagnosis of Health Policy in Poor Countries." *World Bank Research Observer* 15 (2): 199–224.

4. Filmer, D., J. Hammer, and L. Pritchett. 2002. "Weak Links in the Chain II: A Prescription for Health Policy in Poor Countries." *World Bank Research Observer* 17 (1): 47–66.

5. World Bank. 2004. *World Development Report 2004: Making Services Work for Poor People.* Washington, DC: World Bank.

6. Bidani, B., and M. Ravallion. 1997. "Decomposing Social Indicators Using Distributional Data." *Journal of Econometrics* 77 (1): 125–139.

7. Gupta, S., M. Verhoeven, and E.R. Tiongson. 2003. "Public Spending on Health Care and the Poor." *Health Economics* 12 (8): 685–696.

8. Wagstaff, A. 2003. "Child Health on a Dollar a Day: Some Tentative Cross-Country Comparisons." *Social Science Medicine* 57 (9): 1529–1538.

9. Rajkumar, A., and V. Swaroop V. 2002. "Public Spending and Outcomes: Does Governance Matter?" Policy Research Working Paper 2840, World Bank, Washington, DC.

10. Feyzioglu, T.N., V. Swaroop, and M. Zhu. 1996. "Foreign Aid's Impact on Public Spending." Policy Research Working Paper 1610, World Bank, Washington DC.

11. Burnside, C., and D. Dollar. 2000. "Aid, Growth, the Incentive Regime and Poverty Reduction." In *The World Bank: Structure and Policies,* eds. C.L. Gilbert and D. Vines, 210–227. Cambridge: Cambridge University Press.

12. World Bank. 1999. *Peru: Improving Health Care for the Poor.* Washington, DC: World Bank.

13. Ensor, T., A. Hossain, Q. Ali, S. Begum, and A. Moral. 2001. "Geographic Resource Allocation in Bangladesh." Research Paper 21, Ministry of Health and Family Welfare, Health Economics Unit, Dhaka.

14. Diderichsen, F., E. Varde, and M. Whitehead. 1997. "Resource Allocation to Health Authorities: The Quest for an Equitable Formula in Britain and Sweden." *British Medical Journal* 315 (7112): 875–878.

15. World Bank. 2002. *Armenia Public Expenditure Review.* World Bank, Washington, DC.

16. Lambrechts, T., J. Bryce, and V. Orinda. 1999. "Integrated Management of Childhood Illness: A Summary of First Experiences." *Bulletin of the World Health Organization* 77 (7): 582–594.

17. Santos, I., C.G. Victora, J. Martines, H. Goncalves, D.P. Gigante, N.J. Valle, and G. Pelto. 2001. "Nutrition Counseling Increases Weight Gain among Brazilian Children." *Journal of Nutrition* 131 (11): 2866–2873.

18. World Bank. 2003. *Attaining the Millennium Development Goals in India: How Likely and What Will It Take?* Washington, DC: Washington, DC.

19. Jorgensen, S., and J.V. Domelen, 2001. "Helping the Poor Manage Risk Better: The Role of Social Funds." In *Shielding the Poor: Social Protection in the Developing World,* ed. N. Lustig. Washington, DC: Brookings Institution.

20. Newman, J., M. Pradhan, L. Rawlings, G. Ridder, R. Coa, and J.L. Evia. 2002. "An Impact Evaluation of Education, Health, and Water Supply Investments by the Bolivian Social Investment Fund." *World Bank Economic Review* 16 (2): 241–274.

21. Rawlings L, L. Sherberburne-Benz, and J. van Domelen. 2004. "Evaluating Social Fund Performance: A Cross-Country Analysis of Community Investments." World Bank, Washington DC.

22. Soucat, A., W. Van Lerberghe, F. Diop, S. Nguyen, and R. Knippenberg. 2002. "Marginal Budgeting for Bottlenecks: A New Costing and Resource-Allocation Practice to Buy Health Results." World Bank, Washington, DC.

23. Aguilar, A.M,. R. Alvarado, D. Cordero, P. Kelly, A. Zamora, and R. Salgado. 1998. *Mortality Survey in Bolivia: The Final Report.* Basic Support for Institutionalizing Child Survival (BASICS) Project, Arlington, VA.

24. World Health Organization. 1998. *CHD 1996–97 Report.* Geneva: WHO.

25. Ministry of Health and Social Welfare. 2002. *RNTCP Performance Report, India, 3rd Quarter.* 2002. Central Tuberculosis Division, Delhi.

26. Schellenberg, J. 2001. *The MCE-Tanzania Working Group on the 2001 Health Facility Survey.* Health Facility Survey Submitted to the Department of Child and Adolescent Health and Development. Geneva, World Health Organization.

27. MOH BW BASICS/USAID and Sociedad Boliviana De Pediatria. 1999. *Report of the Health Facility Survey in Bolivia.*

28. World Health Organization. 2000. *Health a Key to Prosperity: Success Stories in Developing Countries.* Geneva: WHO.

29. Claeson, M., and E. Bos. 2002. *Health, Nutrition and Population Development Goals: Measuring Progress Using the Poverty Reduction Strategy Framework.* Report of a World Bank Consultation, November 28–29. World Bank, Health, Nutrition and Population Department, Washington, DC.

30. World Bank. 2003. *World Development Indicators 2003.* Washington, DC: World Bank.

31. UNICEF and World Bank. 2003. *Marginal Budgeting for Bottlenecks: How to Reach the Impact Frontier of Health and Nutrition Services and Accelerate Progress towards the MDGS: A Budgeting Model and Application to Low-Income Countries.* New York: UNICEF; Washington, DC: World Bank.

CHAPTER 5

Households—Key but Underrated Actors in the Health Sector

When physician Truong Cong Thang started practicing at the De Ar Commune health clinic in the Central Highlands, he had to take drastic action to win locals' trust. A belief exists in the commune that when childbirth begins a woman must go to the forest by herself, and unaccompanied, deliver her baby, bringing the child home when it is over. A woman following this custom gave birth to a baby girl in the forest. But several days later, she developed a high fever as parts of her placenta were still in her womb. Her desperate parents had asked a traditional healer to pray over her and chase away the forest ghosts, to no avail.

When Thang heard about the woman's predicament, he issued a bold challenge to her family. If he couldn't save her life, he would submit to their punishment, as it is forbidden under local laws for a strange man to see the body of a married woman. Only when commune leaders witnessed and sealed Thang's letter of guarantee did her family let him treat the dying woman. Thirty-year-old Thang's gambit paid off after he saved her life. After this incident, villagers believed their physician was much better than the traditional healers.

When they started working in the commune, the young doctor and nurse Sep went from house to house trying to persuade pregnant women to visit the clinic for check-ups but met a lot of resistance. However, after word spread of Thang's success in treating the woman who nearly died, gradually more women

have come for examinations, and all the commune's women have learned about family planning.

VIETNAM NEWS, *October 19, 2003*

Households matter in the health sector—more than most policymakers acknowledge. Improving the health of households is what the health sector is all about. People rely on their health in their everyday lives, and for poor households, health is one of their major assets. Households are also key actors in the "production" of health. Indeed, they play a dual role—as users of health services delivered by professional providers and as producers of health through the delivery of home-based interventions and in their everyday health behaviors.

In these roles, households are influenced by several factors. The economic resources at their disposal. The woman's control over these resources. The knowledge household members have of health matters. The numeracy and literacy skills that enable them to acquire new knowledge. The accessibility of health facilities. The water, sanitation, and electricity in and around the house. And so on. This chapter shows how communities shape these influences, and how policymakers can modify them. Ten case studies—of child health, maternal mortality, and communicable diseases—illustrate the policy options.

The dual role of households in health

Households play a dual role in health.* They are users of health services delivered by professional providers, and they are producers of health through the delivery of home-based interventions and in their everyday health behaviors. Health is one of the engines of economic growth and poverty reduction. It is also one of the fruits of economic growth—possibly one of the most highly valued. People rely on their health in their everyday lives. As an Egyptian woman put it in *Voices of the Poor,* "We face a calamity when my husband gets ill. Our life comes to a halt until he recovers and goes back to work."[1] And households are where the activities of the health sector are ultimately directed.

If, as in the story from Vietnam, pregnant women do not seek assistance during delivery or do not seek antenatal care during pregnancy, health providers have their hands tied: they cannot deliver care without a client. The same is true when caregivers do not seek assistance when their child falls sick, when patients fail to show up for follow-up visits or do not adhere to the provider's instructions. Weak demand for professional services would appear to be a major obstacle to achieving the Millennium Development Goals. A recent study in Bolivia found that 60 percent of children who died had not been taken to a formal provider in the sickness episode culminating in their death.[2] And yet health planners rarely concern themselves with the factors that hold down demand. The assumption is that if patients need health care they will demand it and the professional provider will then deliver it.

Households are also deliverers of care—especially care directed at children. Mothers breastfeed their children. They and other household members purchase, treat, and use insecticide-treated nets. Caregivers provide timely and appropriate complementary feeding to the growing child, wash their hands before preparing food, safely dispose of feces, administer oral rehydration therapy to children with diarrhea and antimalarials to children with fever. These are not incidental interventions—they are highly effective. The fact is that much of a child's health is—or could be—produced in and by the household through the delivery of interventions or improved household or family practices (box 5.1). The same is true of nutrition outcomes, maternal and reproductive health outcomes, and the prevention of other communicable diseases.

Ten case studies on child health, maternal mortality, and communicable diseases illustrate the policy options (tables 5.1, 5.2, and 5.3); these are located at the end of this chapter.

Households are not islands—health providers and communities help shape health outcomes

Health providers and communities influence the health-related behaviors of households. They, in turn, are influenced—often unwittingly—by policymakers. Health providers influence households' decisions about use of services—providers who deliver care that is perceived as good quality encourage return visits and build faith in the health system. Providers also influence decisions about home-based interventions, providing knowledge about why nutrition matters and how to prepare nutritious meals on a very limited budget.

Through social norms and values, informal networks, and local governance structures, communities influence both household practices and the delivery of services (see chapter 6 on the delivery of services). In some settings the boundaries between households and communities are vague, especially where traditional household structures have broken down, due to civil strife, HIV/AIDS, or other circumstances. AIDS orphans are a case in point. Throughout many countries in Africa the community acts as a safety net that keeps families and households from destitution, providing material relief, labor, and emotional support that would otherwise not be available.[4]

Policymakers can also influence providers and communities. They can affect what providers do, wittingly or unwittingly, to influence household decisions in their dual roles. At the community level, policymakers can encourage or discourage informal networks. Social norms are not immutable: governments can help make communities strong, resilient, and well informed if they choose to do so. Community-based health projects can help, improving household health practices and the delivery of services by professionals.

Consider the World Bank's Comprehensive Rural Health Project in India's Maharashtra State. This project improved the health of more than 250,000 people by helping villagers organize to address health needs and by training local village health care workers. The village health workers in turn organized women's development associations, which initiated credit circles to fund cooperative business enterprises. (The role of the community in service delivery is examined in chapter 6.)

Raising incomes

Low income is a barrier to using most interventions—preventive and curative. Holding constant other influences on

---

* The term "household" is used here to refer to whatever grouping of people share responsibility for health. It is not necessarily limited to biological relatives (stepparents can be caregivers) and can encompass the broad array of kinship and household patters around the world.

Box 5.1 Key family practices for the production of child health and nutrition

Families play a crucial role in keeping their children healthy and well nourished. A recent review summarizing the potential impact of family practices on child mortality, morbidity, growth, and development highlighted the key practices or behaviors that have a significant impact on child health outcomes. Many of them can be delivered by households.

- *Breastfeed infants exclusively for six months.* Breastfeeding is associated with reduced child mortality and morbidity and improved development. Evidence suggests that breastfed infants under two months of age are six times less likely to die of infectious diseases than infants not breastfed. And a protective effect against diarrhea and pneumonia has been observed both in industrial and developing countries.

- *Starting at six months of age, feed children freshly prepared energy-dense and nutrient-rich foods while continuing to breastfeed for two years or longer.* Breast milk continues to be a source of key nutrients and to confer protection against infectious diseases throughout the second year of life. Beginning at six months, however, it is not sufficient to meet nutritional requirements alone. Observational studies indicate that improving feeding practices could save 800,000 lives a year.

- *Ensure that children receive adequate amounts of micronutrients.* Improving the intake of vitamin A, iron, and zinc will have a substantial impact on mortality, morbidity, and development, particularly among poor or micronutrient-deficient populations. Food supplementation or fortification may be necessary.

- *Safely dispose of feces, including children's feces, and wash hands after defecating.* Hand-washing after defecating and before preparing meals and feeding children can reduce diarrheal diseases in children under five by a median of 33 percent (range 11–89 percent). And better access to sanitation is associated with a reduction in all causes of child mortality.

- *Protect children in malaria-endemic areas by ensuring that they sleep under insecticide-treated nets.* A meta-analysis of four African randomized controlled trials showed that treated bednets are associated with a 17 percent reduction in child mortality compared with control populations with no nets or untreated nets.

Households also interact with health care providers, both in seeking care for their children once they fall sick and in following through on care and advice delivered at health facilities. Households can have a crucial impact on child health outcomes in several ways.

- *Take children as scheduled to complete a full course of immunizations (BCG, diphtheria, tetanus, pertussis, oral polio vaccine, and measles) before their first birthday.* Immunizations can prevent an estimated 3 million child deaths each year. Measles vaccination is particularly important.

- *Recognize when sick children need treatment outside the home and seek care from appropriate providers.* Studies examining factors contributing to child deaths have found that poor care-seeking is implicated in 6–70 percent of deaths. A high number of deaths has also been attributed to delays in care-seeking. A median of 23 percent of all fatally ill children are never taken to a health facility.

- *Continue to feed and offer more fluids, including breast milk, to children when they are sick.* Children require more food and fluids during illness, but 16–65 percent of caregivers withhold food, breastmilk, or fluids during illness. Randomized controlled trials have found that feeding nutritionally complete diets to children with diarrhea increases net energy and nutrient absorption. Contrary to many beliefs, feeding locally available foods does not increase the duration of diarrhea.

- *Give sick children appropriate home treatment for infection.* Uncomplicated diarrhea, malaria, and local infections can be managed at home with efficacious treatments. Oral rehydration therapy can prevent death from watery diarrhea in all but the most severe cases. Home treatment of malaria-related fevers by training mothers and increasing access to treatment can have a large impact.

- *Follow health workers' advice about treatment, follow-up, and referral.* Not adhering to treatment and referral recommendations by health workers leads to incomplete treatment, therapy failure, drug resistance, and the later misuse of the left-over medicines.

Source: Reference 3.

demand, higher incomes have been found to increase the likelihood of a pregnant woman receiving antenatal care and skilled care during delivery.[5–9] Higher incomes are also associated with a higher probability of a child being immunized, sleeping under a treated bednet, being given oral rehydration therapy when sick with diarrhea, and being taken to a formal provider when it has fever.[10–13] Income—or rather the ability to buy food with money earned from selling commodities such as crafts—is a key factor in determining whether households have enough food to eat (box 5.2).

Options for raising incomes

Given the link between income and the use of key health interventions, economic growth will be an important source of progress toward the Millennium Development Goals. There is no doubt that economic growth has been a major factor underlying the long-term improvements in health outcomes. And there can be little doubt that slow economic growth has meant slow progress on health outcomes. It has been estimated, for example, that half a million child deaths would have been averted in Africa in 1990

Traditionally, famines have been attributed to a sudden decline in the availability of food. On the face of it this explanation seems plausible—it seems natural to assume that food supply must have declined sharply if people start to starve. The official Famine Inquiry Commission set up by the Indian government following the Bengal famine of 1943, which killed 3 million people, concluded just this—that there had been a sudden decline in the supply of rice, the staple food of the Bengali.

Amartya Sen has shown why a focus on food availability can be misleading. In 1943 there was actually more food available in Bengal than there had been in 1941, when no one went hungry. Sen argues that a household can be plunged into starvation if there is a sudden fall in the price of the commodities it sells relative to the price of food. What marked 1943 as special was a sudden rise in the price of rice. The increase left groups such as barbers, craftspeople, fishers, transport workers, and agricultural

laborers—who saw no appreciable rise in the price of the things they sold—with vastly worse "terms of trade." They were unable to buy enough food to survive. By contrast, peasants and share-croppers (tenant farmers paying their rent with a part of their crop) were hardly affected. What caused the rapid rise in the price of rice in 1943? Part of the explanation lies in the fall of Burma to the Japanese, which brought Bengal close to the war front, causing rapid growth in military and civil construction.

The moral of Sen's argument is not complicated, but it is often overlooked: food production and availability are important, but the key issue from a hunger perspective is the capacity of different groups to afford whatever food is available. The use of public employment programs to increase the purchasing power of vulnerable populations is a key part of a strategy against hunger.

Source: References 14–16.

---

alone if the continent's economic growth in the 1980s had been 1.5 percentage points higher.[17] But economic growth, while important, will not be fast enough to achieve the Millennium Development Goals. Although projected rates of economic growth will leave all but one Bank region (Sub-Saharan Africa) on target for reducing the number of people living on $1 a day, not one Bank region will achieve the required reduction in under-five mortality through economic growth alone.[18] Income transfer schemes provide policymakers with a means of raising the incomes of certain groups more quickly than they would through economic growth. Such schemes are rarely rationalized in terms of improving health outcomes. There is, however, clear evidence that they yield health payoffs. South Africa's old-age pension provides an example. The program was originally a safety net for whites who reached retirement age without an adequate employment-based pension. By the end of 1993 the program had been extended to all racial groups, and it has been an important source of income for non-whites. Recent research finds that the pension improved not only the health of pension recipients but also the health of other members of households in which resources are pooled.[19,20] Among black children under the age of five, the pension is estimated to have led to an eight-centimeter increase in height—equivalent to half a year's growth. And South Africa's pension program has been found to disproportionately benefit poorer households and households with children.[21]

Informal solidarity schemes at the community level often substitute for formal social protection programs (box 5.3). Although a lack of money is an obstacle, communities

can take advantage of social networks to access otherwise inaccessible health services.[22]

Increasing affordability— especially for the poor

The demand for health care, like the demand for almost everything else, depends on price. Out-of-pocket expenditures for professionally delivered health services can be substantial. A normal hospital delivery in Dhaka, Bangladesh,

Formal government mechanisms do not provide adequate access to health services for all people in many countries. In Côte d'Ivoire the imposition of user fees for public services in the 1990s effectively made services inaccessible to the poorer segment of the population. Yet many poor people use modern health care services that have become quite expensive. Solidarity among parents, friends, and members of community social networks allows them to do so.

Many factors at the household level are significantly associated with using financial solidarity to gain access to health services. The number of children born to the head of the household to which the ill person belongs was found to be the strongest. Households with no children were less likely to benefit from financial solidarity than households with children. Gender is also a determining factor: women have a better chance of receiving financial support for illness than men.

Source: Reference 22.

costs the equivalent of one-quarter of the average monthly income.[23] A single hospital visit for a Vietnamese in the poorest fifth of the population in 1998 entailed fees and drug costs equivalent to 22 percent of that person's annual discretionary income (income after deducting food expenses).[24]

In many cases out-of-pocket payments are informal rather than formal. In Armenia in 1999, 91 percent of health service users made an informal payment to a health care provider.[25] In Azerbaijan and Poland the figure was 78 percent. In nearly all developing countries tuberculosis treatment is officially provided free of charge, but indirect costs and informal illegal payments mean that the real prices of care are much higher, and can diminish early and full help-seeking, and increase transmission of disease.

It is not just the fees paid to health providers that matter—households incur other money costs in using health facilities, including the cost of transportation. A study of referral and follow-up recommendations based on the Integrated Management of Childhood Illness strategy in Sudan found that only about half the children judged in need of urgent referral were taken for such care within 24 hours. The cost of getting to the hospital was the reason most frequently cited for not getting the needed care.[26] *Voices of the Poor* identifies other money costs.[27] A young woman in Muynak, Uzbekistan, said: "We do not go to hospital because it is necessary to bring your own bed linen, dishes, sometimes even a bed."

Higher money prices tend to reduce demand—especially among the poor—unless accompanied by improvements in service quality.[28] Cost is one of the main reasons sick people give for not seeking care. In Georgia in 1997, 94 percent of those who did not seek care when ill said it was the high cost that prevented them doing so.[25] In China, when tuberculosis treatment was made free, demand for it increased significantly. Informal payments deter as much as formal payments. Informal payments were identified as one of the factors underlying the low use of community hospitals and health centers in Thailand in the 1970s.[29]

The demand for preventive home-delivered interventions also depends on price. High food prices, for example, tend to be associated with low nutrient intake and low levels of child survival and nutrition.[30–33] The nutritional status and nutrient intake of the poor are particularly sensitive to changes in the price of food.[31,33] In a recent study, affordability was the most frequently cited reason for not owning a mosquito net, especially among the poorest group.[34]

Reasons to reduce the price of health care

Many interventions relevant to the health Millennium Development Goals are activities that generate externalities—the benefits of the intervention "spill over" to people who do not receive the intervention. For example, an individual can reduce the probability of contracting malaria through a variety of preventive interventions, including the use of insecticide-treated nets. Once a person is infected, the use of an antimalarial will eliminate the malaria in the blood. By reducing the reservoir of infected people, the use of both preventive and treatment interventions reduces the probability of mosquitoes becoming infected, which in turn reduces the probability of other people being bitten by an infected mosquito.

Immunization is another intervention that generates a positive externality. If person A gets vaccinated against a particular disease, persons B and C benefit through the lower risk of transmission from person A. The benefits of vaccination to person A spill over to other people. Subsidizing the use of such interventions makes economic sense. In the absence of subsidies the use of immunization and preventive and treatment interventions against malaria would be at inefficiently low levels.

The same case can be made for the interventions listed in figure 3.2 in chapter 3 for all but two of the other leading causes of childhood deaths (the exceptions are birth asphyxia and preterm delivery). And it can be made for the interventions for tuberculosis, malaria, and HIV/AIDS and for several interventions to reduce maternal mortality.

Even where there are no spillovers, an equity case can be made for reducing prices. The equity concern is likely to relate to poorer groups, who cannot afford care at the regular price or would risk being plunged into—or further into—poverty if they paid for it. Price reductions should, in principle, target such groups.

Reductions in the price of care at the point of use may also come about as part of an expansion in insurance coverage. Risk aversion coupled with the unpredictability of illness provides a motivation for pooling risks through an insurance scheme. Revenues are collected from those at risk—or at least from a large number of them—and then used to pay the costs incurred by people if and when they fall ill. To counter moral hazard—the tendency for insured people to increase use beyond an efficient level when they get sick—insurance programs often require a copayment by the insured at the time services are used. Such insurance schemes range from private insurance to community-based schemes to social security schemes and tax-financed programs.

From blanket to targeted subsidies

General revenues are often used to finance all government health services for everyone. These blanket subsidy schemes suffer from two drawbacks: they are not targeted on interventions that produce externalities, and for the most part they are not well targeted on the poor. Although the poor appear to benefit disproportionately in cost terms from subsidies to the health sector in some countries and states in the developing world (Costa Rica, Malaysia, Kerala), the better off generally benefit most (box 5.4, figure 5.1).[35-42]

Focusing subsidies on specific interventions (immunizations) or on certain groups (the poor) is in principle a more attractive approach. Subsidies for specific interventions can be implemented through differential charging (setting a zero fee for, say, immunizations in government clinics) or through a system of vouchers that allows the holder to obtain the intervention free of charge from any approved facility.

As part of a deliberate policy to improve maternal and child health, especially among the poor, the government of Malaysia introduced free antenatal care and home deliveries by government midwives.[43] Bolivia's Maternal and Child Health Insurance program, introduced in 1996, covers the cost of antenatal care, care received during labor and delivery, postpartum and newborn care, and management of all obstetric and newborn complications.[44] The program appears to have increased the use of antenatal care and skilled birth attendants, especially among the poorest fifth of the population, which saw nearly a doubling in pregnant women receiving two or more antenatal visits (figure 5.2). In Ifakara, Tanzania, vouchers were used to provide a 17 percent subsidy on the cost of a mosquito net for pregnant women and children under five. In combination with social marketing to increase the knowledge and availability of bednets, these subsidies led to increased use of bednets.[45-47] One attraction of an explicit voucher scheme is that it ensures that the provider gets paid for treating the patient in question (box 5.5). A zero fee may simply leave providers out of pocket, creating incentives for them to deliver unsubsidized interventions.

The use of entitlement cards provides a means of focusing government subsidies on specific groups. A health card scheme introduced in Indonesia during the crisis of the

---

Box 5.4 Blanket subsidies often benefit the better off most

Benefit-incidence analysis provides a means of seeing how different income groups benefit from public subsidies to a particular sector. For each income group the analysis examines the use of different types of facilities and the amount of subsidy per visit (or inpatient day). The subsidy may vary across income groups if, say, the better off are charged higher fees.

In most countries the better off benefit most from government subsidies to the health sector (see figure 5.1). (Colombia, Costa Rica, Malaysia, and Sri Lanka are exceptions.) In Guinea the richest 20 percent of the population receives nearly 50 percent of the government's subsidy. The failure of blanket subsidies to benefit the poor disproportionately stems from the upper income groups' above-average use of government-subsidized services, especially services provided by hospitals, where much of the typical government subsidy is spent. This skewed pattern of use could in principle be offset by linking user fees to income. Although this happens in some countries, the results make it clear that if it does happen, the user fee gradient is not steep enough to offset the higher use rates among the better off.

Source: World Bank staff.

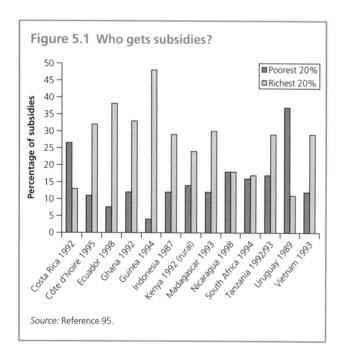

Figure 5.1 Who gets subsidies?

Source: Reference 95.

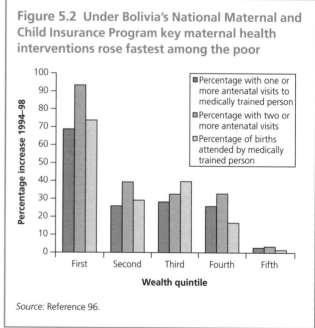

Figure 5.2 Under Bolivia's National Maternal and Child Insurance Program key maternal health interventions rose fastest among the poor

Source: Reference 96.

Box 5.5 Vouchers for sex workers in Nicaragua

In Managua, Nicaragua, a voucher scheme has been used to increase the uptake of reproductive health services among female sex workers.[50] Every three to five months, fieldworkers and nongovernmental organizations (NGOs) at prostitution sites distribute about 1,200 vouchers, depending on the estimated number of sex workers operating in the city at any given time. The vouchers entitle the sex workers to free services at one of 8–10 private, NGO, and public clinics, contracted to the voucher agency by competitive tender. Approved providers must follow a set treatment protocol and receive training. Contracts are reviewed after each round of voucher distribution and renewed subject to an assessment of quality of care. The clinics return the vouchers to the voucher agency, which reimburses the provider an agreed fee per voucher.

Sex workers were involved in the design of the program and have opportunities to express their preferences and complaints. In each round 10 percent of recipients are interviewed about their experience. Initially, sex workers reported that the gatekeepers to care (nurses and receptionists) lacked sensitivity: training and sensitization of this group helped improve their attitudes toward these clients. The technical quality of care (as assessed by an examination at the outset of the project) was lower than expected, so training and treatment protocols were introduced.

Although the prevalence of sexually transmitted infections is only slightly lower than at the beginning of the project (possibly due to the high turnover of female sex workers), incidence among women who used vouchers more than once dropped by 65 percent in the first three years of the program. Following a recommendation by the sex workers, they now receive vouchers to give to their regular partners and clients as well. Sex workers appreciated the fact that they could choose which clinic to attend and made their choices on the basis of distance and staff friendliness. The clinics reported that their main benefit was improvement in the technical quality of their services and that the lessons learned were applied to all of their clients. They felt their reputation was enhanced by being contracted by a prestigious public health agency (the Central American Health Institute).

Source: World Bank staff.

Some recent programs—especially in Latin America—have pushed these ideas even further. Rather than simply reducing the cost of using specific interventions, these programs provide cash payments to users. Receipt of cash payments is linked to the use of specific interventions, and participation is restricted to certain groups—often poor mothers and their children. The experience with these programs, in targeting and impact, is encouraging (box 5.6). Financial inducements—including negative copayments—have also been used to induce people to seek treatment of particular illnesses, such as tuberculosis.

Empowering women

It is not just a household's total income that matters—women's control over its use also makes a difference to health outcomes. In some countries the proportion of women who can decide how to spend their own money is staggeringly small (figure 5.3). Poor women are likely to be particularly disadvantaged. Research shows that women who exert relatively little control over household financial resources are, all else constant, less likely to receive antenatal care, less likely to have antenatal visits, and less likely to have visits in the first trimester of pregnancy.[57] It seems likely that part of the effect of the South African pension program on child health stems from the fact that it is paid to women (grandmothers) rather than to men. Britain decided to make child benefit payments to women rather than to men for similar reasons.

Microcredit programs aimed at poor women are thought to be one way of increasing women's financial autonomy, and they may have increased the use of maternal health services. The evidence is somewhat mixed, but it seems likely that the impact varies from one scheme to the next.[58] Box 5.7 provides an encouraging case of women's empowerment for better health.

It is not just women's financial independence that is important. Their ability to take decisions more generally—including those that do not have major financial consequences—also matters. For example, in India, although contraceptives are readily available in retail shops, community pressure or the disapproval of husbands often prevents women from using them.

Improving information and knowledge

Affordability—the price paid relative to discretionary income—is undoubtedly one important barrier preventing the use of health services. But it is not the only one. Knowledge—or a lack of it—is another.

A lack of knowledge can result in people not seeking care when they need it, despite the absence of price barriers. In Bolivia a large fraction of poor babies are not deliv-

late 1990s was targeted toward the poor.[48] In Egypt a school health insurance program was introduced covering all school-attending children. Although coverage rates are higher among the better off (simply because better-off children are more likely to be enrolled in school), the program is likely to have increased coverage more among the poor than among the better off (many of whom were already covered under other schemes).[49] In addition to being fairly well targeted, both the Indonesia and Egypt programs have had a considerable impact.[48,49]

Box 5.6 Increasing coverage of key interventions through demand-side incentives

A convincing body of evidence is beginning to accumulate on the potential role of cash transfer programs in bringing about the behavior changes necessary to achieve the Millennium Development Goals. Used as a means of combating short-term poverty, cash transfer programs have been seen as vulnerable to political manipulation and ill suited for promoting longer-term development. But a new generation of programs being implemented in Brazil, Colombia, Honduras, Jamaica, Mexico, and Nicaragua makes receipt of the cash payments conditional on household behaviors that foster the development of human capital, such as using preventive health care services or keeping young children in school.

These programs tend to be well targeted to the poor.[51] The mechanisms for achieving this propoor targeting vary greatly from program to program. Honduras' Family Allowance Program (PRAF-II) used a height census of all first-grade school children in the country to identify municipalities at risk of malnutrition. Mexico's PROGRESA program (now Oportunidades) supplemented geographic targeting with a household screening tool to estimate each family's standard of living from a limited number of readily verifiable indicators. Despite these differences, PRAF, PROGRESA, and Nicaragua's Social Protection Network (RPS) pilot program each managed to ensure that more than 50 percent of beneficiary households (more than two-thirds for Honduras and Nicaragua) were from the poorest 30 percent of all households.

These programs have in most cases invested heavily in impact evaluation, providing important lessons about their strengths and weaknesses. Most of the programs have conducted thorough assessments of levels of development in their areas of influence before phasing in the program benefits, allowing investigators to track changes over time.

In Nicaragua vaccination rates (complete vaccination in one-year-old children) increased by 18 percentage points.[52] In Honduras opportune delivery of early infancy immunization increased by 7–10 percentage points, but later vaccinations, already at high coverage levels, were not affected.[53] In Brazil,[54] Honduras,[53] Mexico,[55] and Nicaragua,[52] health service use increased substantially. In Honduras the proportion of women receiving antenatal care five or more times during their pregnancy increased by 18–20 percentage

Operational characteristics of conditional cash transfer programs in Latin America and the Caribbean

Payment method	Condition for payment	Enforcement
Brazil, Bolsa Alimentação Magnetic debit card can be used to withdraw cash at an automatic teller machine or from a lottery ticket seller	Six antenatal care visits during pregnancy; monthly well-child checkups, including complete immunization coverage and growth monitoring	Compliance with preventive health care undertakings supposed to be reviewed by local health team after six months; no information on number of beneficiaries suspended
Colombia, Familias en Acción Cash payment by bank	Regular attendance of child at growth-monitoring sessions	Attendance monitored; no information on number of beneficiaries suspended
Honduras, Family Allowance Program (PRAF) Phase II Freely exchangeable voucher distributed through primary schools or by program directly	Five antenatal care visits during pregnancy, perinatal checkup within 10 days of delivery, monthly well-child checkups	Beneficiaries deposit bar-coded coupons at health center on attendance; no exclusions implemented as of mid-2003
Jamaica, PATH Cash payment at "pay agency"	Regular preventive health care checkups for children under six years, pregnant and lactating women, elderly, disabled, and destitute adults	Intended; no information about current operation
Mexico, PROGRESA/Oportunidades Cash distributed directly	Regular preventive health care checkups for the entire family, attendance at health education sessions	Conditions monitored and apparently enforced
Nicaragua, Social Protection Network (RPS) Cash distributed directly	Growth promotion for young children, complete immunization coverage, no more than two consecutive months of inadequate growth, attendance at health education sessions	All conditions rigorously monitored and enforced

points. In Nicaragua the poorest residents of the program area bene-fited from the intervention more than the less poor. Similar findings were reported in Honduras.[56]

Although conditional cash transfers are a powerful way of changing the behaviors of poor families, thought needs to be given to identifying the precise behavioral responses that need to be fostered in order to achieve life-transforming impacts. In gen-eral, household-level incentives are probably best combined with measures that improve the quality of services offered by schools and clinics in poor communities. The Honduras program explic-itly aims to evaluate the synergies between these two approaches, but the impact of the supply-side interventions will not be known until the final evaluation round planned for 2004.

Source: Saul Morris.

Figure 5.3 Poor women have less of a say in spending their own money

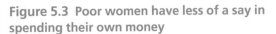

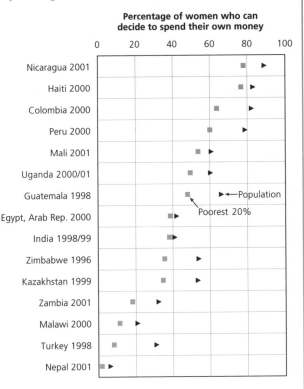

Source: World Bank tabulations and reference 97.

Box 5.7 Helping poor women protect themselves—India's SEWA

The Self-Employed Women's Association (SEWA), an organi-zation of poor self-employed women in Gujarat, India, helps women attain full employment and makes them self-reliant. An Integrated Social Security Scheme provides life insurance, medical insurance, and asset insurance. The premium is the equivalent of $1.70, just under half of which is earmarked for medical insurance that covers hospital care up to a ceiling of $28 a year. Several preexisting conditions, and diseases caused by addiction, are excluded from coverage. There is no restric-tion on the choice of provider—members can use public, pri-vate, and nonprofit providers. Members make claims for reimbursement after discharge, on presentation of specified documentation. In 1999–2000, 23,214 women participated in SEWA's medical insurance fund, in 10 districts of Gujarat.

A recent study found that women making claims were poorer than the general population, suggesting that the scheme was including the poor.[59] This may have been due to the embedding of the insurance plan within a scheme that targeted poor employed women and the fact that the premium was rela-tively low (0.4 percent of median income among claimants). Insurance significantly reduced the financial cost of hospitaliza-tion. On average, 76 percent of hospital costs were reimbursed. Without reimbursement, hospital costs would have been "cata-strophic" (more than 10 percent of annual household income) for 36 percent of claimants. It was estimated that 15 percent of claimants faced expenses that were catastrophic even after reim-bursement. The poorest groups were found more likely to be protected by the fund from catastrophic expenses. The fairly low reimbursement ceiling limited the degree of coverage but also reduced "adverse selection" (the tendency of below-average risks to self-insure because premiums reflect average risks).

Source: World Bank staff.

ered by a trained attendant even though the mothers are eligible for free care under the Maternal and Child Health Insurance program.[44] In India, where immunization is free, 60 percent of children have not been fully immunized. Asked why they had not immunized their child, 30 percent of mothers said it was because they were not aware of the benefits. Another 30 percent said they did not know where to get their child vaccinated.[60]

A lack of knowledge can also result in people seeking and receiving inappropriate care—and paying for it. The infor-mation asymmetry between patient and provider gives providers scope to induce demand for their services. In India

the poor—like the better off—report a large number of short-duration illnesses, but unlike the rich they tend to visit a doctor immediately, usually a private one.[61] They end up spending a large proportion of their income on these short-duration illnesses, often without getting the cause diagnosed.

Furthermore, the medication they receive is often inappropriate or contraindicated. A poor child in Indonesia gets more than four (often useless) drugs per diarrhea attack—instead of oral rehydration therapy. Many studies find that female education is an important determinant of coverage of key Millennium Development Goal interventions. The use of almost all child health interventions is higher in households with better-educated mothers, typically the better off (figure 5.4). The list includes intake of complementary foods among infants, hand-washing, appropriate disposal of excreta, the likelihood of receiving antenatal care, the likelihood of choosing formal rather than traditional care, the timing of antenatal consultations, the likelihood of a baby being delivered away from home and by a trained person, the use of well-baby clinics, the likelihood of a child being immunized, the use of oral rehydration therapy, and the likelihood of a caregiver seeking care for a child with fever.[5–11,13,62–66]

A lack of knowledge and skills may also result in people not getting the full health gain from inputs they have available to them and use. Many women, for example, do not know that piped water often requires further purification and that hand-washing confers much of the health benefit of piped water. It is scarcely surprising in the light of this

that piped water in India has a substantially greater impact on the prevalence of diarrhea among the better-off and better-educated.[67] Likewise, malnutrition is often caused—at least in part—by the lack of knowledge about how and how much to feed infants and young children.[68]

In many societies, inaccurate knowledge based on traditional beliefs or popular notions of modernization—often influenced by mass media advertising—can have a significant influence on health behavior. In The Gambia poor breastfeeding practices, including prelacteal feeding and failure to practice exclusive breastfeeding, were found to be due to traditional beliefs and perceptions—among women and men—that bottle feeding was part of modernization.[69] Some women do not use chloroquine tablets to prevent malaria because they believe the pills induce abortion.[70]

Girls'—and boys'—education

Increasing education—especially among girls—is likely to yield health payoffs. But there are two caveats. First, the payoffs will be felt on the health of the next generation of children: efforts under way today to increase primary school completion rates among girls will not yield health payoffs in lower rates of under-five mortality and child malnutrition for at least another 5–10 years. Second, the health benefits to increased primary education for girls—in better health outcomes for their children—may not be as large as previously thought. A recent study found that once confounding factors were taken into account, primary education of the mother had a statistically significant impact on child survival in only 3 of 23 countries studied.[71] The effect appears to be especially muted in Sub-Saharan Africa.[71,72]

Another recent study[73] sheds light on how mother's education influences child health and suggests why the effect appears to be small. It finds that it is not schooling, literacy, or numeracy that leads to better child health but the fact that better-educated women tend, on average, to have more health knowledge. The study also finds that girls acquire this knowledge after leaving school, using the general literacy and numeracy skills they acquired at school.

This points to the need to ensure high-quality education at the primary level. If the quality of primary education is low, girls will fail to acquire sufficient numeracy and literacy skills to enable them to develop the health knowledge later in life that will help their children remain healthy. Low school quality, coupled with a more hostile health environment, may be part of the reason for the small and largely insignificant effects of primary schooling on child survival in Africa. Where school quality is low, it may make sense for girls and boys to be taught health education at the primary level.

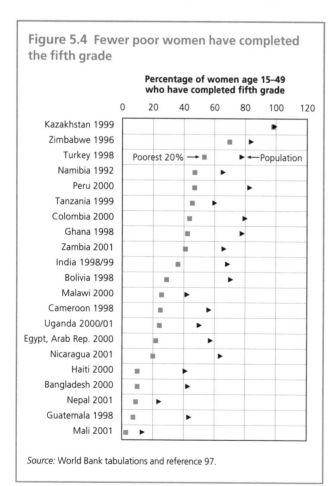

Figure 5.4 Fewer poor women have completed the fifth grade

Source: World Bank tabulations and reference 97.

Conveying health knowledge through the health sector

Conveying health knowledge through public facilities has a long history. A recent example is the lactation management clinic opened five years ago at the Children's Hospital in Islamabad. The program's aims were to promote exclusive breastfeeding—rare in Pakistan—until four to six months of age and to try to solve mothers' breastfeeding difficulties. Mothers receive one-on-one consultation with trained health professionals on the benefits and proper techniques of exclusive breastfeeding. So far, more than 4,000 mothers have been counseled at the clinic. Preliminary results show that 67 percent of mothers had solved their breastfeeding difficulties. More than 60 percent were exclusively breastfeeding, and another 25 percent were breastfeeding and giving other fluids. Only 9 percent of those followed were no longer breastfeeding.[74]

This commonly used approach can be effective for those who participate, but its impact is limited by the fact that many people—including many poor people—do not use the public sector when they fall ill. And in many cases they do not seek care from a formal provider at all. Programs based in the community—where the conveyers of knowledge actively seek out target groups—seem likely to have a better chance of reaching a broader catchment group and of reaching the poor.

There are several success stories here. Health workers in Brazil trained in the Integrated Management of Childhood Illness (IMCI) provided information and counseling at health facilities and in the community.[75] Health knowledge among mothers improved, as did feeding practices. After only 18 months the nutritional status of children in the area improved. In India a counseling strategy was devised jointly by government, NGOs, community volunteers, and health workers in eight villages in rural Haryana.[76] Compared with the control areas (where no community volunteers or health workers were trained), the intervention areas achieved longer breastfeeding durations, a higher quality of complementary feeding provided to children after six months, and increased hand-washing before feeding children.

Killing two birds with one stone—social marketing

Social marketing is proving a promising approach to the design and delivery of both health messages and products (box 5.8). It aims at promoting new or modified behaviors that are acceptable and feasible to most people. It actively involves key actors in designing and implementing activities.[68]

Social marketing refers not only to the marketing of socially valuable products (contraceptives, vitamins) but to the promotion of key behaviors. It integrates communica-

---

Box 5.8 Working with the private sector to improve hygiene behaviors

A recent review found that 12 hand-washing interventions in nine countries achieved a median reduction in diarrhea incidence of 35 percent.[77] Many of the most successful interventions provided soap to mothers, explained the oral-fecal route for disease transmission, and asked mothers to wash their hands before preparing food and after defecating.

One promising approach to the delivery of these interventions is social marketing, using private-public partnerships. Such an initiative was implemented in 1996–99 in Costa Rica, El Salvador, and Guatemala.[78] The objective was to improve hand-washing habits in order to reduce diarrheal disease among children under five. The approach was to combine the expertise and resources of the soap industry with the facilities and resources of governments to promote hand-washing with soap. Four private soap companies launched hand-washing campaigns in collaboration with the public sector. The key features of the project were behavioral research to identify consumers' baseline hand-washing habits; mass media coverage (both education and commercial); community activities through the public sector, NGOs, and foundations; and monitoring and evaluation.

The private-public partnership succeeded in improving hand-washing behaviors and reducing the incidence of diarrheal disease. The results included a 30 percent increase in hygienic hand-washing behavior in mothers, with an estimated 300,000 fewer cases of diarrhea a year in poor children under five in Guatemala. Including USAID, the BASICS project, soap manufacturers, the Pan American Health Organization, and the World Bank, the initiative leveraged resources and sustained the involvement of the private sector in social programs.

Source: World Bank staff.

---

tions, training, policy change, and product development and marketing into an overall strategy to achieve the desired sustainable behavior change. When the focus is on product marketing, social marketing organizations are often nonprofit firms or associations, but the products tend to be distributed through various for-profit outlets and NGOs.

Social marketing has been applied to such diverse interventions as family planning, the treatment of sexually transmitted infections, the use of insecticide-treated mosquito nets, the use of soap for hand-washing, water purification, improved weaning and breastfeeding practices, and increased consumption of foods rich in vitamin A. A recent evaluation of Tanzania's social marketing of mosquito nets—which included an element of subsidy as well as commercial marketing—found that coverage increased substantially in all project areas and that socioeconomic differentials in net ownership narrowed.[45,46]

Media and behavior change

The media often play a role in communication efforts aimed at behavior change. Under government leadership, messages on AIDS were broadcast frequently during the peak of the epidemic in Thailand, a key element in the campaign to reduce the spread of HIV/AIDS.[79] The well-designed and culturally sensitive radio communication project in Nepal appears to have promoted positive health outcomes (box 5.9).[80] But many of the poor do not have access to a radio. In Bolivia, India, Morocco, and Mozambique less than 30 percent of the poorest fifth of the population has access to the media.

The influence of providers on demand

The way health services are organized (hours of operation, waiting time), their amenities and facilities, the disposition and integrity of staff, and the cultural appropriateness of services all make a difference to the household's demand for professionally delivered health care. *Voices of the Poor* is full of complaints by poor people about the lack of friendliness of facilities and health service staff.[27]

- A woman in Los Juries, Argentina, remarked: "You go to the hospital, you have to get a number, you go to the guard, the nurses are chatting. You have to wait until they fancy giving you a number . . . 'Is the doctor here?' 'No, the doctor isn't here,' they lie."

- A young woman in Muynak, Uzbekistan, said: "We do not go to hospital because it is necessary to bring your own bed linen, dishes, sometimes even a bed."

- In Tanzania, people complain of being treated "worse than dogs" by rude health staff and of being "yelled at, told they smell bad, and called lazy and good for nothing."[81]

- People complain about corrupt health staff, who demand unofficial "fees" or expect small "gifts."

- Indigenous people in Ecuador complain of staff who mistreat patients because of their lack of knowledge of Spanish, and women everywhere are reluctant to seek care for maternal health problems from male staff. (Making provider organizations more responsive to patients' legitimate concerns is discussed in chapter 6.)

People's perceptions of the technical quality of the service they receive also matters. They may, of course, not be the best judges of technical quality, but the fact is that perceptions of quality influence demand. From a policy perspective the challenge is not just to improve the quality of care but to provide methods for patients to better judge whether specific providers are delivering quality care. (These issues are also taken up in chapter 6.)

Roads, transport, and accessibility

Transportation systems, road infrastructure, and geography influence the demand for care delivered by formal providers—through their impact on time costs, which can be substantial.[6,30–32,82] In rural Senegal only 42 percent of the population live within 30 minutes of a health facility, and 43 percent live more than an hour away.[83] In rural communities, where the roads are poor and transportation unreliable, the time spent waiting for transportation may be as great as—if not greater than—the time spent traveling to the facility. Time costs tend to be a major issue for maternal mortality—health centers cannot provide essential obstetrical care for a complicated delivery, and women would have to travel to distant hospitals to get such care. In *Voices of the Poor* a Togo resident observed: "If a woman has a difficult delivery, a traditional cloth is tied between two sticks and we carry her for seven kilometers to the health center. You know how long it takes to walk like that?"[84]

Road and transportation improvements support the health sector

Better access to health facilities is rarely the primary goal of road rehabilitation projects—or even an explicit objective at all. But a recent road rehabilitation project in Vietnam cut the average walking time to the local hospital by 17

> **Box 5.9 Radio dramas to promote contraception**
>
> The Radio Communication Project uses the radio to satisfy the large unmet need for contraception in Nepal, strengthen the quality of services and service delivery, and increase client demand for quality reproductive health services. It produced two complementary radio serial dramas, one for service providers and one for community members. Education through radio had a positive impact on both groups.
>
> On the client side 81 percent of the women who listened to the drama were using modern family planning, compared with 33 percent of the women who did not listen. Exposure to radio was also linked to greater spousal communication about family planning: 87 percent of men who listened to the serial drama discussed family planning with their wives, compared with the 64 percent of men who did not listen. The program linked positive attitudes toward family planning, discussion of family planning with health workers, and perceived policy support for family planning.
>
> *Source:* Reference 80.

Public water companies serving about one-third of Argentina's municipalities and covering almost 60 percent of the population were transferred to private control between 1991 and 1999.[94] The largest privatization was the 1993 transfer of the federal company Obras Sanitarias de la Nácion (OSN) to the private consortium Aguas Argentinas, led by the French company Lyonnaise des Eaux. The concession required that 100 percent of households be connected to piped water by the end of the 35-year concession and 95 percent of households be connected to the sewerage system. Quality standards were also imposed for service and waste treatment. Use fees and connection charges were regulated, and—in response to protests over a large increase in the connection fee—a fixed fee was introduced for all customers. The new revenues subsidized the cost of new connections. Aguas Argentinas cut the old OSN labor force and dramatically increased invest-

ment in new equipment. Connections increased and quality improved on a number of fronts, including the speed of repairs, water leakages, sewerage blockages repaired, and percentage of clients with appropriate water pressure.

A recent study assesses the impact of privatization.[94] In the country as a whole and especially in Buenos Aires, access grew at a faster rate between 1991 and 1997 in municipalities in which water had been privatized than in municipalities in which it had not (see figure). The expansion of coverage was pronounced among poorer households. The study also finds a beneficial effect of privatization on child mortality, especially for poorer municipalities. The study finds that mortality decline was faster for causes of death that are common among the poor (infectious, parasitic, and perinatal disease).

Source: World Bank staff.

Water privatization in Argentina reduced child mortality for the extremely poor by more than 25 percent

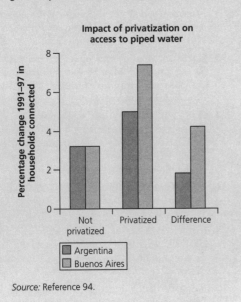

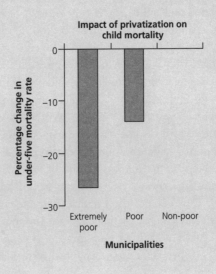

Source: Reference 94.

minutes and by 22 minutes for the poorest 40 percent of the population.[85] The benefits of using existing roads to improve transportation to and between health facilities are also evident. Malaysia and Sri Lanka provide free or subsidized transportation to hospitals in the case of emergencies.[43] Brazil recently made major investments in ambulances to facilitate rapid referral from a primary care facility to the hospital. In Sierra Leone focus group discussions made it clear that poor transportation was a major impediment to emergency obstetric care. So the city hospital in Bo acquired a four-wheel drive vehicle and two-way radios to link the hospital, the primary care units, and the vehicle.[86] The number of women with major obstetric

complications arriving at the hospital from the project area increased from 0.9 to 2.6 a month, and the case fatality rate dropped from 20 percent to 10 percent.

Other options exist for increasing accessibility

Upgrading and improving roads and improving transportation between existing facilities are options for improving accessibility to health facilities. But other options may be cheaper and more effective. Providers could take services to clients through an outreach program using existing facilities. Governments could construct new public facilities where access to existing facilities is limited. They could form partnerships with NGOs, private providers, or community organizations to provide additional services in underserved areas. Or they could contract with NGOs, private providers, and community organizations to provide publicly financed services to underserved communities. (These service delivery options are discussed in chapter 6. The role of roads and transportation is discussed in chapter 8.)

Water and sanitation

Hygiene and the quality and quantity of drinking water depend on infrastructure. Hand-washing is easier if the household has piped water that provides readily available quantities of safe water. The safe disposal of feces is easier if the household has an improved form of sanitation (a connection to a public sewer or septic system, a pour-flush, ventilated-improved, or a simple pit latrine). The hygienic storage of food is easier if the household has electricity. And so on. Not surprisingly, therefore, the availability of plenty of water and improved sanitation are associated with better maternal and child health outcomes, at least among the better educated, even after controlling for other influences.[30,32,67,87–92]

The developing world lags well behind the industrial world in water and sanitation: 1.1 billion people live without access to safe drinking water, and 2.4 billion live without access to improved sanitation.[93] In the 1990s the least developed countries saw a decline in safe water coverage, and in Sub-Saharan Africa there was no increase in the coverage of improved sanitation. Asia lags behind in improved sanitation, with coverage rates of 34 percent in South Asia and 48 percent in East Asia and the Pacific. Although East Asia and the Pacific has a higher coverage rate for safe water than Sub-Saharan Africa, it has the largest number of people who lack access. Poor people fare especially badly: they are less likely to be connected to a network, and the sources they rely on tend to be more costly per liter than the networked services used by the better off.[18]

The issues of increasing access to water and sanitation have recently been examined in the World Bank's *World Development Report 2004: Making Services Work for Poor People*.[18] The report notes the need for provider organizations to be accountable to policymakers, for policymakers to be accountable to households, and for front-line providers to be accountable directly to households through user charges and competition. Publicly managed water and sanitation networks sometimes seem more directed at serving the interests of politicians than households, while unregulated private providers have sometimes been criticized for delivering low-quality services and ignoring the poor.

Changes that improve accountability along one or more of the lines suggested by the *World Development Report* can improve access—for everyone. In Argentina the provision of water services was privatized under a regulatory regime that laid down strict rules for quality, access, and price. The regime was revised after pressure from the community, which saw the price rises authorized as harmful to the interests of the poor. The *World Development Report* observes that "community involvement is essential in the regulatory process but has not been sufficiently encouraged." It notes with approval the consultations that preceded the concession processes in Manila and South Africa. And it reports the results of a survey showing how a majority of Peruvians would have favored the privatization of the electric utility if the process had been transparent and tariff increases had been under the control of the regulator. (The intersectoral synergies of water and health are discussed in chapter 8.)

References

1. Narayan, D., R. Patel, K. Schafft, A. Rademacher, and S. Koch–Schulte. 2000. *Voices of the Poor: Can Anyone Hear Us?* New York: Oxford University Press.

2. Aguilar, A.M., R. Alvarado, D. Cordero, P. Kelly, A. Zamora, and R. Salgado. 1998. *Mortality Survey in Bolivia: The Final Report.* Basic Support for Institutionalizing Child Survival (BASICS) Project, Arlington, VA.

3. Hill, Z., B. Kirkwood, and K. Edmond. 2003. *Family and Community Practices that Promote Child Survival, Growth, and Development: A Review of the Evidence.* London School of Hygiene, Department of Epidemiology and Population Health, Public Health Intervention Research Unit.

4. Foster, G., and J. Williamson. 2000. "A Review of Current Literature on the Impact of HIV/AIDS on Children in Sub-Saharan Africa." *AIDS* 14 (Suppl. 3): S275–S284.

5. Barbhuiya, M.A., S. Hossain, M.M. Hakim, and S.M. Rahman. 2001. "Prevalence of Home Deliveries and Antenatal Care Coverage in Some Selected Villages." *Bangladesh Medical Research Council Bulletin* 27 (1): 19–22.

6. Wong, E., B. Popkin, D. Guilkey, and J. Akin. 1987. "Accessibility, Quality of Care and Prenatal Care Use in the Philippines." *Social Science and Medicine* 24 (11): 927–944.

7. Panis, C., and L. Lillard. 1994. "Health Inputs and Child Mortality." *Journal of Health Economics* 13 (4): 455–489.

8. Guilkey, D., and R. Riphahn. 1998. "The Determinants of Child Mortality in the Philippines: Estimation of a Structural Model." *Journal of Development Economics* 56 (2): 281–305.

9. Schwartz, J., J. Akin, and B. Popkin. 1988. "Price and Income Elasticities of Demand for Modern Health Care: The Case of Infant Delivery in the Philippines." *World Bank Economic Review* 2 (1): 49–76.

10. Steele, F., I. Diamond, and S. Amin. 1996. "Immunization Uptake in Rural Bangladesh: A Multilevel Analysis." *Journal of the Royal Statistical Society*. Series A 159 (2): 289–299.

11. Gage, A.J., A.E. Sommerfelt, and A.L. Piani. 1997. "Household Structure and Childhood Immunization in Niger and Nigeria." *Demography* 34 (2): 295–309.

12. Rashed, S., H. Johnson, P. Dongier, R. Moreau, C. Lee, R. Crepeau, J. Lambert, V. Jefremovas, and C. Schaffer. 1999. "Determinants of the Permethrin Impregnated Bednets (PIB) in the Republic of Benin: The Role of Women in the Acquisition and Utilization of PIBs." *Social Science and Medicine* 49 (8): 993–1005.

13. Filmer, D. 2000. "Fever and Its Treatment among the Poor and Less Poor in Sub-Saharan Africa." World Bank, Washington, DC.

14. Sen, A.K. 1981. *Poverty and Famines: An Essay on Entitlement and Deprivations.* Oxford: Clarendon Press.

15. Drèze, J., and A.K. Sen. 1989. *Hunger and Public Action.* Oxford: Clarendon Press.

16. Sen, A.K. 1994. "The Political Economy of Hunger." In *Overcoming Global Hunger: Proceedings of a Conference on Actions to Reduce Hunger Worldwide,* eds. I. Serageldin and P. Landell–Mills. Washington, DC: World Bank.

17. Pritchett, L., and L.H. Summers. 1996. "Wealthier Is Healthier." *Journal of Human Resources* 31 (4): 841–868.

18. World Bank. 2004. *World Development Report 2004: Making Services Work for Poor People.* Washington, DC: World Bank.

19. Case, A. 2001. "Does Money Protect Health Status? Evidence from South African Pensions." Center for Health and Wellbeing Working Paper, Woodrow Wilson School, Princeton University, Princeton, NJ.

20. Case, A. 2001. "Health, Income, and Economic Development." Paper presented at the Annual World Bank Conference on Development Economics, Washington, DC.

21. Case, A., and A. Deaton. 1998. "Large Cash Transfers to the Elderly in South Africa." *Economic Journal* 108 (450): 1330–1361.

22. Ayé, M, F. Champagne, and A.P. Contandriopoulos. 2002. "Economic Role of Solidarity and Social Capital in Accessing Modern Health Care Services in the Ivory Coast." *Social Science and Medicine* 55 (11): 1929–1946.

23. Nahar, S., and A. Costello. 1998. "The Hidden Cost of 'Free' Maternity Care in Dhaka, Bangladesh." *Health Policy Planning* 13 (4): 417–422.

24. World Bank, SIDA, AusAID, Royal Netherlands Embassy, Ministry of Health of Vietnam. 2001. *Vietnam. Growing Healthy: A Review of Vietnam's Health Sector.* Hanoi: World Bank.

25. Lewis, M. 2000. "Who Is Paying for Health Care in Eastern Europe and Central Asia?" World Bank, Washington, DC.

26. Al Fadil, S.M., S.H.A. Alrahman, S. Cousens, F. Bustreo, A. Shadoul, S. Farhoud, and S.M. El Hassan. 2003. "Integrated Management of Childhood Illnesses Strategy: Compliance with Referral and Follow-Up Recommendations in Gezira State, Sudan." *Bulletin of the World Health Organization* 81 (10): 708–716.

27. Dodd, R., and L. Munck. 2001. *Dying For Change: Poor People's Experience of Health and Ill-Health.* Geneva: World Health Organization; Washington, DC: World Bank.

28. Alderman, H., and V. Lavy. 1996. "Household Responses to Public Health Services: Cost and Quality Tradeoffs." *World Bank Research Observer* 11 (1): 3–22.

29. Roemer, M.I. 1981. "The Health Care System of Thailand: A Case Study." Report No. 11, World Health Organization Regional Office for Southeast Asia, Manila.

30. Lavy, V., J. Strauss, D. Thomas, and P. De Vreyer. 1996. "Quality of Care, Survival and Health Outcomes in Ghana." *Journal of Health Economics* 15 (3): 333–357.

31. Thomas, D., V. Lavy, and D. Strauss. 1996. "Public Policy and Anthropometric Outcomes in the Côte d'Ivoire." *Journal of Public Economics* 61 (2): 155–192.

32. Benefo, K., and T. Schultz. 1996. "Fertility and Child Mortality in Côte d'Ivoire and Ghana." *World Bank Economic Review* 10 (1): 123–158.

33. Alderman, H. 1993. "New Research on Poverty and Malnutrition." In *Including the Poor,* eds. M. Lipton and J. Van Der Gaag. Washington, DC: World Bank.

34. Hanson, K., and E. Worrall. 2002. "Report on the Analysis of SMITN2 End-of-Project Survey." London School of Hygiene and Tropical Medicine.

35. Peters, D.H., A.S. Yazbeck, R. Sharma, G. Ramana, L.H. Pritchett, and A. Wagstaff. 2002. *A Better Health Systems for India's Poor: Findings, Analysis, and Options.* Washington, DC: World Bank.

36. Wagstaff, A. 2001. "Inequalities in Health in Developing Countries: Swimming against the Tide?" Policy Research Working Paper 2795, World Bank, Washington, DC.

37. Castro-Leal, F., J. Dayton, L. Demery, and K. Mehra. 1999. "Public Social Spending in Africa: Do the Poor Benefit?" *World Bank Research Observer* 14 (1): 49–72.

38. Castro-Leal, F., J. Dayton, L. Demery, and K. Mehra 2000. "Public Spending on Health Care in Africa: Do the Poor Benefit?" *Bulletin of the World Health Organization* 78 (1): 66–74.

39. Filmer, D., J. Hammer, and L. Pritchett. 2000. "Weak Links in the Chain: A Diagnosis of Health Policy in Poor Countries." *World Bank Research Observer* 15 (2): 199–224.

40. Filmer, D., J. Hammer, and L. Pritchett. 2002. "Weak Links in the Chain II: A Prescription for Health Policy in Poor Countries." *World Bank Research Observer* 17 (1): 47–66.

41. Sahn, D., and S. Younger. 2000. "Expenditure Incidence in Africa: Microeconomic Evidence." *Fiscal Studies* 21 (3): 329–348.

42. Yaqub, S. 1999. "How Equitable Is Public Spending on Health and Education?" Background Paper for the *World Development Report 2000/2001: Attacking Poverty* World Bank, Washington, DC.

43. Pathmanathan, I., J. Liljestrand, J.M. Martins, L.C. Rajapaksa, C. Lissner, A. De Silva, S. Selvaraju, and P.J. Singh. 2003. "Investing in Maternal Health: Learning From Malaysia and Sri Lanka." World Bank, Health, Nutrition, and Population Department, Washington, DC.

44. Koblinsky, M.A., and O. Campbell 2003. "Factors Affecting the Reduction of Maternal Mortality." In *Reducing Maternal Mortality: Learning from Bolivia, China, Egypt, Honduras, Indonesia, Jamaica, and Zimbabwe,* ed. M.A. Koblinsky. Washington, DC: World Bank.

45. Schellenberg, J.R., S. Abdulla, R. Nathan, O. Mukasa, T.J. Marchant, N. Kikumbih, A.K. Mushi, H. Mponda, H. Minja, H. Mshinda, M. Tanner., and C. Lengeler. 2001. "Effect of Large-Scale Social Marketing of Insecticide-Treated Nets on Child Survival in Rural Tanzania." *Lancet* 357 (9264): 1241–1247.

46. Abdulla, S., J.A. Schellenberg, R Nathan., O. Mukasa, T. Marchant, T. Smith, M. Tanner, and C. Lengeler. 2001. "Impact on Malaria Morbidity of a Programme Supplying Insecticide-Treated Nets in Children Aged under 2 Years in Tanzania: Community Cross-Sectional Study." *British Medical Journal* 322 (7281): 270–273.

47. Armstrong Schellenberg, J., A. Mushi, H. Mponda, and C. Lengeler. 2002. "Discount Vouchers for Treated Nets in Tanzania: Targeted Subsidy for Malaria Control." Paper presented at a meeting on malaria and equity organized by the World Bank and the London School of Hygiene and Tropical Medicine, London.

48. Saadah, F., M. Pradhan, and R. Sparrow. 2001. "The Effectiveness of the Health Card as an Instrument to Ensure Access to Medical Care for the Poor During the Crisis." World Bank, Washington, DC.

49. Yip, W., and P. Berman. 2001. "Targeted Health Insurance in a Low Income Country and Its Impact on Access and Equity in Access: Egypt's School Health Insurance." *Health Economics* 10 (3): 207–220.

50. Gorter, A., P. Sandiford, Z. Segura, and C. Villabella. 1999. "Improved Health Care for Sex Workers: A Voucher Program for Female Sex Workers in Nicaragua." *Research for Sex Work* 2: 11–14.

51. Mesoamerica Nutrition Program Targeting Study Group. 2002. "Targeting Performance of Three Large-Scale, Nutrition-Oriented Social Programs in Central America and Mexico." *Food Nutrition Bulletin* 23 (2): 162–174.

52. International Food Policy Research Institute. 2002. *Final Report: Nicaragua Social Protection Network, Pilot Evaluation System, Impact Evaluation.* Washington, DC: IFPRI.

53. International Food Policy Research Institute. 2003. *Sexto informe. Proyecto PRAF/BID Fase II: Impacto intermedio.* Washington, DC: IFPRI.

54. International Food Policy Research Institute. 2003. *Estudo de avaliação de impacto para o Programa Bolsa Alimentação. Relatório 3: ánalise de impacto final.* Washington, DC: IFPRI.

55. Gertler, P., and S. Boyce. 2001. "An Experiment in Incentive-Based Welfare: The Impact of PROGRESA on Health in Mexico." University of California, Berkeley.

56. Morris, S., R. Flores, P. Olinto, and J. Medina. 2003. "A Randomized Trial of Conditional Cash Transfers to Households and Peripheral Health Centers: Impact on Child Health and Demand for Health Services." Paper presented at the Fourth International Health Economics Association World Congress, San Francisco.

57. Beegle, K., E. Frankenberg, and D. Thomas. 2001. "Bargaining Power within Couples and Use of Prenatal and Delivery Care in Indonesia." *Studies in Family Planning* 32 (2): 130–146.

58. Pitt, M.M., S.R. Khandker, S.M. Mckernan, and M Abdul Latif. 1999. "Credit Programs for the Poor and Reproductive Behavior in Low-Income Countries: Are the Reported Causal Relationships the Result of Heterogeneity Bias?" *Demography* 36 (1): 1–21.

59. Ranson, M. 2002. "Reduction of Catastrophic Health Care Expenditures by a Community-Based Health Insurance Scheme in Gujarat, India: Current Experiences and Challenges." *Bulletin of the World Health Organization* 80 (8): 613–621.

60. Pande, R.P., and A.S. Yazbeck. 2003. What's in a Country Average? Wealth, Gender, and Regional Inequalities in Immunization in India." *Social Science and Medicine* 57 (11): 2075–2088.

61. Das, J., and C. Sánchez-Párano. 2003. "Short But Not Sweet: New Evidence on Short Duration Morbidities from India." Policy Research Working Paper 2971, World Bank, Washington, DC.

62. Cebu Study Team. 1991. "Underlying and Proximate Determinants of Child Health: The Cebu Longitudinal Health and Nutrition Study." *American Journal of Epidemiology* 33 (2): 185–201.

63. Pebley, A.R., N. Goldman, and G. Rodriguez. 1996. "Prenatal and Delivery Care and Childhood Immunization in Guatemala: Do Family and Community Matter?" *Demography* 33 (2): 231–247.

64. Gertler, P., O. Rahman, C. Feifer, and D. Ashley. 1993. "Determinants of Pregnancy Outcomes and Targeting of Maternal Health Services in Jamaica." *Social Science and Medicine* 37 (2): 199–211.

65. Galvao, C.E., A.A. Da Silva, R.A. Da Silva, S.A. Dos Reis Filho, M.A. Novochadlo, and G.J. Campos. 1994. "Oral Rehydration Therapy for Acute Diarrhea in a Region of Northeastern Brazil, 1986–1989." [In Portugese.] *Revista de Saude Publica* 28 (6): 416–422.

66. Coreil, J., and E. Genece. 1988. "Adoption of Oral Rehydration Therapy among Haitian Mothers." *Social Science and Medicine* 27 (1): 87–96.

67. Jalan, J., and M. Ravallion 2001. "Does Piped Water Reduce Diarrhea for Children in Rural India?" Policy Research Working Paper 2664, World Bank, Washington, DC.

68. Favin, M., and M. Griffiths. 1999. *Communication for Behavior Change in Nutrition Projects.* Washington, DC: World Bank.

69. Semega-Janneh, I.J., E. Bohler, H. Holm, I. Matheson, and G. Holmboe-Ottesen 2001. "Promoting Breastfeeding in Rural Gambia: Combining Traditional and Modern Knowledge." *Health Policy Plan* 16 (2): 199–205.

70. Ndyomugyenyi, R., S. Neema, and P. Magnussen. 1998. "The Use of Formal and Informal Services for Antenatal Care and Malaria Treatment in Rural Uganda." *Health Policy Plan* 13 (1): 94–102.

71. Desai, S., and S. Alva. 1998. "Maternal Education and Child Health: Is There a Strong Causal Relationship?" *Demography* 35 (1): 71–81.

72. Hobcraft, J. 1993. "Women's Education, Child Welfare and Child Survival: A Review of the Evidence." *Health Transition Review* 3 (2): 159–175.

73. Glewwe, P. 1999. "Why Does Mother's Schooling Raise Child Health in Developing Countries?" *Journal of Human Resources* 34 (1): 124–59.

74. Abbas, K.A. 1995. "Counselling in a Hospital Setting. Breastfeeding." *Dialogue Diarrhoea* (59): 3.

75. Santos, I., C.G. Victora, J. Martines, H. Goncalves, D.P. Gigante, N.J. Valle, and G. Pelto. 2001. "Nutrition Counseling Increases Weight Gain among Brazilian Children." *Journal of Nutrition* 131 (11): 2866–2873.

76. Bhandari, N., R Bahl, J. Martines, and M.K. Bhan. 2002. "A Community-Based Randomized Controlled Intervention to Improve Breast Feeding and Complementary Feeding Practices through Nutritional Counselling in Rural Haryana, India." Presentation at the WHO Regional Advisers Meeting.

77. Hill, Z., B. Kirkwood, and K. Edmond. 2001. "Family and Community Practices that Promote Child Survival, Growth, and Development: A Review of the Evidence." London School of Hygiene, Department of Epidemiology and Population Health, Public Health Intervention Research Unit.

78. Saade, C., M. Batemen, and D.B. Bendahmane. 2001. *The Story of a Successful Public-Private Partnership in Central America.* Arlington, VA: BASICS II, EHP, UNICEF, USAID, and World Bank.

79. Ainsworth, M., C. Beyrer, and A. Soucat. 2003. "AIDS and Public Policy: The Lessons and Challenges of 'Success' in Thailand." *Health Policy* 64 (1): 13–37.

80. Heerey, M., and M.A. Kols. 2003. "Improving the Quality of Care: Quality Improvement Projects from the Johns Hopkins University Bloomberg School of Public Health Center for Communication Programs." Center Publication No. 101, Johns Hopkins University, Baltimore..

81. Alubo, O. 2001. "The Promise and Limits of Private Medicine: Health Policy Dilemmas in Nigeria." *Health Policy Plan* 16 (3): 313–321.

82. Mwabu, G., M. Ainsworth, and A. Nyamete. 1993. "Quality of Medical Care and Choice of Medical Treatment in Kenya: An Empirical Analysis." *Journal of Human Resources* 28 (4): 838–862.

83. Diop, F., A. Soucat, A. Wagstaff, and F. Zhao. 2002. "Health and the Poor in Senegal." Draft chapter for Senegal Country Economic Memorandum. World Bank, Washington, DC.

84. Narayan-Parker, D., and P.L. Petesch. 2002. *From Many Lands: Voices of the Poor*. Washington, DC: Oxford University Press and World Bank.

85. Van De Walle, D., and D. Cratty. 2002. "Impact Evaluation of a Rural Road Rehabilitation Project." World Bank, Washington, DC.

86. Samai, O., and P. Sengeh. 1997. "Facilitating Emergency Obstetric Care through Transportation and Communication, Bo, Sierra Leone." Bo PMM Team. *International Journal of Gynaecology and Obstetrics* 59 (Suppl. 2): S157–S164.

87. Merrick, T.W. 1985. "The Effect of Piped Water on Early Childhood Mortality in Urban Brazil, 1970 to 1976." *Demography* 22 (1): 1–24.

88. Ridder, G., and I. Tunali. 1999. "Stratified Partial Likelihood Estimation." *Journal of Econometrics* 92 (2): 193–232.

89. Lee, L.–F., M. Rosenzweig, and M. Pitt. 1997. "The Effects of Improved Nutrition, Sanitation, and Water Quality on Child Health in High-Mortality Populations." *Journal of Econometrics* 77 (1): 209–235.

90. Esrey, S.A., and J.P. Habicht. 1988. "Maternal Literacy Modifies the Effect of Toilets and Piped Water on Infant Survival in Malaysia." 1988. *American Journal of Epidemiology* 127 (5): 1079–1087.

91. Wolfe, B., and J. Behrman. 1982. "Determinants of Child Mortality, Health and Nutrition in a Developing Country." *Journal of Development Economics* 11 (2): 163–93.

92. Behrman, J., and B. Wolfe. 1987. "How Does Mother's Schooling Affect Family Health, Nutrition, Medical Care Usage and Household Sanitation? *Journal of Econometrics* 36 (1): 185–204.

93. UNICEF. 2001. *Progress Since the World Summit for Children: A Statistical Review*. New York: UNICEF.

94. Galiani, S., P. Gertler, and E. Schargrodsky. 2002. "Water for Life: The Impact of the Privatization of Water Services on Child Mortality." Working Paper No. 154, Stanford University Center for Research on Economic Development and Policy Forum, Stanford, CA.

95. Filmer D. 2003. "The Incidence of Public Expenditures on Health and Education." Background note for the *World Development Report 2004: Making Services Work for Poor People*. World Bank, Washington, DC.

96. Gwatkin, D., S. Rutstein, K. Johnson, R. Pande, and A. Wagstaff. 2000. "Socioeconomic Differences in Health, Nutrition and Population." Health, Nutrition and Population Discussion Paper. World Bank, Washington, DC. http://www.Worldbank.Org/Poverty/Health/Data/index.Htm.

97. ORC Macro. 2003. Demographic and Health Surveys. http://www.Measuredhs.Com/.

Table 5.1 Reducing barriers facing households in the use of effective child health interventions

Item	Bolivia: National Maternal and Child Insurance Program	Brazil, Egypt, Mexico, Philippines: Promotion of oral rehydration therapy in National Control of Diarrheal Diseases Programs	Costa Rica, El Salvador, Guatemala: Central American Hand-Washing Initiative	Honduras: Integrated Child Care Program
Background to policy shift	High maternal and child mortality have plagued Bolivia for decades. In 1994 the under-five mortality rate was 132 per 1,000 live births and the maternal mortality rate 390 per 100,000 live births. Both indicators were among the highest in the region. Use of health services was very low in the mid-1990s. In 1996 only 53 percent of pregnancies received medical attention, less than 45 percent of births occurred in health facilities, and only 36 percent of women in labor were attended by skilled medical personnel. The cost of health services was considered one of the most important barriers to utilization.	In 1980 diarrhea was the leading cause of child mortality in the world, accounting for 4.6 million deaths a year. Diarrhea accounted for 41 percent of infant mortality in Brazil and was the second-leading cause of under-five mortality, accounting for 8.5 deaths per 1,000 population. Oral rehydration therapy was introduced in 1979 as an intervention to treat diarrhea. Consisting of the oral administration of sodium, a carbohydrate, and water, oral rehydration therapy has been described as potentially the most significant medical advance of the twentieth century. It was recognized in 1980 that barriers to utilization included lack of knowledge and availability and accessibility concerns.	In 1995 diarrhea was the cause of 45 percent of under-five mortality in Guatemala and 20 percent in El Salvador. Hand-washing with soap can have an important impact on the incidence of diarrhea. But 78 percent of mothers in Guatemala used inadequate hand-washing practices in 1996. Lack of knowledge constituted an important barrier to utilization.	In the late 1980s international and local research prompted key actors in the Ministry of Health to emphasize that malnutrition imposes a severe burden on the population, that malnutrition is the underlying cause of more than half of the deaths in children under five, and that inadequate weight gain rather than nutrition was the best early warning sign of a sick child.
Policy shift	Decentralization of the government structure in 1994 changed the financing and delivery of health services. Twenty percent of government revenues were shifted to the country's municipalities, and a certain proportion of those funds was to be earmarked for the health sector. This shift significantly improved equity, since it was the first time that rural municipalities were given access to these funds. Ownership of health facilities and responsibility for financing of equipment and basic inputs were also decentralized to the municipalities. Management of human resources was decentralized to the Ministry of Health's regional administrations. In 1996 it was determined that a portion of the central government's funds should be targeted to a new special program, aimed exclusively at pregnant women and children under five. The new program, called the National Maternal and Child Insurance Program, aimed to reduce maternal and child mortality rates by removing fees for key health interventions. Because it allocated funds on a per capita basis, it constituted a propoor financing mechanism. Historically, financing had been biased toward richer urban municipalities.	In recognition of the severe burden of disease imposed by diarrhea and the fact that effective interventions such as oral rehydration therapy had become available, a number of countries introduced National Control of Diarrheal Diseases Programs in the early 1980s. The programs aimed to reduce morbidity and mortality from dehydration associated with acute diarrhea in children under five. National Control of Diarrheal Diseases Programs were operational in 35 countries by 1983 and in 80 countries by 1990. The experience of Brazil, Egypt, Mexico, and the Philippines is highlighted here because the impact in these countries has been evaluated in detail.	The Central American Hand-Washing Initiative was implemented in Costa Rica, El Salvador, and Guatemala between 1996 and 1999. The initiative's goal was to reduce morbidity and mortality among children under five by promoting proper hand-washing with soap.	Honduras began to reform its health sector in the early 1990s, with decentralization a main goal. The strategy emphasized the critical role of communities in the health sector. As part of these reform efforts, in 1994 the Ministry of Health established the Integrated Child Care Program as a critical component of its child health strategy. The program had been successfully pilot tested in 1992–93. By 1994 the focus of the program had shifted from interventions at the facility level to interventions at the household and family level through increased community participation. At the same time, the malnutrition paradigm changed from disease treatment to health promotion.

Item	Bolivia: National Maternal and Child Insurance Program	Brazil, Egypt, Mexico, Philippines: Promotion of oral rehydration therapy in National Control of Diarrheal Diseases Programs	Costa Rica, El Salvador, Guatemala: Central American Hand-Washing Initiative	Honduras: Integrated Child Care Program
Programmatic action	The program provided key health interventions, such as antenatal and neonatal care and treatment of acute respiratory infections and diarrhea free of charge to pregnant mothers and children under five on a universal basis. Both public and private institutions were included in the program. The participating institutions included Ministry of Health facilities, social security hospitals, and private nonprofit organizations.	The program focused on making oral rehydration therapy available on a large scale, through primary care facilities, for example. This effort was combined with extensive training of health workers and information campaigns, including mass media, to inform the general public about the availability and benefits of oral rehydration therapy.	This public-private partnership included the ministries of health and education, soap producers, NGOs, the media, and the project facilitator, the U.S. Agency for International Development (through Basic Support for Institution Child Survival and the Environmental Health Project). The initiative began by analyzing the hand-washing behavior of the targeted population. Public health messages about hand-washing (when and how to wash) were then delivered through the mass media and NGOs, while soap producers used their marketing skills to sell soap by promoting hand-washing with soap.	The program aims to improve health by promoting the healthy growth of children. The main focus is on monthly growth-monitoring and promotion sessions. During the sessions, community volunteers (*monitoras*) weigh each child under two, assess the growth rate relative to the expected weight gain, and provide counseling to the caregiver. Seriously ill children are referred to health centers, where they also receive immunizations. Training is provided to nurses of the health centers and the *monitoras*.
Affordability	The program explicitly aimed to promote demand by reducing the cost barriers for users and guaranteeing free access to services.		Mobile units distributed free soap samples to households.	The government subsidizes the main components of the program, though community leaders and mothers incur some costs. A recent cost analysis of the program found that it is both inexpensive and effective.
Women's autonomy		Women's autonomy was increased, as the program enabled them to treat many episodes of diarrhea themselves, thereby avoiding costly visits to health centers and admissions to hospitals.		The program empowers women to prevent malnutrition by making small changes in behavior using existing resources within the household. It builds women's confidence because monthly feedback on the changes in child growth show them that they can make a difference by themselves.
Knowledge	Through promotional efforts, such as public announcements on radio and television and in community *charlas* (informal discussions), the government succeeded in informing the public about the program and, therefore, about health services in general.	Efforts to educate the public significantly increased knowledge of the availability and appropriate use of oral rehydration therapy. An evaluation of the National Control of Diarrheal Diseases Program in Egypt showed that most mothers were able to mix oral rehydration therapy correctly.	The main barrier to utilization addressed by the initiative was knowledge. To increase demand for soap, the initiative stressed the importance of washing hands with soap at critical times and in appropriate ways and stressed that hand-washing reduces the incidence of diarrhea.	During the counseling sessions, caregivers are trained in how to maintain or improve the growth of their children. Key messages include breastfeeding, child feeding, care for sick children, and hygiene.
Accessibility	Decentralization and the program increased accessibility by bringing health services closer to the people. Increased coverage reached not only the urban rich but also rural and poor populations. In addition, since primary-level facilities had more control over funds, they were better able to stock the facilities with drugs and supplies.	Accessibility was affected by increasing the supply of oral rehydration therapy and bringing it closer to clients. Local production and imports of supplies increased substantially. In Mexico the availability of oral rehydration salts increased from 7.6 in 1984 to 79.7 million packets in 1993. Extensive promotion of oral rehydration therapy in primary care facilities made therapy available closer to the population.	Accessibility was increased by mobile units distributing free soap samples and by school programs.	Coverage of growth monitoring and promotion was deemed critical to the program's success. As the government realized that adequate coverage could not be achieved if these services were available only at the health-facility level, the program focuses on the household and community level, bringing services closer to the people. The *monitoras* make home visits to children who were not present during the monthly sessions and to sick children or children with inadequate weight gain.

Item	Bolivia: National Maternal and Child Insurance Program	Brazil, Egypt, Mexico, Philippines: Promotion of oral rehydration therapy in National Control of Diarrheal Diseases Programs	Costa Rica, El Salvador, Guatemala: Central American Hand-Washing Initiative	Honduras: Integrated Child Care Program
User-friendliness				User-friendliness is built into the basic design of the program, since the development of counseling messages is conducted through trials of improved practices in the homes of beneficiaries.
Water and sanitation				Water and sanitation is addressed indirectly through quarterly community meetings, at which community problems and solutions, including water and sanitation issues, are discussed.
Impact of policies on utilization	Introduction of the program resulted in substantial increases in the utilization of key maternal and child health interventions, particularly among the poor. Skilled birth attendance increased from 37 percent to 60 percent in nonindigenous municipalities between 1996 and 2001; in indigenous municipalities, it doubled, rising from 18 percent to 36 percent. Treatment of pneumonia in children also increased significantly. Many of the people served under the program were people who had previously not used modern health services.	Utilization of oral rehydration therapy increased in all four countries. In Mexico use of oral rehydration therapy increased from 47.5 percent of all diarrhea episodes in 1986 to 80.7 percent in 1993. In the Philippines the access rate increased from 60 percent to 85 percent between 1989 and 1992.	Hand-washing behavior improved as a result of the initiative, both in terms of hand-washing at critical times and hand-washing technique. A recent evaluation of the initiative in Guatemala found that inadequate hand-washing practices of mothers decreased from 78 percent to 68 percent between 1996 and 1999. Intermediate and optimal practices increased from 22 percent to 32 percent.	A recent mid-term evaluation of the program found significant improvements in the knowledge and behavior (caregiving and feeding practices) of caregivers in the program. Program coverage is almost universal (92 percent) in the communities surveyed by the evaluation. Compared with control communities, program caregivers were significantly more likely to have received counseling on breastfeeding, care of sick children, hygiene, and iron and vitamin A supplementation. Immunization coverage, iron supplementation, use of oral rehydration therapy, and vitamin A intake were also much better in program communities. The program has also contributed to more rational use of health facilities: nurses say that they no longer see patients whom they do not need to see, allowing them to focus more attention on people with severe disease.
Impact of policies on health outcomes	The under-five mortality rate was reduced from 132 in 1994 to 99 in 1998, an average annual decrease of about 6 percent. Maternal health also improved: by 2000 the maternal mortality rate had dropped to 234. There is evidence that these achievements are linked to the policy shift in 1994 and the improved access made possible by public health insurance. A survey on the use of public health insurance revealed that the probability that women receive skilled birth attendance (which increased during the time of the insurance) is linked to the maternal mortality rate.	Evaluations of the four countries show significant improvement in health outcomes. In Brazil the proportion of infant mortality caused by diarrhea decreased from 41 percent in 1980 to 25 percent in 1989. In Egypt infant mortality caused by diarrhea fell by an annual average of 15.9 percent between 1984 and 1990, a more rapid decline than for mortality attributed to other causes. In Mexico the proportion of under-five deaths caused by diarrhea declined from 26.4 percent in 1983 to 11.0 percent in 1993. In the Philippines both infant and under-five mortality rates associated with diarrhea fell by about 5 percent annually between 1975 and 1993. Although other factors may explain these improved health outcomes, it seems that the National Control of Diarrheal Diseases Program had an important impact. A simulation model performed in Brazil indicated that factors other than oral rehydration therapy explained only about a third of the actual decline.	In Guatemala the prevalence of diarrhea among children under five fell about 4.5 percent, affecting almost 1.6 million children under five.	A case study found that malnutrition had been reduced by 10 percent in most communities by 1999.

Source: World Bank staff.

Table 5.2 Reducing barriers to the use of effective maternal health interventions by households

Item	China, Yunnan Province	Honduras	Sri Lanka
Background to policy shift	Although China has recorded impressive reductions in the maternal mortality ratio since 1950 (when it was as high as 1,500 per 100,000 live births), the ratio was still about 100–200 in rural areas in China in 1980. In 1989 it was 149 in Yunnan Province.	In 1990 the maternal mortality ratio was 182 per 100,000 live births.	In 1950, two years after independence, the maternal mortality ratio was as high as 555 per 100,000 live births.
Policy shift	While policies are formulated at the national level, strategies to translate policies into action are determined at the provincial level or below. Since 1980 Yunnan Province has implemented several policy actions, such as decentralization to increase local ownership and accountability and skills enhancement to reduce maternal deaths.	The report of the high maternal mortality ratio in 1990 alarmed the government and triggered a massive effort to reduce maternal mortality. The government focused its efforts strategically on areas with high maternal mortality ratios.	Reducing maternal deaths was one of the goals of the Ministry of Health of the new government that took office after independence. Several decisions reveal the importance it placed on maternal health. In the 1950s the government increased access and coverage to basic maternal and child health services by expanding the health unit system. The system emphasized preventive and health promotion services at the community level, delivered by skilled attendants and field workers with guaranteed professionalism. The management and infrastructure of maternal health programs was improved with an effective monitoring and supervisory system. Transportation and communications were improved to provide safe transportation and referral of women with complications.
Programmatic action	In the 1970s "barefoot doctors" staffed village clinics in the province. Since 1982 government regulations have required that doctors take an exam on applied aspects of maternal health (attending clean delivery and identifying risk factors and complications before and during delivery). If they pass, they become "village doctors" and receive on-site training. Career growth of village barefoot doctors is thus linked to demonstrated ability to provide maternal health care. Yunnan Province launched the Systematic Management of Pregnant Women (SMPW) in 1985. The program provides every woman with a management booklet, at least five antenatal care checkups, a minimum of three postnatal visits in her home, and modern delivery methods. The Emergency Referring System for Pregnant Women was formed in Tonghai County in Yunnan Province in 1990. It aims to ensure that women with complications are moved from the village clinic to the county maternal and child health station or hospital. The Emergency Referring System consists of eight strategies: coordination, ensuring functioning phones at all levels, equipping emergency facilities (including vehicles), improving skills, enhancing the referral network, supervising and evaluating, and focusing on meeting targets. Provider accountability is built into the schemes; facility grants, continuation of employment, and promotion of managers are determined on the basis of achievement of set targets.	To lower the maternal mortality ratio, the government implemented a two-pronged approach: ensuring that women who develop obstetric emergencies are referred to the hospital and identifying women at high risk for complications and encouraging them to deliver in a health facility. To support this approach, the government built seven new rural area hospitals and, with community input, new maternity waiting homes and birthing centers. The maternity waiting homes are fully managed by the local communities. The number of health staff, especially auxiliary nurses, was increased. Skills of clinical staff and community health workers, including traditional birth attendants, were enhanced through training, which focused on recognizing risks in pregnancy and danger signs in childbirth and make appropriate referrals. The Ministry of Health also produced new technical manuals in this area.	Efforts to reduce maternal mortality took place in three phases. The first phase focused on making services accessible to the majority of the population and improving antenatal coverage, midwifery services, and detection and early referral of complications. A public health midwife is responsible for all pregnant women in her jurisdiction, covering a population of 4,000–5,000. The second phase involved monitoring the field maternal and child health program through improved reporting systems. The third phase emphasized quality-of-care considerations, particularly by using the findings of maternal death inquiries to identify deficiencies in the system and address those deficiencies through new initiatives. Provider accountability and skill enhancement are critical components in the efforts to improve maternal health in Sri Lanka.

Item	China, Yunnan Province	Honduras	Sri Lanka
Affordability	A maternal and child health prepayment scheme was piloted and is now available throughout the province. Households pay a modest fee and are covered if complications associated with delivery or diseases of the child arise. Those who have joined this scheme have sought maternal and child health services more actively, though whether this reflects adverse selection or moral hazard is unclear. The scheme does not include delivery charges.		Sri Lanka has a very high level of government commitment to, and popular support for, the welfare state, including universal free access to health care. Although user fees were introduced early on, it appears that patients are rarely charged for health services, including drugs and supplies.
Women's autonomy			The autonomy of women was enhanced through the promotion of women's rights and empowerment by cross-sector initiatives.
Knowledge	Knowledge as a barrier to utilization was addressed by providing every woman with the SMPW booklet and at least five antenatal care checks and by creating community awareness and demand for the SMPW package. The government also provided health education to pregnant women.	In focus group sessions, women in areas where traditional birth attendants were trained acknowledged the risk of going to an untrained traditional birth attendant.	Special efforts were made to reach Indian Tamils living and working on estates, who had not benefited from social change, including improvements in education and health. Following nationalization of the estates in 1972, medical officers with transportation facilities were appointed to establish a network of estate health clinics. The clinics provided maternal and child health and family planning services to the estate population. Through this program, knowledge and skills of the estate health staff were improved. This is a good example of a strategy for improving access to underserved and neglected population groups.
Accessibility	To improve accessibility, the SMPW provides every woman with access to antenatal care and at least three postnatal visits in her home. Access to facilities offering emergency services was improved by providing vehicles.	Accessibility was explicitly addressed by building maternity waiting homes, with community assistance, alongside several hospitals. It had been recognized that it was sometimes difficult for women living in remote rural areas to get to a hospital when labor began. The waiting homes provided a way to ensure that women were already near the hospital when labor began. Construction of new birthing homes brought skilled attendance at birth closer to women in hard-to-reach areas.	Accessibility was addressed by expanding the health service infrastructure to cover the whole country and by rapidly educating and training health staff. Transportation was supported through a system of ambulance services. Most facilities had ambulances by 1950. In addition, the government reimburses health staff for the cost of alternative modes of transportation, enabling them to better reach the population.
User-friendliness			
Water and sanitation and other cross-sector linkages			Following the acceptance by estate management of the initiative to reach estate workers with health interventions, the two government estate agencies implemented a series of interventions to improve water and sanitation on the estates. In Sri Lanka as a whole, efforts were made to improve sanitation.
Impact of policies on utilization	In Tonghai an already high rate of hospital delivery in 1990 (70 percent) was increased to 92 percent. In a poorer county, Huaning, the rate increased from 49 percent in 1990 to 62 percent in 1999.	Skilled attendance increased from 46 percent in 1987–91 to 54 percent in 1997. Maternity waiting homes increased the likelihood that high-risk women (older women and women who had already given birth several times) delivered in a hospital.	Attended deliveries by personnel in government facilities increased from 33 percent in 1950 to 87 percent in 1995, while deliveries in the home decreased from 25 percent to 2 percent. Today 95 percent of births are attended by a skilled practitioner, with the majority taking place in hospitals. For estate women, deliveries in government facilities increased from 20 percent in 1986 to 63 percent in 1997, deliveries in estate maternity units rose from 29 percent to 42 percent, and deliveries in the home decreased from 37 percent to 8 percent.

Table 5.2 Reducing barriers to the use of effective maternal health interventions by households *(continued)*

Item	China, Yunnan Province	Honduras	Sri Lanka
Impact of policies on health outcomes	In Tonghai county in Yunnan, an already high rate of hospital delivery in 1990 (70 percent) was increased to 92 percent. In a poorer county, Huaning, the rate increased from 49 percent to 62 percent between 1990 and 1999. Between 1989 and 1998, the maternal mortality ratio in Yunnan decreased from 149 to 101.	Skilled attendance increased from 46 percent in 1987–91 to 54 percent by 1997. Maternity waiting homes increased the likelihood that high-risk women (older women and women who had had several births previously) delivered in a hospital. Between 1990 and 1997, the maternal mortality ratio fell from 182 to 108.	The maternal mortality ratio in Sri Lanka declined from 555 in 1950 to 24 in 1995.

Source: World Bank staff.

Table 5.3 Reducing barriers to the use of effective interventions for malaria, HIV/AIDS, and tuberculosis by households

Item	Home-based treatment of malaria in Tigray region of Ethiopia	Home-based care of people with HIV/AIDS in northern Thailand	Strengthening national tuberculosis control interventions in China
Background to policy shift	Malaria is a leading killer of children under five in Africa. Almost a million children die in Africa from malaria every year. Eighty percent of childhood malaria cases are treated outside of the public sector. Most treatment is provided at home, with drugs purchased from informal drug sellers or pharmacists. The drugs purchased through drug sellers are often of poor quality or counterfeit. Dosages purchased are frequently inadequate to fully treat infection.	Two-thirds of the approximately 1 million people living with HIV/AIDS reside in the northern part of Thailand. Historically, rates of infection have been high among women who are or were sex workers, but in the late 1990s the highest rates of increase were among women in stable relationships. At that time, HIV prevalence among women attending antenatal clinics was 4–8 percent. The Sanpatong area was one of the hardest hit by the epidemic. Government hospitals were hard-pressed to provide care, with as many as 60 percent of hospital beds occupied by people with HIV/AIDS.	Unlike in most developing countries, tuberculosis treatment in China was not exempt from the shift to fee-for-service care. Case detection and cure rates were low, and drug-resistant disease was emerging.
Policy shift	It was recognized in the Tigray region of Ethiopia that an effective strategy for ensuring that children receive rapid and effective treatment for malaria would have to focus on improving treatment practices in the household. This would include improving mothers' ability to detect fever and malaria symptoms and to correctly treat their children with antimalarial drugs.	Volunteers from the faculty of medicine at Chiang Mai University, Chiang Mai public health staff, and nurses from the Sanpatong Red Cross health center, all with extensive community experience, decided to pool their practical and academic experience to develop a new community-based holistic model of care to provide "bio-psycho-social support" to help people living with HIV/AIDS be treated at home. The bio component involved treatment of symptoms, the psycho component helped people deal with stress and problems, and the social component helped improve the ability to cope with, participate in, and be accepted by the community.	The World Bank–financed DOTS program has provided free tuberculosis treatment for infectious tuberculosis patients in parts of 16 provinces since 1992. Village doctors and tuberculosis dispensaries provide DOTS care; hospitals are supposed to refer patients. Providers receive payment from the Ministry of Health for each infectious case detected and each case cured.
Programmatic action	Selected "mother coordinators" from the community were trained to provide education to other mothers in their community on the symptoms and sign of fever and malaria. Mother coordinators were also supplied with chloroquine, which they provided to mothers with sick children along with information on how to administer the drug.	The project provided education and skills training to family members, volunteers from the community, and village leaders. It recruited volunteer medical personnel and people living with HIV/AIDS through the community.	The National TB Control Program within the new Center for Disease Control was strengthened to support capacity-building, monitoring, and supervision of providers in the provinces and counties participating in the DOTS program. The logistics system was overhauled, and an efficient national drug procurement and supply system was developed.

Table 5.3 Reducing barriers to the use of effective interventions for malaria, HIV/AIDS, and tuberculosis by households *(continued)*

Item	Home-based treatment of malaria in Tigray region of Ethiopia	Home-based care of people with HIV/AIDS in northern Thailand	Strengthening national tuberculosis control interventions in China
Affordability	The program provided mothers with free chloroquine, which costs about $0.08 per child treatment dose.	With an orientation toward building partnerships and alliances, the project has created strong referral services from the home to the health center to the district hospital and vice versa. Partnerships between the public health system and the private sector have reduced the cost of care to both individual families and the government health services. Material support for school fees, food, and clothing has been obtained from private donations for needy families.	With free drug provision and consults, there was a dramatic improvement in the affordability of six-month therapy—especially important given evidence of the higher prevalence of tuberculosis in poorer counties and marginalized communities.
Women's autonomy	Mothers are the primary caregivers of sick children, who suffer most from malaria in Africa. This strategy empowered mothers to take actions to effectively treat their children in the home.	In northern Thailand, HIV infection has often resulted in the illness of women who are wives and mothers. Caregiving in these situations falls to the grandparents, particularly grandmothers. Although Thai grandmothers have always had an important role in the care and upbringing of children, this unexpected burden in their later years is a heavy one. The project has sought to improve the ability of grandmothers to function as home caregivers through training, financial support from the Social Welfare Ministry, and emotional support.	Tuberculosis case detection rose for both male and female patients by increasing access to care in local communities and improving support systems.
Knowledge	A key component of this intervention was improving mothers' knowledge and ability to detect fever and malaria and to provide their sick children with proper treatment.	Training and education for family and community members is conducted on home care, ways to decrease stigma, and spirituality, using local Buddhist monks to teach meditation.	There were no mass campaigns about the new service, but information was rapidly disseminated, as increased demand revealed.
Accessibility	This approach dramatically increased access to effective treatment in the home, where most malaria treatment is provided.	Services have been brought to the household level for hundreds of infected people and their families.	Access to tuberculosis care increased as a result of the proximity of village doctors to patients and the provision of free care.
User-friendliness	The approach used was very straightforward, with simple messages and skills promoted by the mother coordinators.	Providers got whole villages to accept and participate in the care of people living with HIV/AIDS and their families and to adopt a holistic approach to health care.	Ambulatory care provided as part of the DOTS strategy offers a better alternative to hospitalization.
Water and sanitation			
Impact of policies on utilization	This approach can be expected to alleviate the burden of severe malaria cases on hospitals.	The model has relieved pressure on government hospital beds and strengthened the referral between community health centers and central hospitals. It has also been replicated and recognized as a "model" community-based service throughout Asia.	Utilization increased and more than 1 million patients were treated. Patients were still seeking diagnosis in hospitals that were not referring patients for DOTS care. Some poorer provinces and counties had difficulty covering costs to participate. Both challenges are addressed in a follow-up project.
Impact of policies on health outcomes	The under-five mortality rate was reduced by 40 percent in intervention areas. The approach was also expected to alleviate the burden of severe malaria cases on hospitals.	Most people living with HIV/AIDS experienced substantial weight gain after three months in the project. Compared with the mid-1990s, fewer families and people living with HIV/AIDS asked that confidentiality be maintained.	More than 1 million patients were cured between 1991 and 2000. DOTS areas experienced a 35 percent reduction in tuberculosis prevalence over 10 years, compared with a 3 percent reduction in non–DOTS areas. The case detection rate almost doubled between the first and fifth years of implementation (from 14 to 26 per 100,000) in areas covered by the project, indicating significant demand among prevalent cases.

Source: World Bank staff.

CHAPTER 6

Improving Service Delivery

I was assigned to Puskesmas Tanjung Aru, East Kalimantan, five hours from the district capital by boat through river and sea. It was staffed by two nurses, one midwife, one immunization officer, and one sanitation overseer. Unexpected problems confronted me on arrival. The 52-year-old senior nurse tried to persuade the other staff that I was unable to run the health center and that I would rigidly control their day-to-day activities. He might have been correct. I was not at all confident about my management ability. Later, I learned he was worried my presence might disturb his private practice, which he had developed since the last doctor left six years before. Nobody knew about the budget except him.

The health center's workload and achievements were baffling. There were only three to five patients a day. The latest data, aside from the registers, were from two years before. Guidelines could not be found. They were taken by the last doctor when he left. Four months later we received photocopies of the guidelines from the District Health Office. They were not too helpful for managerial matters. There was no money left for operational tasks even though the year had three months to go. The doctor's house was dirty and unfurnished. The previous doctor took the furniture when he left. A request for replacement was sent to the District Health Office, but six years had passed with no response. Staff suggested I take a spare examination bed from the health center. I did this because I could not afford to buy a bed. The staff lacked initiative. No one came to work before 10 a.m., and everyone left before 1 p.m. They said that there was little to do.

Source: *World Bank staff, Indonesia.*

Health providers in both the public and private sectors, and in both the formal and informal sectors, play a key role in delivering interventions of relevance to the Millennium Development Goals. Many are efficient, deliver high-quality care, and are responsive to their patients. But many are not. As a result, resources—public and private—are wasted, and facilities sit underused. Patients often receive care that is inappropriate to their needs, paying for it out of very limited means. They may also receive care that is downright dangerous.

Two things can make a difference. One is the quality of management. Better management means a clearer delineation of responsibilities and accountabilities inside organizations, a clearer link between performance and reward, and so on. The first part of the chapter reviews these and other elements of good management, providing examples of where better management has made a difference.

Something else can also make a difference. Management means getting accountabilities right within an organization. Equally important—if not more so—are accountabilities between the organization and the public. These can be improved along one or both of two routes.[1] The short route, leading directly from the patient to the provider, can be strengthened through a variety of schemes, including vouchers, report cards, and citizen management groups. The long route, leading from the citizen to the policymaker and then to the provider, can be strengthened at two points—the citizen-policymaker relationship (making policymakers more responsive to citizens) and the policymaker-provider relationship (making providers more responsive to policymakers).

The World Development Report 2004: Making Services Work for Poor People[1] provides a thorough discussion—for several sectors—of ways to strengthen both routes and both elements of the long route. The focus here is on just one sector (health) and within it on services and service providers of special relevance to the Millennium Development Goals for health. The focus is also on just two relationships—the link between the patient and the front-line provider and the link between the policymaker and the provider organization. The interested reader is referred to the *World Development Report* for ways of strengthening the citizen-policymaker link, a generic rather than health-specific issue.

Another area of service delivery is only partially covered in this chapter. This is the delivery mode—where different services should be delivered and by which medical staff (see box 6.1 and chapter 7).

Who's who in the health sector— and the challenges that face them

Anyone attempting to improve service delivery has to wrestle with the fact that a variety of providers deliver care of relevance to the Millennium Development Goals, often to the same person in the same illness episode. The array of relevant providers is bewildering (box 6.2).

The boundaries between the different sets of actors—especially between public and private—can seem confusing, because a provider may be, say, private on one dimension but public on another.

- *Payment* can be public or private, regardless of who provides the services.

- *Ownership of the business or activity.* Ownership refers not to the ownership of the premises but to the ownership of any leftover funds (or debts) at the end of the year, after all costs have been paid. When clinics or hospitals are publicly owned, leftover funds belong to the treasury or public purse. When clinics or hospitals are privately owned, the organization itself or a private person has a legal claim to all leftover revenue. For a nonprofit entity, the profits cannot be distributed outside the organization.

- *Ownership of premises.* Public clinics are almost always located in publicly owned buildings. Private clinics, and even hospitals, however, often do not own their premises but rather rent them. Sometimes private clinics are even run in publicly owned buildings. This does not

---

Box 6.1 The changing mix of cure and care: Who treats what—and where?

Throughout the twentieth century, service institutions have responded—albeit slowly—to rapid changes in health technology. Countries choose combinations of "delivery modes" based on costs and international standards but also on country-specific characteristics, such as geographic and density constraints, transport and infrastructure capacity, existing health infrastructure inherited from previous technological innovations, labor market characteristics, training and orientation of providers, and so on. What is delivered as inpatient treatment, outpatient hospital, health center or home visits—and by whom—is far from standard across countries.

Technological progress triggers modifications in the nature, type, and quantity of services required. Hospital tuberculosis treatment (the sanatorium) was replaced by outpatient clinical care thanks to antibiotics. Screening followed by treatment—DOTS (directly observed treatment, short-course)—were later standardized to allow delivery through community outreach. Similarly, new treatments for HIV and cancer cut long hospitalization requirements. The care and cure functions of the hospital also evolve. Hospitals are being transformed into long-term care centers for the elderly, while more complex procedures are conducted in ambulatory clinics. Home-based nursing care is being revived.

Countries at similar levels of technology have opted for different models with comparable success. Independent practitioners developed first in Western countries and have been the cornerstone of Western systems. The hegemony of hospitals in the Western world is no older than the twentieth century. In contrast, hospitals have played a much larger role in the provision of outpatient care in Eastern Europe and Central Asia, Latin America, Sri Lanka, and Vietnam. In Africa health systems developed through hospitals and mobile clinics since the beginning of the twentieth century, with primary health care emerging only in the 1980s. Different skill levels are also used for similar interventions. Health technicians and nurses have performed caesarean sections in Mozambique, while other countries use general practitioners or skilled obstetricians.

Source: Reference 1.

make the business, or operation, any less "private," since the leftover revenue still remains with the organization or its owners.

- *Employment.* Health professionals can work in the public sector, the private sector, or both. Sometimes this is legal. Sometimes it is not. Sometimes people employed in the public sector "steal" the time they are supposed to devote to public employment and sell it privately, in much the same way that they sometimes steal drugs and sell them privately. It is not difficult to distinguish what is public and private in this case. When employees work for a public organization and steal time, they are stealing from a public employer. When employees sell what they have stolen—be it drugs or time—it is a private transaction (they are selling something they own, even if they obtained it by stealing).

By being clear about which aspect of health services delivery is being discussed, it is easy to distinguish whether it is public or private. Such distinctions are critical in understanding the organization of health services and the incentives associated with the organization.

The public sector

Many of the problems associated with the public sector are rooted in the more general structural problems related to the broader public sector:

- service commitments greatly in excess of allocated funds, undermining the accountability relations between policymakers and service providers

- weak public sector accountability arrangements and limited capacity for core administrative and policymaking tasks

- managers who are judged not on performance but on "political merit"

- managers who are appointed not on their technical merits but through cronyism

- budgets that are unpredictable and funds that leak out of the public sector

---

Box 6.2 Who delivers which care for the Millennium Development Goals for health?

The answer to the question "Who delivers which care for the health Millennium Development Goals?" is simple—a bewildering variety.

Public providers include primary health clinics, health centers, and hospitals. Public providers of potential relevance for achieving the Millennium Development Goals include rural and urban clinics and health posts, as well as first-level referral hospitals. Public facilities are almost always arranged as a hierarchy of facilities—of decreasing sophistication as one gets farther into rural areas. Facilities are formally staffed by qualified medical staff, who are salaried civil service employees (and managed largely from outside the facility).

Services are often officially free or subsidized. Public funds flow to facilities based on installed capacity and centrally established norms. Accountability for performance is through administrative oversight, usually by the Ministry of Health, less often by local government bodies. Oversight typically focuses on appropriate use of funds and adherence to rules related to personnel. The largest facilities—referral hospitals—are often integrated into the political realm, in that senior management is appointed and dismissed following changes in government.

Private providers come in three broad guises:

- For-profit formal providers include registered self-employed doctors, clinics, hospitals, and diagnostic clinics, as well as registered, organized, formally trained traditional healers (ayurvedic healers, traditional Chinese medicine healers, midwives).

- Nonprofit formal providers or nongovernmental organizations often operate primary health care facilities as well as district—and sometimes referral—hospitals. They often include organizations undertaking outreach activities, such as information, education, and communication programs and social marketing.

- For-profit informal providers include traditional healers, drug sellers, pharmacists (who offer informal diagnosis and recommendations on medications to take), unqualified practitioners of allopathic medicine, and traditional birth attendants.

All play a role in delivering services and interventions relevant to the Millennium Development Goals. And there is a striking degree of heterogeneity within a country for the same type of intervention or service. One woman might have her baby delivered by a traditional birth attendant. Another might have hers delivered by a midwife at home. A third might have hers delivered by a doctor at a hospital. One child with diarrhea might be taken to a public facility, while another might be taken to a private provider. To complicate matters further, the same person may visit several types of provider within the same illness episode—some in the public sector, some in the private.

Source: World Bank staff.

- self-selection into the public sector of staff who prefer a work environment not based on performance

- an inappropriate wage structure

While important, these problems are generally best addressed through interventions that cover the entire public sector.

Other problems can be addressed within the health ministry or sector. These include:

- low wages

- leakages of funds from the ministry of health to facilities

- weak external accountability arrangements for service delivery tasks

- a lack of management skills and training on the part of health facility management; managers who do not manage staff (civil service) and who cannot therefore be held accountable or make required cost savings or quality-enhancing changes

- significantly higher costs to deliver services in rural areas (people educated in cities prefer not to live in rural areas)

- unclear objectives and responsibilities of provider organizations

- the fact that the services produced are valued by individuals and can be sold privately, which, coupled with weak management, leads to dual practice and absenteeism

- the perception that the work (such as treating people with HIV/AIDS) is dangerous

- general skills that are valued elsewhere, leading to emigration and loss of staff to the private sector

The private sector

Various structural features create service delivery problems for the nonprofit sector as well. Its dependence on donations and other inputs tied to philanthropy or altruism limits its opportunity to expand. Many nonprofits operating in developing countries rely extensively on international nonprofits for funding, making their funding unpredictable. Some nonprofits undertake religious or political activities or are closely associated with organizations that do. This sometimes contributes to a lack of trust by governments and the population, hampering their activities and growth prospects.[2] The absence or weakness of mechanisms or forums for regular communication and coordination with other nonprofits and with policymakers reduces the efficiency of nonprofits.

The formal for-profit sector also exhibits certain structural features that can cause problems. The bottom-line focus discourages the sector from cross-subsidizing patients or services, and the desire for return customers can lead for-profit providers to deliver unneeded or inappropriate care when patients want it. In developing countries, mutual distrust, and often animosity, between the government and the private health care sector is common, meaning that interaction with the public system is minimal. Even where common interests exist, the lack of mechanisms or forums for interaction and coordination makes working together very difficult.

The informal private sector can also be weakened by various underlying structural issues. In developing countries, regulation usually has very little influence on informal private providers. They tend to be weakly organized, making it hard for policymakers to reach them with any policy intervention, and there is little or no professional support for quality improvement. Informal providers are almost always organized as solo practices, a setting known to undermine the quality of care. They are also isolated from the public sector and the formal private sector, further constraining coordination and the quality of care. Animosity from the formal allopathic medical profession keeps them isolated and excluded from most policy dialogue.

Better management—improving accountability within provider organizations

The Malaysian state of Sarawak and the Indonesian province of West Kalimantan face one another across the Malaysia-Indonesia border. They share language, ethnicity, and religious characteristics (box 6.3). Yet the approach to management in their public health facilities is markedly different. Sarawak health workers are highly committed to quality and client satisfaction. They work in teams in a cooperative fashion, and they are encouraged to set priorities in the light of local circumstances, to take initiative, and to be innovative. Their attitude reflects a deliberate policy in Malaysia to encourage local initiative, right down to the individual staff member. The aim is to instill, through training and the use of health systems research as a management tool, strong problem-solving and decisionmaking skills in management teams—at the facility, district, and provincial levels. Initiative is rewarded: each year a health worker is chosen to receive a prestigious national award recognizing personal initiative.

Across the border in West Kalimantan, things work differently. The Indonesian government imposes detailed guidelines, activity schedules, and workload norms on staff, leaving no room for local decisionmaking and initiative.

These two sets of facilities provide examples of two entirely different perspectives on management. The Indonesian approach has its roots in the hierarchical command-and-control model. Initiative and decisionmaking are exercised only at the highest level. Problems encountered

Box 6.3 Different management styles, different countries—but just miles apart

In March 1999 a team that included Indonesian and Malaysian experts and an expatriate medical anthropologist spent a month visiting health facilities and assessing service delivery in Sarawak (Malaysia) and the adjacent Kalbar Province of West Kalimantan (Indonesia), areas that share some language, ethnicity, and religious characteristics. Both Indonesia and Malaysia are committed to the Health for All vision. But discussions with staff, patients, community leaders, and others revealed important differences in approach—differences that probably account for much of the strikingly different results observed in these adjacent provinces. For example, the estimated infant mortality rate in Sarawak, 9 deaths per 1,000 live births, is roughly a fifth of the rate thought to prevail in Kalbar.

Facilities

In Sarawak clinics are spacious and clean, and they provide a healthy environment in a well-maintained setting. Local attendants are hired to maintain each facility. Every clinic has a delivery room. Clean water is available, and the latrines and furniture are superior to those in Indonesia. In Kalbar the team encountered filthy unused rooms with equipment in disrepair and patients who needed to be referred to other facilities. But it also found a pristine clinic with a healing herb garden, patients happy with services, and staff whose only complaint was that they weren't paid enough.

Uniformity or innovation

Conditions and services of the same level in Sarawak are standardized and predictable regardless of where facilities are located. Only three staff are posted in each rural clinic, with consistency of effort and skill maintained. The health care provided may not stray from that guaranteed by the system. The medical assistant is permitted to follow up a complex case only after the doctor receiving the referral has established the treatment regimen. But the state health department encourages personnel to be innovative. A prestigious award goes every year to staff who develop new ways to accomplish their tasks.

Program activities

Sarawak's clinics, unlike Kalbar's, provide only outpatient and mother and child health services. Health education is integrated into every activity. Outreach activities are done by village health teams and the Flying Doctor Service, each based in the divisional health office. The only outreach handled by clinics is the updating of the village health survey every two years. This census identifies

villages with low health status, a key step in Sarawak's initiative to decentralize priority-setting to clinics.

Quality issues

Quality-related slogans and pictures appear on office walls in facilities throughout Sarawak. Almost everyone, from the director in Kuching (the state capital) to medical assistants at Klinik Desa, talks about quality. Quality is their culture, influencing the way they think and deliver services. Starting with top managers, everyone in the system is trained in quality. This contrasts starkly with the situation in Indonesia, where efforts to improve quality started at the grass roots without preparing managers. The Sarawak Health Department's vision, mission, and client charter are displayed to staff and the public. Every service and support unit must develop and exhibit its client charter.

Competence of staff

Medical assistants, who perform the same tasks as nurses in Indonesia's *Puskesmas,* were trained to diagnose and treat certain diseases. Their training—senior high school plus three years of nursing school—is equivalent to *Akademi Perawat* in Indonesia. New staff also receive training on quality assurance and corporate culture before they are deployed. Staff receive briefs about field activities and the obstacles they may encounter. Motivational and corporate culture courses are held annually. The Sarawak Health Department also provides staff with technical guidelines. All staff concerned use the guidelines, unlike Kalbar, where most staff said they had never read or referred to the guidelines. Sarawak's technical and administrative guidelines are readable, clear, well-structured, and comprehensive. And implementation of the guidelines is closely monitored through quarterly quality checks. Staff performance, linked to salary increments, is assessed yearly.

Teamwork and management

Teamwork is demonstrated at all levels in Sarawak. Two key elements are dedication to quality and customer value and an environment of cooperation with rewards for the success of teams rather than individuals. An informal and professional atmosphere exists, with staff throughout the state having met each other or even worked together. In Kalbar interpersonal and interorganizational communication is poor, community acceptance of services is limited, and effort and imagination in training personnel is minimal.

Source: Reference 6.

at lower levels are passed up to higher levels for a decision. There are no managers in the true sense of the word. Instead, administrators execute decisions according to previously agreed protocols and rules, with little or no scope for autonomous decisionmaking at the facility level.

The Malaysian approach, by contrast, has more in common with the new public sector management philosophy.[3,4] Responsibility for tasks and decisionmaking is delegated to specific parts of the organization and to specific individuals. Individual accountability is emphasized, and there is a focus on performance—not inputs and processes but outputs and outcomes.[5] Good performance is rewarded, financially or in some other way. There is a focus on clients and a belief that an organization is ultimately accountable to its clients. A client-oriented strategy emphasizes customer choice and satisfaction. Business techniques enhance performance and are a standard part of strategic planning.

Elements of the philosophy are evident in successful nutrition and child health programs. In Tamil Nadu's Integrated Nutrition Program (box 6.4), community nutrition workers were given clearly defined duties. Information on outputs enabled the community to keep workers accountable, and it enabled the workers to see how their programs were working. In Céara's Programa de Agentes de Saúde (box 6.5), credited with a substantial reduction in child mortality, health agents and nurse-supervisors were assigned clear tasks and given clear responsibilities, and the intended outcomes of the program were emphasized throughout to both health workers and members of the public. Good performance by a team (high immunization rates) was rewarded with a prize. And health agents were held accountable for their performance through a community-based monitoring process.

World Health Organization guidelines in developing national Integrated Management of Childhood Illness (IMCI) programs stress clear definitions of the roles of central and district levels, strengthening existing management structures, involving staff with good clinical skills in supervision, and using management information to solve problems and improve planning.[7] Performance feedback, which is also emphasized, has been found in Niger to have a "significant and consistent" impact on provider performance among those with previously low compliance.[8]

In maternal health, too, successful programs include elements of the new public sector management philosophy. China has a multilevel management strategy to achieve maternal health goals. Management plans for maternal and reproductive health care are developed at the lower levels, and those managers are rated on specific tasks, which also serve as a basis for promotion. Greater autonomy and accountability through this system have helped promote preventive measures and increase referral rates among high-risk pregnant women.[9]

In other settings, audits and evidence-based standards have improved the quality of obstetric care. In Indonesia the government committed itself to systematized, district-level audits to monitor performance and ensure quality of care. Malaysia intensifies management attention to underperforming districts identified through such procedures, revising protocols for personnel and facilities on the basis of data it collects.[10,11]

Performance-oriented measures have been shown to be effective. In Ecuador quality assurance measures significantly increased provider compliance with clinical standards for maternal health, even without additional resources to implement the initiative.[12] In Ghana and Jamaica the introduction of audits as a monitoring and nonpunitive educational tool was associated with better processes for obstetric care (more use of protocols), with feedback identified as crucial to successes.[13] In South Africa an adolescent services program links achievement of national standards and criteria to accreditation of public sector "adolescent-friendly" clinics. Using a combination of quality improvement methods, external assessment, and a rating system, the program has been integrated into a broader sexual health program, with promising results.[14,15]

Institutional reform—strengthening the accountability of provider organizations

Public providers

Attempts to improve the performance of public providers—most often focusing on productivity and quality—are the most common service delivery reforms in developing countries. The mechanisms applied in the health sector typically seek to alter institutional arrangements to create better incentives for public providers—either by increasing the leverage of patients (the short route of accountability) or by improving the effectiveness of supervision (part of the long route). Mechanisms to increase patient leverage and supervisory effectiveness often rely on financial incentives by seeking to tie payments to provider organizations (not necessarily individual providers) more closely to performance. Some initiatives also seek to reduce organizational constraints associated with public sector ownership that block responses to existing incentives. Some are in the realm of public sector reform more broadly (civil service reform, budget management and execution reform, improved human resource policies) and are not reviewed here.

PERFORMANCE-BASED PAYMENT (INTERNAL CONTRACTS) Public sector organizations in developing countries are typically neither recognized nor rewarded for better performance. So performance-based payment is a common strategy to improve performance. It consists of formal agreements between a government supervisory agency and public providers linking remuneration to specific aspects of performance. This funding arrangement for public services, widespread in industrial countries, is now more common in middle-income countries. The agreements typically focus on increasing productivity (and sometimes quality) by clarifying related organizational objectives and responsibilities, thereby strengthening policymakers' accountability relationship with the provider(s). When applied to primary care, the

Box 6.4 Management in India's Tamil Nadu Integrated Nutrition Program

The Tamil Nadu Integrated Nutrition Program, started in 1980, was converted to the Integrated Child Development Services Program in 1997. Core features of the program were growth monitoring, nutrition education, and food supplementation programs, implemented in community nutrition centers by community nutrition workers. The program was successful in several respects. It reduced severe malnutrition in the program areas. It has been sustained for a long period. And it operates on a large scale. Reductions in moderate malnutrition were lower than expected, but the results have been attributed to unrealistic targets rather than the level of achievement.

How did the management of human resources contribute to the positive results of the program? Changes in staffing and job design, training and supervision, and monitoring made a difference.

Staffing and job design

The program implemented well-designed procedures for staffing and job design:

- *Recruitment.* Individuals were eligible to become community nutrition workers if they resided in the village, had at least eight years of schooling, and were acceptable to the community. Special efforts were made to recruit women who were both poor and had healthy and well-nourished children. The rationale for this approach was that there would be no social barrier between the community nutrition workers and their poor clients and that they would be credible, since they had already managed to raise well-nourished children despite their low socioeconomic status.

- *Duties and work routines.* To help community nutrition workers focus on priority issues, their job description included a limited number of clearly defined duties, to be performed according to a specific work schedule. Village registration of women and children was to be conducted once every three months. Growth monitoring took place during three days a month. The supplementary feeding program was implemented between set hours in the morning. Home visits were conducted in the afternoon.

- *Rewards.* The community nutrition workers received a low monthly wage, but their compensation was still higher than they would have earned as agricultural workers. Community nutrition workers were also motivated by factors other than income: the satisfaction of helping others and the higher status that came from being associated with a program that improved the lives of their peers in the community.

Training and supervision

The community nutrition workers received training and supervision support in two main areas:

- *Preservice training.* Community nutrition workers and community nutrition supervisors received training that lasted two months, a significant amount of time for this kind of program. Training groups were kept small, enabling a strong emphasis on role-playing exercises.

- *Supervision and in-service training.* The high supervisor-to-worker ratio (one community nutrition supervisor supervised 10–15 community nutrition workers) meant that community nutrition supervisors had time to adequately supervise the community nutrition workers. In addition to routine supervision, joint home visits were made to families who failed to bring their children to weighing and feeding or whose children did not gain weight after 90 days of food supplementation. The community nutrition supervisors were in turn supervised by community nutrition instructors.

Monitoring

The monitoring system generated timely and good-quality data, although too much information was sometimes collected. Monitoring information was used for two purposes:

- *Information for workers and clients.* Special efforts were made to collect data not only for managers but for frontline workers and their clients in the communities as well. Every month data collected by the community nutrition workers were displayed outside the community nutrition centers. The data included information on the number of children who had been weighed, the number of children of different nutritional status, and the number of children who received supplementary feeding. These data provided community members with an idea of how the program was doing.

- *Information for management.* Community nutrition supervisors and instructors collated information from the community nutrition workers during monthly meetings. The data were sent to the project coordination office, to be converted into key performance indicators and used for overall management of the program.

Source: Reference 16.

payment often flows to providers based on patient choice. In these cases, the strategy also relies on increasing the leverage of patients to improve accountability. Another key element of the improved incentives is the enhanced enforceability of the agreement—that is, the ability to verify when responsibilities have been fulfilled or not on both

sides and the fact that at least part of the funding flows are tied to some measurable aspect of performance.

Does it work? Evidence on impact in developing countries is mixed. Performance-based payment appears to work fairly well in middle-income countries and less well

Although it is one of the poorest states in Brazil, the northeastern state of Céara has achieved impressive improvements in child health. The infant mortality rate fell from about 100 per 1,000 live births in the mid-1980s to 65 in 1992, a 36 percent reduction. A rural preventive health program, Programa de Agentes de Saúde (health agent program, PAS), has been credited with much of the improvement.

A central feature of the program was the use of health agents, who visited households to provide advice and assistance on oral rehydration therapy, vaccination, antenatal care, breastfeeding, and growth monitoring. The agents also collected data for health monitoring purposes. By 1993 the health agents were making monthly home visits to 850,000 families—roughly 65 percent of the state's population. Even though health agents did not earn more than the minimum wage and worked under temporary contracts without job security or fringe benefits, they performed well and helped achieve important health gains.

How did Céara achieve this? Effective public management of human resources played a large role, in a variety of areas, including addressing concerns about clientelism, the hiring process, motivation, supervision, and community monitoring.

Addressing concerns about clientelism

Before PAS was initiated in 1987, most municipalities had no public health program. At most, the mayor had an ambulance at his disposal and kept a small stock of prescription medicines at his home. Medicines and ambulance rides were usually given to

relatives and friends in return for political loyalty. The new Brazilian constitution of 1988 increased mayors' access to revenues for health expenditures, as it increased federal transfers to the municipalities. The planners of the PAS had to work within this context of decentralization. They feared that hiring a large number of health agents and nurse-supervisors would be vulnerable to clientelism. The state addressed the problem in three main ways. First, it hired workers based on merit and offered them temporary contracts, not job tenure. Second, the health agents' salaries were paid directly from the governor's office. Third, the state health department appropriated the responsibility for hiring the health agents, while leaving the hiring of nurses to supervise the health agents to each municipality.

Hiring

The state-level coordinating committee placed strong emphasis on hiring people based on merit. It required all applicants to submit written applications, from which it selected candidates to interview. Two members of the selection team (usually a nurse and a social worker) then traveled to each town for interviews, followed by a group meeting. The group meeting was often followed by a second round of individual interviews with candidates likely to be selected. The visits of the hiring team created a sense of excitement in the towns and added to the prestige of being selected. Although the jobs paid only the minimum wages and came with no fringe benefits, many people found the position

---

in low-income countries.[18–23] In both settings the evidence is relatively strong that the strategy leads to increases in output, access, productivity, and responsiveness.[18–24] Quantifiable positive impact on health care quality is less easy to identify, partly because it is so rarely measured.

Performance-based payment appears easier to apply for primary care services than for acute care, probably because it is more feasible to tie the payment allocation to patient choice of provider. (It is widely accepted that patients can judge the quality of primary care services, and hence providers, better than they can judge hospitals and hospital service quality.)

There is more evidence from middle-income countries, especially from Latin America and Central and Eastern Europe. In both regions there is stronger evidence of positive impact for performance-based payments at the primary care level than at higher levels of care. Such evidence comes from Croatia, Estonia, Latvia, Lithuania, Peru, Poland, and Romania.[18,23,25,26] In Argentina and Nicaragua social security institutes have increased productivity by establishing capitation payments for an integrated package

of inpatient and ambulatory services.[27] In Central Europe, where capped, case-based payments cover inpatient services, increases in the volume of services and declining average lengths of stay—in Bulgaria, the Czech Republic, Estonia, Hungary, Latvia, Lithuania, Poland, Romania, and the Russian Federation—suggest increases in productivity.[18]★ Deterioration in quality (due to skimping on costly nonobservable aspects of quality) has not arisen as a serious concern. Elsewhere in the former Soviet republics, and in Latin America, the results are more ambiguous. This lack of response is typically attributed to insufficient provider autonomy and a weak link between performance and pay (insufficient funds relative to service commitments).

When does it work best? Key influences on the success of the approach include whether the public provider has the ability to respond (see the discussion of

---

★ Since other systemic changes have been implemented along with performance-based payment in Central Europe, it is not possible to attribute the results to any single aspect of the reforms (such as the payment mechanism).

desirable, particularly as it was a year-round rather than a seasonal job. The newly hired workers began their jobs with a strong sense of prestige for having been selected.

Motivation

The positive effects of the hiring process were enhanced during the implementation period. The program received much publicity, in large part thanks to funding from private firms for radio and television campaigns. Municipalities that achieved the highest immunization coverage were awarded prizes, further adding to the prestige of agents in the communities. The program provided three months of full-time training to the health agents, a strong motivating factor. Access to this kind of training was unimaginable to most people in the interior of Céara. Health agents were also motivated by the fact that their jobs were more diverse and satisfying than most other jobs in the area.

Supervision

Supervision of the health agents by nurses was a critical part to the program's success. In urban clinics and hospitals, where many of the nurse-supervisors had previously worked, they had a subordinate status and performed much more administrative work rather than actual nursing duties. They often felt alienated from their work and ignored as professionals. In the program in Céara, their status changed dramatically. Each nurse supervised and trained 30 health agents and was considered a very important person in the community. The nurses were also paid more than

they had been paid in their previous jobs. These factors helped the state ensure good supervision of its health agents.

Community monitoring

In addition to effective supervision by nurses, the community made sure that health agents performed well. During the hiring process, the program linked prestige not just to those who passed the rigorous selection process but to the whole program and its mission of reducing infant mortality and morbidity. A special message was given to applicants who were not chosen for the job. They were encouraged to make sure that the health agents followed the rules of the program. The rules, constantly repeated, were that the health agents had to live in the area in which they worked, work eight hours a day, visit each household at least once a month, and attend all training and review sessions.

To avoid turning disgruntled job-seekers into overzealous watchdogs, the selection committee conveyed the message to the applicants in a way that made them feel involved in the program. Indeed, community members reported to the nurse-supervisors when they felt satisfied about the job a particular agent was doing, not only when they perceived that the agent had done something wrong. This socialization of all job applicants to the program's mission created an informal but powerful monitoring presence in the communities, adding to a sense of collective responsibility for the program.

Source: Reference 17.

---

autonomization below), whether service commitments are congruent with funding levels, whether output and key components of performance expectations are easily measurable (as in primary healthcare), and how far capacity strengthening of the payer or funder is addressed as a central part of the initiative.

Other factors are important, too. Positive impacts are more likely when the potential bonuses to be gained by better performance are sufficient to justify substantial effort by the provider. And responses are greater when the provider organization can retain and allocate the extra revenues. Schemes in which this is not the case have little or no impact. Can the patient choose the provider and in the process direct funding flows? For hospitals it appears that the threat to take away funding is usually perceived as hollow. So reforms are more successful when performance pressure relies not on pressure from competition for market share but on the possibility of bonuses.†

---

† Public providers rarely perceive the threat of not receiving a contract as credible, even where alternative providers exist.[28]

AUTONOMIZATION The weak impact of performance-based payment strategies in public hospitals is frequently attributed to the lack of decisionmaking authority and flexibility to respond to incentives. That is why another strategy—autonomization—is used, often in conjunction with or following those just described. Autonomization consists of delegating additional decisionmaking authority to hospitals. It aims to improve productivity by giving providers the flexibility to respond to performance incentives, especially to manage labor and production, to pay staff based on performance, and to undertake cost-saving or quality-enhancing changes.[28] Autonomization also often seeks to create some risk-bearing for the provider to motivate performance (residual claimant status). In low-income countries autonomization is most often driven by fiscal crises and a desire to shift more care toward the primary level. There is usually a focus on mobilizing resources in the autonomized facilities from user fees. Autonomization does not work through improving the accountability relations for policymakers or patients—it seeks to increase the ability of providers to respond to whatever incentives—created primarily by the public payment system and the choices of private payers—exist.

Does it work? No rigorous evaluation of autonomization has been conducted in low-income settings. The assessments that have been done have produced mixed results.[29] Efficiency and sometimes quality have improved when labor management is delegated—as they did in India and Kenya.[30,31] But the emphasis on revenue generation from fees has undermined access for the poor in a number of countries, including Indonesia and Malaysia.[32,33] Results in middle-income countries are better, with evidence of efficiency gains in Colombia[34] and efficiency gains combined with quality improvements in Tunisia.[32] The greater capacity of the funder or payer in middle-income countries allows the use of payments as performance leverage for providers.

When does it work best? A variety of factors influence the success of autonomization. Are services for the poor paid for or otherwise supported and monitored? Are agreements about maintenance of important but money-losing services explicit and monitored? Is there explicit support for central government and other administrative officials to shift the nature of their oversight? The reform time horizon for autonomization is long (three to five years). Management capacity needs to be in place in the provider unit before the reform is imitated—or at least strengthened as a central part of reform. There has to be an explicit and focused effort to create accountability mechanisms that are not based on day-to-day administrative control (oversight boards, regulation, accreditation). The organization's mandate has to be narrow and clear. And output-based or performance-based funding has to be in place before the provider reforms.

PRIVATIZATION Like autonomization for hospitals, privatization has been applied at the primary level to give public providers the freedom and the high-powered incentives that come from being the owner (residual claimant). Privatization at the primary level converts a salaried publicly employed physician into a self-employed independent contractor, with a service contract with a public payer (such as a social insurance organization). The strategy was implemented to different degrees in almost all Central European countries following the establishment of social insurance systems (95 percent of primary healthcare providers in the Czech Republic and 80 percent in Estonia have been privatized). In Croatia, Estonia, and Romania the capitation payment is allocated based on patients' choice of provider.

Does it work? Privatization of primary healthcare, in conjunction with capitation-based payment and training in family medicine, is associated with positive results in three assessed cases in Central Europe. In Estonia the annual num-

ber of visits per doctor and the number of visits per inhabitant rose. Immunization coverage, which is paid for separately, rose from 74 percent to 88 percent.[20] In Romania the use of primary healthcare—a key goal of the initiative—increased significantly.[23] Efficiency also increased. And as in Estonia, significant increases in immunization rates were observed. In Croatia efficiency was not assessed in the privatized practices, but physicians were more accessible and patient satisfaction had increased.[22]

The reform appears to generate two sources of accountability: pressure to please patients enough to maintain registered patients and requirements for pricing, professional licensing, facility adequacy, and other staffing to maintain the contract with the insurer. But privatization in these three countries, and others in the region, has been associated with fragmentation (such as reduced practice size), raising concerns about reduced efficiency and a possible decline in clinical quality.

When does it work best? Privatization of health services in developing countries has been assessed only at the primary healthcare level. It appears to work well when there is an established, solvent purchaser in place and capitation payments are combined with patient choice. The tendency toward fragmentation may be reduced by contract processes that promote group practice (price-setting) and by provisions to promote access to capital and premises.

DECENTRALIZATION Decentralization is intended to improve the quality of services and the productivity of providers by strengthening the policymaker's accountability relations with providers (the local government supervisor is closer). Indirectly, decentralization may increase patient leverage, as patients are likely to be able to exert more pressure on local governments to improve health services than they could on the central government, partly because information on preferences and performance is easier to obtain at the local level.

Does it work? The impact of decentralization has been mixed in low-income countries. The health services element of broad decentralization initiatives has been particularly poorly designed and implemented, often driven by political or fiscal considerations. In Tanzania decentralization improved the efficiency of and access to primary healthcare services, but in Ghana efficiency declined.[35] There have been notable examples of deterioration in the provision of public goods, such as disease surveillance and preventative services (Ghana, Indonesia, Tanzania), and in the equity of access (Uganda). There is less evidence on the impact of decentralization in middle-income countries, though it has generated improvements in responsiveness and equity in Colombia.[36]

When does it work best? Adequate resources to operate services have to be allocated along with new service responsibilities. Local political institutions have to be relatively functional (voters need to have influence—another element of the long route of accountability). Health authorities have to be integrally involved in designing and implementing the decentralization initiatives for health services. Concerted efforts to build local government capacity—planning, supervision, budgeting, and expenditure and financial management—have to be part of the initiative. Mechanisms also need to be in place to ensure capacity to cover the core public functions outlined in chapter 8 (disease surveillance and control, funding for and attention to preventive services and services that promote health, human resource planning, interregional coordination). Adequate time has to be allocated to design and implementation, especially for building the capacity of local authorities to perform new oversight tasks.

GOVERNANCE PARTICIPATION Participation is intended to improve productivity and the quality of services by involving representatives of community interests in the governance of local facilities. It relies on directly strengthening the leverage of patients (the short route of accountability), or at least their representatives, in provider oversight. Patients' first-hand knowledge and influence shorten the "feedback" loop of supervisory accountability.

Does it work? Some governments have had difficulty establishing meaningful participation, but there have been positive changes where it has been established. In Burkino Faso participation of community representatives in public primary healthcare clinics increased immunization coverage and the availability of essential drugs.[37] The percentage of women with two or more antenatal visits also increased. But the resources spent increased as well, so it is not possible to assess the impact on efficiency. In Peru participation is associated with reduced absenteeism of staff, reduced waiting times, and the perception of higher quality by patients.[26,38]

When does it work best? No formal evaluation of participation has been conducted, but several characteristics seem to contribute to success. Better results are achieved where the selection process for representatives is transparent and involves community members rather than appointed representatives. Governance participation is more likely to improve service provision where reasonably strong community organizations already exist and motivated community members are present. Supervisory responsibilities need to be well defined and focused (as in the allocation of revolving drug funds in the Bamako initiative and elsewhere). Governance participation probably works better for primary care than for hospitals—the greater complexity of the services and organization of hospitals appears to undermine the influence of community representatives in oversight processes. And strong technical and advisory support has to be provided to community representative bodies.

ACCREDITATION OF HOSPITALS Accreditation initiatives are becoming more common in developing countries. Under this strategy, public hospitals are motivated to improve quality standards as assessed by external reviewers in order to receive "accredited" status. This approach does not directly use either policymaker oversight or patient leverage, though it often relies on those forces indirectly by linking accreditation to eligibility for public funds or by directing patients to accredited facilities.

Does it work? Only two developing countries that have implemented accreditation for health services providers have been assessed. The accreditation initiative in South Africa has improved process quality, though there is no evidence on the impact on outcomes.[39] In Zambia there has been no demonstrable impact.[40]

When does it work best? Accreditation works best when it is linked to financial leverage—when it adds to the provider's "bottom line." It is most successful when provider associations are productively engaged and involved in developing standards. Substantial facilitation or consulting services are required to help hospitals implement needed improvements.[41,42]

Nonprofit providers

When governments work with nonprofit providers to achieve sector objectives, their efforts usually focus on expanding services or increasing efficiency through better coordination. Several approaches are commonly used, including informal arrangements for in-kind subsidies and public-private partnerships. But the only strategy that evidence suggests may work is service contracting.

Contracting initiatives for health and nutrition services have been implemented in several countries. Most initiatives work through nonprofit organizations seeking to build on their comparative advantage (efficiency, quality, willingness to cross-subsidize) and focus (slum dwellers, malnourished children, poor socially excluded groups). Implicitly, the initiatives also build on the close alignment of the providers' organizational objectives and the policymakers' goals. This alignment is believed to reduce the need for oversight and general capacity of the government in interacting with them. Such initiatives are rarely rigorously evaluated, because little emphasis is placed on collecting information or monitoring providers, whom policymakers tend to trust. This lack of rigorous evaluation makes evaluating the impact difficult.

HEALTH SERVICE CONTRACTING Government, it is argued, gets more value for money from public spending by paying a nonprofit provider to provide priority services, such as basic services for maternal and child health, and communicable diseases, or by serving priority population groups in which they have a comparative advantage than they would by providing services directly. Services for which governments commonly contract include outreach for health promotion or education in urban slums, outreach to stigmatized or hard-to-reach groups, and social marketing of priority health goods or services (box 6.6).

Box 6.6 Contracting health services in Cambodia, Guatemala, and Pakistan

Cambodia

In Cambodia the government contracted with nongovernmental organizations (NGOs) in two ways.[43] The first was a contracting-out model, in which contractors had responsibility for delivering specified services, directly employed their own staff, and had full management control. The second was a contracting-in model, in which contractors managed the district health care system within the Ministry of Health. The government met recurrent operating costs through normal channels, although a small supplement was provided, which the contractors could spend as they saw best. In a control group, services were delivered under the existing Ministry of Health system and the same small supplement was provided.

Twelve districts, covering about 1.5 million people, were randomly assigned to one of the three groups (contracting-out, contracting-in, or control), and baseline household and health facility surveys were administered before the contracts started. The surveys were repeated two and a half years after the contracts began.

What were the results? Much larger improvements in immunization coverage, antenatal care, and other indicators were observed in the contracting-out and contracting-in districts than in the control districts, although all districts were quite similar at the outset. The increases were especially pronounced in the contracting-out districts. The poor appear to have benefited disproportionately. Vitamin A supplementation increased faster among the poorest half of the population. And treatment of illness among the poorest half of the population increased several times faster in contracted districts than in the control districts. The results show that contracting with NGOs can improve service delivery in a short period.

What about cost? Cost was considerably higher for contracting out than for contracting in or the control groups, but contracting out led to a considerable savings in out-of-pocket expenditures for people in the communities. The cost difference between the contracting-in and the control districts ($0.96 per capita per year) was smaller, reflecting almost entirely the cost of the contract with the NGO. Because the two groups thus had the same amount of resources to spend on actual service delivery, extra resources do not explain the performance difference. Overall, contracting was considerably more successful than government delivery of the same services.

Guatemala

The government of Guatemala contracted with NGOs to deliver primary healthcare services to indigenous populations in mountainous areas using three models: a direct model, which involved giving NGOs considerable autonomy to run existing clinics (similar to contracting out in Cambodia); a mixed model, which required the NGOs to keep the same staff and so gave them less autonomy (closely resembling contracting in); and the traditional model, which was essentially the usual way the government delivered services.

Municipalities covering some 190,000 people were assigned to one of the approaches, and a household survey was undertaken after about two years. No baseline survey was available.

The household survey found that the mixed approach achieved the best results in antenatal care, immunization, and receipt of oral rehydration salts by young children with diarrhea. But the areas in which the direct model was implemented had more isolated households with considerably less access to health facilities. The traditional and mixed samples appeared quite similar.

The mixed model appears more successful than the traditional model, with a difference in coverage of services of 5–16 percentage points. The absence of a baseline makes it difficult to be sure that this is the true size of the effect, but it appears that contracting with NGOs had a real impact. It is also difficult to conclude much about the direct approach because it was implemented in more remote and difficult areas.

Pakistan

In a poorly performing district of Punjab, an NGO was allowed to run all the primary health care facilities and implement changes in organization and management. The NGO was given the same budget previously provided to the district. The NGO nearly tripled the salaries of selected doctors and had them cover three different basic health units instead of the usual one. The NGO also improved the supply of drugs available without increasing the budget.

An interrupted time series was used to assess the intervention. Information from the routine reporting system on the number of outpatient visits in the district was tracked over time. No data from other nearby districts are available yet. The district comprises 104 basic health units for about 2 million people.

How were patients affected? Once the NGO started running the system, outpatient visits to the basic health units enjoyed nearly a fourfold increase.

The intervention took place in one medium-size district. No household survey data are available, nor are data available on any other aspect of health service delivery, such as immunization. But the sudden dramatic increase in outpatient visits suggests that the NGO was more successful than the government in operating the services with managerial autonomy.

Source: World Bank staff and references 43–45.

Does it work? Contracting with NGOs is used most often in low-income countries. In most cases that have been evaluated, positive impacts were observed on target outcome or output variables. In Bangladesh, for example, contracts with nonprofit providers for the planning and implementation of an expanded immunization program were credited with increasing coverage from 25 percent in 1985 to 80 percent in 1990.[46] Contracting for a primary healthcare package in Haiti also generated significant increases in immunization coverage.[47] Nutrition services also appear to be amenable to contracting in low-income countries. In Bangladesh, Madagascar, and Senegal, significant reductions in nutrition rates were attributed to contracting initiatives.[48]

Only a small number of cases assess efficiency. One found that the contracted provider (Prosalud) in Santa Cruz, Bolivia, outperformed the Ministry of Health facilities on productivity, use, efficacy, and cost-effectiveness in outpatient care.[49] Many social marketing initiatives rely on contracted nonprofit organizations to market bednets, oral rehydration salts, fortified foods, and the like.

When does it work best? Nonprofit providers need to be strong, with well-functioning accountability arrangements and internal motivation to perform—as those in Bangladesh and Bolivia are. The government needs to be capable of assessing, selecting, and managing the ongoing relationship with the providers. It must also fulfill its end of the deal (contractual agreements on funding are genuine) and not interfere with the running of the nonprofit providers, which need full control of the operation (box 6.6).

For-profit formal providers

The past 10 years have seen greater efforts to harness the formal for-profit sector to improve the quality of care it provides, to use it to serve certain populations in exchange for public funding, and to reduce the cost to poor people for for-profit services.

HEALTH SERVICE CONTRACTING Contracting in developing countries is most often used to try to mobilize for-profit providers, usually to increase access or efficiency. In exchange for public funds, private providers deliver services of a specified type and quality, in agreed quantities, to agreed recipients, and over agreed periods. Like performance-based payment of public providers, contracting strengthens accountability relations between the policymaker and the provider and emphasizes financial incentives. But the for-profit orientation of these providers means that more rigorous tendering and contract management process are required to bring about desired improvements. Contracting with for-profit providers often focuses on primary care services and on procuring services in areas in which the public sector lacks capacity and equipment, such as diagnostic services and high-tech services.

Does it work? The results are mixed. Contracting with formal for-profit providers is frequently effective in increasing access, use, and responsiveness. In many cases it appears that for-profit providers can also produce contracted services at lower cost. What is not clear is whether the government captures any of the efficiency gains or whether the cost savings come at the expense of clinical quality or access by high-cost patients. Efficiency increased through contracting for high-tech diagnostic services in Thailand.[50] Contracts for high-tech services in India improved some aspects of quality (availability of services, frequency of functioning equipment), though private payment for the services almost certainly constrained access for poor patients. In Zimbabwe inpatient and outpatient services were tendered, and the cost per service decreased.[51] But the lack of volume control led to an increase in total cost. In South Africa the cost of hospital services declined, but the cost to government did not.[52]

A weak contracting capacity on the part of the government often allows the provider to capture any efficiency gains or to expand volume to generate more income. In Brazil contracting with for-profit hospitals led to increases in access.[53] But it also led to cream-skimming to avoid costly patients, as well as fraud (false billing for services).

Contracting with formal for-profit providers for primary healthcare services appears to succeed more often. In El Salvador and Peru, social insurance institutes contracted with private primary healthcare providers to serve their clients, which increased access, choice, and consumer satisfaction.[54] Contracting with (privatized) self-employed physicians in Croatia, Estonia, and Romania has improved efficiency, quality, and use.[20,22,23]‡

When does it work best? Investment in developing capacities for managing the contracting process clearly needs to be a central part of such initiatives.[55] And quality in the private sector has to be at least as good as in the public sector (since ability to monitor quality is usually low). Such contracting probably works best for primary care or other relatively observable services (diagnosis).

ENHANCING THE REGULATORY FRAMEWORK TO IMPROVE QUALITY Given widespread concern with the quality of health care services in developing countries, there have been many attempts to improve the effectiveness of the regulatory framework for health services and

---

‡ Contracting in these cases was introduced at the same time as the conversion from public to private practice and the introduction of the "family doctor" model of practice. Hence it is not possible to attribute these results to any one factor.

facilities. Strategies typically consist of enacting or updating laws or regulations related to minimum standards, especially for inputs and starting a profession or business. These efforts are sometimes accompanied by efforts to strengthen the capacity of the relevant regulatory agency.

Does it work? There is no documented case in a developing country of a successful initiative to improve the effectiveness of the regulatory framework for health services broadly. Targeted regulatory initiatives (for pharmacies) have, however, improved targeted practices.[56,57] The role of professional and provider organizations in such initiatives appears to have been very small—in marked contrast to industrial countries.

When does it work best? Regulatory initiatives have to target a specific group of providers and a well-defined set of behaviors (overprescribing antibiotics, mixing pharmaceuticals). And they have to be accompanied by an effective information dissemination strategy and enhanced inspection (the Lao People's Democratic Republic),[57] reinforced by education and peer influence (Vietnam)[56] and by the dissemination of information (on, say, the use of oral rehydration therapy rather than antimotility drugs for children's diarrhea [Pakistan]).[58]

DISSEMINATING INFORMATION TO PATIENTS AND CAREGIVERS One of the biggest problems with formal for-profit providers is their willingness to accede to patients' requests for inappropriate treatment, including prescriptions. Some countries have tried to address this problem by improving patient knowledge of appropriate treatment and thus changing their demand in targeted areas. Easy-to-understand information is disseminated on appropriate treatment and care-seeking. The intention is that providers will then deliver better-quality care because the demand for inappropriate care declines.

Does it work? Some positive results have been reported, though only from a small number of experiences. In Bangladesh a 10-year campaign to inform mothers about oral rehydration therapy led to a sharp increase in the number of rural drug sellers prescribing it. Physicians also increased their recommendation of oral rehydration therapy, albeit by less.[59]

When does it work best? A key issue is whether the problem is grounded in inappropriate patient demand or in financial benefit to the provider. The information provided needs to be easy to understand.

SOCIAL MARKETING AND COMMERCIALIZATION Social marketing and commercialization consists of a two-part initiative to increase the use of important

health goods (condoms, oral rehydration salts, fortified foods): conducting a marketing campaign for the branded good and commercializing the sale of the branded good for target providers. Sometimes the strategy is applied to shift consumption from lower-quality goods to better ones. It uses the (existing) market-based accountability of sellers to purchasers to influence retailers and producers of goods. It has been widely successful in increasing the use of important public health goods.[60–62]

More recently, it has been applied to health services, such as reproductive health services and treatment of sexually transmitted diseases (STDs).

Does it work? In Uganda a social marketing-commercialization initiative improved the quality of STD treatment offered by formal for-profit providers in three rural districts. Targeted retailers stocked and prescribed prepackaged STD drugs, increasing treatment compliance from 87 percent to 93 percent, cure rates from 47 percent to 84 percent, and condom use during treatment from 17 percent to 36 percent.[62] Another such initiative created a "branded" reproductive health service, which attracted 11,000 providers. The use of the branded providers increased significantly, providing contraceptive services to one Pakistani couple in five at a cost of less than $4 a year per person.[63] As with health goods, social marketing and commercialization of services is more sustainable than contracting because it relies on patient payment and is implemented through commercial organizations. But the focus on cost recovery makes this strategy less effective in reaching the very poor.

When does it work best? Adequate attention needs to be paid to market segmentation to reduce "crowding out."§ Goods or services need to be homogeneous, so that consumers can easily distinguish the targeted goods, services, or providers. Other provisions such as targeted subsidies and vouchers are needed to promote use by the poor.

Informal private providers

Given the significance of informal private providers for people in developing countries, especially the poor, it is unfortunate (to say the least) that very few attempts have been made to improve the quality of their services. It is widely accepted that the quality of care they provide is low, but little has been done to improve it. In the few instances in which initiatives have been taken to improve the quality of care of informal

---

§ Subsidizing consumption has no effect if buyers shift from commercial to subsidized sources of supply. This is the case when subsidized suppliers "crowd out" existing commercial suppliers, so that there is no overall increase in purchase (or use) of the good.

providers, the focus has been mostly on training. Several of these efforts have been successful (chapter 7).

Some limited attempts have been made to regulate informal providers. One such initiative, which focused on improving the quality of services offered by drug vendors, was assessed in the Lao People's Democratic Republic.[57] Changes in regulations were reinforced by more frequent inspections, with feedback provided to vendors. Information about the regulations was also disseminated. Results included greater availability of essential drugs, more appropriate information given to customers, and less mixing of drugs in the same package.

What works? What doesn't? Why?

Six key lessons emerge from the assessment of service delivery:

- The evidence on management and broader institutional reforms is not strong. Debate is often guided more by political prejudice than by hard evidence. In part, this is because too little effort has been invested in strengthening the evidence base.

- Limited but encouraging evidence suggests that application of some of the key ingredients of the new public sector management philosophy seems to improve performance. Going down the Sarawak road (see introduction) can, in the right circumstances, lead to gains.

- Institutional reforms may be most effective when more than one approach is used—coupling autonomization with performance-based payment, for example, or regulation with information for providers or patients, or social marketing with commercialization.

- Efforts need to focus on the most relevant providers, not the ones policymakers may prefer or the ones easiest to reach. This implies a need to focus reform efforts much more on informal providers, who continue to be a major supplier of services in the developing world.

- The effectiveness of contracting with for-profit providers differs across types of services and organizations. Most success has been with primary healthcare providers. Success has been limited with specific high-tech diagnostic services. And success has so far been very limited with hospitals.

- Despite the lack of broader regulatory initiatives in developing countries, there is no alternative to governments wrestling more successfully with this critical role in the health sector. A concerted effort to help developing country governments in this effort is warranted.

References

1. World Bank. 2003. *World Development Report 2004: Making Services Work for Poor People.* Washington, DC: World Bank.

2. Dejong, J. 1991. *Non-Governmental Organizations and Health Delivery in Sub-Saharan Africa.* WPS 708. World Bank, Washington, DC.

3. Flanagan, H. 1996. *Public Sector Management Effectiveness: Theory and Practice in the National Health Service.* Buckingham, United Kingdom: Open University Press.

4. Mintzberg, H. 1994. *The Rise and Fall of Strategic Planning: Reconceiving Roles for Planning, Plans, Planners.* New York: Free Press.

5. Shaw, P. 2002. "New Public Sector Management in Health." *HNP Discussion Paper,* ed. A.S. Preker. World Bank, Washington, DC.

6. World Bank. 2000. "Health Strategy in a Post-Crisis, Decentralizing Indonesia." Report No. 21318-IND, World Bank, Washington, DC.

7. Lambrechts, T., J. Bryce, and V. Orinda. 1999. "Integrated Management of Childhood Illness: A Summary of First Experiences." *Bulletin of the World Health Organization* 77 (7): 582–594.

8. Kelley, E., C. Geslin, S. Djibrina, and M. Boucar. 2001. "Improving Performance with Clinical Standards: The Impact of Feedback on Compliance with the Integrated Management of Childhood Illness Algorithm in Niger, West Africa." *International Journal of Health Planning and Management* 16 (3): 195–205.

9. Koblinsky, M.A. 2003. "Reducing Maternal Mortality: Learning from Bolivia, China, Egypt, Honduras, Indonesia, Jamaica, and Zimbabwe." World Bank, Washington, DC.

10. Pathmanathan, I. 2003. " Investing in Maternal Health in Malaysia and Sri Lanka." World Bank, Washington, DC.

11. Ronsmans, C. 2001. "What Is the Evidence for the Role of Audits to Improve the Quality of Obstetric Care?" In *Safe Motherhood Strategies: A Review of the Evidence,* ed. W. Van Leberghe, 203–223. London and Antwerp: Centre for Sexual and Reproductive Health; UON Network Unmet Need for Major Obstetric Interventions.

12. Hermida, J., and M.E. Robalino. 2002. "Increasing Compliance with Maternal and Child Care Quality Standards in Ecuador." *International Journal for Quality in Health Care* 14 (Suppl. 1): 25–34.

13. Wagaarachchi, P.T., W.J. Graham, G.C. Penney, A. Mccaw-Binns, K. Yeboah Antwi, and M.H. Hall. 2001. "Holding Up a Mirror: Changing Obstetric Practice through Criterion-Based Clinical Audit in Developing Countries." *International Journal of Gynaecology and Obstetrics* 74 (2): 119–130.

14. Harrison, D. 2002. "Lovelife Appears to Be an Effective Prevention Program for South African Youth." Press release, American Medical Association, Barcelona, July 7.

15. Dickson-Tetteh, K., A. Pettifor, and W. Moleko. 2001. "Working with Public Sector Clinics to Provide Adolescent-Friendly Services in South Africa." *Reproductive Health Matters* 9 (17): 160–169.

16. Heaver R. India's Tamil Nadu nutrition program: lessons and issues in management and capacity development. HNP Discussion Paper. Washington, DC: World Bank, 2002.

17. Tendler, J., and S. Freedheim. 1994. "Trust in a Rent-Seeking World: Health and Government Transformed in Northeast Brazil." *World Development* 22 (12): 1771–1791.

18. Langenbrunner, J. 2003. "Resource Allocation and Purchasing in ECA Region: A Review." World Bank, Washington, DC.

19. Naimoli, J.F. 2003. "Performance-Based Management in an Evolving Decentralized Public Health System in West Africa: The Case of Burkina Faso." Background paper prepared for the *World Development Report 2004*. World Bank, Washington, DC.

20. Koppel, A., K. Meiesaar, H. Valtonen, A. Metsa, and M. Lember. 2003. "Evaluation of Primary Health Care Reform in Estonia." *Social Science and Medicine* 56 (12): 2461–2466.

21. Howard, K. 2002. "Lessons from Poland on the Private Provision of Primary Health Care." London, London School of Economics.

22. Hebrang, A., N. Henigsberg, V. Erdeljic, S. Foro, S. Turek, and M. Zlatar M. 2002. "Privatization of the Croatian Health Care System: Effect on Indicators of Health Care Accessibility in General Medicine." *Lijec Vjesn* 124 (8–9): 239-243.

23. Vladescu, C., and S. Radulescu. 2001. "Primary Health Services: Output-Based Contracting to Lift Performance in Romania." *Public Policy for the Private Sector* 239.

24. Eichler, R., P. Auxilia, and J. Pollock. 2001. "Promoting Preventive Health Care: Paying for Performance in Haiti." In *Contracting for Public Services: Output-Based Aid and its Applications*, eds. P.J. Brook and S. Smith. Washington, DC: World Bank International Finance Corporation.

25. Chawla, M., P. Berman, A. Windak, and M. Kulis. 1999. "Provision of Ambulatory Health Services in Poland: A Case Study from Krakow." Harvard School of Public Health, International Health Systems Group, Boston.

26. Cotlear, D. 1999. "Peru: Improving Health Care for the Poor." Human Development Department (LCSHD) Paper Series 57, World Bank, Washington, DC.

27. Bitran, R. 2001. *Paying Health Providers through Capitation in Argentina, Nicaragua and Thailand: Output, Spending, Organizational Impact and Market Structure*. PHR Project, USAID, Washington, DC.

28. Preker, A.S., and A. Harding. 2003. "Innovations in Health Service Delivery." World Bank, Human Development Network, Washington, DC.

29. Pearson, M. 2000. *International Experience of Hospital Autonomy.* London: Institute for Health Sector Development.

30. Chawla, M., and A. George. 1996. "Hospital Autonomy in India: The Experience of APVVP Hospitals." Project supported by USAID. Harvard University, Cambridge, MA.

31. Collins, D., G. Njeru, J. Meme, and W. Newbrander. 1999. "Hospital Autonomy: The Experience of Kenyatta National Hospital." *International Journal of Health Planning and Management* 4 (2): 129–153.

32. Harding, A., and A. Preker. 2003. "Private Participation in Health Services." World Bank, Human Development Network, Washington, DC.

33. Bossert, T., S. Kosen, B. Harsono, and A. Gani. 1997. "Hospital Autonomy in Indonesia." Project supported by USAID. Harvard University, Cambridge, MA.

34. Mcpake, B., F.J. Yepes, S. Lake, and L.H. Sanchez. 2003. "Is the Colombian Health System Reform Improving the Performance of Public Hospitals in Bogota?" *Health Policy Planning* 18 (2): 182–194.

35. Gilson, L., and A. Mills. 1995. "Health Sector Reforms in Sub-Saharan Africa: Lessons of the Last 10 Years." *Health Policy* 32 (1–3): 215–243.

36. Londono, B., I. Jarmillo, and J. Uribe. 1999. *Decentralizaiton and Reforms in Health Services: The Colombian Case.* World Bank, Washington, DC.

37. Eichler, R. 2001. "Improving Immunization Coverage in an Innovative Primary Health Care Delivery Model: Lessons from Burkina Faso's Bottom Up Planning, Oversight and Resource Control Approach that Holds Providers Accountable for Results." World Bank, Washington, DC.

38. Ewig, C. 2003. "The Contributions of Community-Based Decentralization to Democracy: Peru's Local Health Administration Committees." Paper presented at the annual meeting of the American Political Science Association.

39. Bukonda, N., P. Tavrow, H. Abdallah, K. Hoffner, and J. Tembo. 2002. "Implementing a National Hospital Accreditation Program: The Zambian Experience." *International Journal for Quality in Health Care* 14 (Suppl. 1): 7–16.

40. Tavrow, P., J. Heavens, J. Warren Salmon, and C. Lombard. 2003. *The Impact of Accreditation on the Quality of Hospital Care: Kwazulu-Natal Province, Republic of South Africa* Quality Assurance Project, USAID, Bethesda, MD.

41. Whittaker, S., R.W. Green-Thompson, I. Mccusker, and B. Nyembezi. 2000. "Status of a Health Care Quality Review Programme in South Africa." *International Journal of Quality in Health Care* 12 (3): 247–250.

42. Whittaker, S., C.D. Shaw, A. Bruwer, D. Green, J.J. Taljaard, and A. Skibbe. 1994. "The South African Pilot Hospital Accreditation Programme. Part II. The Development of Standards." *South African Medical Journal* 84 (4): 193–194.

43. Bhushan, I., S. Keller, and B. Schwartz. 2002. "Achieving the Twin Objectives of Efficiency and Equity: Contracting Health Services in Cambodia." ERD Policy Brief Series 6, Asian Development Bank, Manila.

44. Loevinsohn, B. 2000. "Contracting for the Delivery of Primary Health Care in Cambodia: Design and Initial Experience of a Large Pilot Test." *WBI Online Journal*. Washington, DC, World Bank.

45. Loevinsohn, B, and A. Harding. 2004. *Contracting for Health Service Delivery: A Review of Developing Country Experience and Results.* Health Nutrition, Population Discussion Paper, World Bank, Washington, DC.

46. Loevinsohn, B. 2002. "Practical Issues in Contracting for Primary Health Care Delivery: Lessons From Two Large Projects in Bangladesh." *WBI Online Journal*. World Bank, Washington, DC.

47. Eichler, R., P. Auxilia, and J. Pollock. 2001. *Output-Based Health Care: Paying for Performance in Haiti.* World Bank, Washington, DC.

48. Marek, T., I. Diallo, B. Ndiaye, and J. Rakotosalama. 1999. "Successful Contracting of Prevention Services: Fighting Malnutrition in Senegal and Madagascar." *Health Policy Planning* 14 (4): 382–389.

49. Richardson, P. 1992. *Quality, Costs and Cost Recovery: A Comparative Study of the Unidad Sanitaria of the Ministry of Health (MOH) and PROSALUD in Santa Cruz, Bolivia.* University Research Corporation and International Science and Technology Institute, Washington, DC.

50. Tangcharoensathien, V., and N. Khongsawatt Nas. "Private-Sector Involvement in Public Hospitals: Case Studies in Bangkok." In *Private Health Providers in Developing Countries: Serving the Public Interest?* ed. A. Mills. London: Zed Books.

51. Mcpake, B., and C. Hongoro. 1995. "Contracting Out of Clinical Services in Zimbabwe." *Social Science and Medicine* 41 (1): 13–24.

52. Broomberg J., P. Masobe, and A. Mills. 1977. "To Purchase or to Provide? The Relative Efficiency of Contracting Out versus Direct Public Provision of Hospital Services in South Africa."

In *Private Health Providers in Developing Countries,* ed. A. Mills. London: Zed Books,

53. Slack K., and W. Savedoff. 2001. "Public Purchaser-Private Provider Contracting for Health Services: Examples from Latin America and the Caribbean." Sustainable Development Department Technical Paper Series 111, Inter-American Development Bank, Washington, DC.

54. Fiedler, J.L. 1996. "The Privatization of Health Care in Three Latin American Social Security Systems." *Health Policy Planning* 11 (4): 406–417.

55. Mills, A. 1998. "To Contract or Not to Contract? Issues for Low and Middle Income Countries." *Health Policy Planning* 13 (1): 32–40.

56. Chuc, N.T., M. Larsson, N.T. Do, V.K. Diwan, G.B. Tomson, and T. Falkenberg. 2002. "Improving Private Pharmacy Practice: A Multi-Intervention Experiment in Hanoi, Vietnam." *Journal of Clinical Epidemiology* 55 (11): 1148–1155.

57. Stenson, B., L. Syhakhang, C.S. Lundborg, B. Eriksson, and G. Tomson. 2001. "Private Pharmacy Practice and Regulation: A Randomized Trial in Lao P.D.R." *International Journal of Technology Assessment in Healthcare* 17 (4): 579–589.

58. Bhutta, T.I., and C. Balchin 1996. "Assessing the Impact of a Regulatory Intervention in Pakistan." *Social Science and Medicine* 42 (8):1195–1202.

59. Chowdhury, A.M., F. Karim, S.K. Sarkar, R.A. Cash, and A. Bhuiya. 1997. "The Status of ORT (Oral Rehydration Therapy) in Bangladesh: How Widely Is It Used?" *Health Policy Planning* 12 (1): 58–66.

60. Schellenberg, J.R., S. Abdulla, H. Minja, and others. 1999. "KINET: A Social Marketing Programme Of Treated Nets And Net Treatment For Malaria Control In Tanzania, With Evaluation Of Child Health And Long-Term Survival." *Trans R Soc Trop Med Hyg* 93 (3): 225–231.

61. Abdulla, S., J.A. Schellenberg, R. Nathan, and others. 2001. "Impact on Malaria Morbidity of a Programme Supplying Insecticide Treated Nets in Children Aged under 2 Years in Tanzania: Community Cross-Sectional Study." *British Medical Journal* 322 (7281): 270–273.

62. Jacobs, B., F.S. Kambugu, J.A. Whitworth, M. Ochwo, R. Pool, A. Lwanga, S. Tifft, J. Lule, and J.R. Cutler. 2003. "Social Marketing of Pre-Packaged Treatment for Men with Urethral Discharge (Clear Semen) in Uganda." *International Journal of STD and AIDS* 14 (3): 216–221.

63. Agha, S., C. Squire, and R. Ahmed. 1997. *Evaluation of the Green Star Pilot Project.* Population Services International, Washington, DC.

CHAPTER 7

Tackling Human Resource
and Pharmaceutical Constraints

Joytsna Neopane, an anesthesiologist from Nepal based in New York City, has just completed her medical residency and expects to make $225,000–$250,000 a year once she is hired. "Compare that with less than $100 a month I used to make at a government hospital in Kathmandu, and you have the answer why thousands of doctors from the Indian Subcontinent end up here," she says.

"We observe it—we cannot lie about it. Not respecting working hours is a problem that we got used to, and this has created problems for the patients. During teatime, for example, people go to other places—to work in the private sector, for personal commitments, etc. Even that small amount of time we have in the facility we do not use effectively, and patients complain about that," says a health assistant in Ethiopia.

"The effect of HIV/AIDS on health workers has been totally ignored. It is difficult to differentiate between patients who are infected with the virus and those who are not. Health workers are exposed to difficult situations. It is like sacrificing your life. This is serious at lower levels and in rural areas. There are several emergencies that do not allow much time to look for gloves, and this forces health workers to treat a patient with bare hands. And we know the risks we are taking. A lot of colleagues have died of AIDS," reports a health assistant in Ethiopia.

Source: *References 1 and 2.*

Health systems rely on two key sets of inputs—human resources and drugs. Weaknesses in policies and practices in both areas undermine progress toward the Millen-

nium Development Goals. Stocks of human resources for health systems in low-income countries are small—and in some countries emigration and HIV/AIDS are making them smaller. Poor management and inappropriate human resources policies often cause flows from the public sector to the private, and from rural areas to urban, increasing internal imbalances. The motivation and productivity of health workers are often low. Problems with drugs include national shortages, lack of affordability for the poor, counterfeiting and substandard quality, inappropriate prescribing and use, and inefficient logistics systems.

Policies need to be broad-based. For human resources they need to address compensation issues but also nonpecuniary factors that motivate staff. Training needs to focus on skills of relevance to the Millennium Development Goals, in part to reduce skill marketability. Skills also need realignment. Relocating low-skilled staff willing to work in rural areas offers considerable scope for expanding the coverage of key Millennium Development Goal interventions. Public policy also needs to come to grips with issues related to drugs and consumables. A combination of sound policies on pricing, procurement, and logistics management and better information for consumers and healthcare providers could significantly increase stocks of drugs, vaccines, and consumables, accelerating progress toward the Millennium Development Goals.

This chapter sets out the key issues and pulls together what is known about the causes of the problems and the effectiveness of policies to deal with them.

Human resources for health

An increasingly common lament in international health is that faster progress toward the health-related Millennium Development Goals is being impeded by a variety of human resources problems. A recent United States Agency for International Development (USAID) report argued that there is already a "grave and complex human resource crisis" in the health sector in Sub-Saharan Africa that threatens achievement of the child survival and other Millennium Development Goals.[3] A recent World Bank study found that 26 of 28 Poverty Reduction Strategy Papers (PRSPs) from Sub-Saharan Africa identify the performance of the health workforce as an important issue. Of the 22 high-burden countries that account for 80 percent of the world's tuberculosis cases, 17 have reported that staffing problems are hampering their efforts to reach the 2005 targets.[4]

What are the issues?

STOCKS OF MEDICAL HUMAN RESOURCES ARE LOW, AND IN SOME COUNTRIES THEY ARE FALLING In Europe and Central Asia there are an average of 3.1 physicians per 1,000 people (figure 7.1). In Sub-Saharan Africa there is just 0.1. Within Africa are large differences (figure 7.2), with Namibia and Nigeria relatively well endowed with doctors, and Eritrea and Liberia having very few.

Human resource stocks are not constant. In the 1990s the Middle East and North Africa saw its physician stock

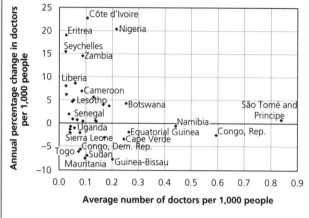

Figure 7.2 Doctors across Sub-Saharan Africa in the 1990s—how many and how much change

Source: Reference 96.

increase considerably, while South Asia saw its stock decline (see figure 7.1). Within Africa, changes in stocks varied, with Côte d'Ivoire and Nigeria seeing their stocks increase and Sierra Leone and Sudan seeing their stocks fall. Hard data are difficult to come by, but the situation in Sub-Saharan Africa seems to have worsened considerably at the end of the 1990s (e.g., see box 7.1). Tanzania's health workforce is projected to fall from 49,000 in 1994 to 36,000 in 2015.[5] Between 1998 and 2001 the number of nurses working in the public sector in The Gambia fell from 784 to 655.[6]

Do low stocks matter for Millennium Development Goal outcomes? Do falling stocks jeopardize progress? The answer is presumed to be "yes" to both questions, but the evidence is scant. A study of infant mortality in Malaysia found that, holding other factors constant, a lower population per doctor ratio was associated with a lower infant mortality rate.[8] But the population per *public* doctor was not found to be significantly related to the infant mortality rate, leading the authors to conclude that increases in the number of public doctors is partly offset by decreases in the number of doctors working in private practice.

Two other studies—one of Ghana[9] and one of Côte d'Ivoire[10]—found ambiguous evidence. Having more doctors in local facilities was associated, other things equal, with taller children, but the estimated effect was very small: raising the average number of doctors in a facility to the national average would raise the mean height-for-age by only 0.04 (the national average is −1.32). Further, the estimated impact of human resource stocks on Millennium Development Goal outcomes was highly sensitive to the focus—urban or rural, nurse or doctor, malnutrition or child survival.

Such ambiguity and sensitivity of results is not reassuring. This evidence—together with the widespread evidence on

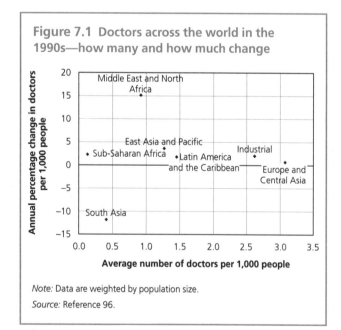

Figure 7.1 Doctors across the world in the 1990s—how many and how much change

Note: Data are weighted by population size.

Source: Reference 96.

The *State of Ghanaian Economy Report 2002* reports that 31 percent of trained health personnel, including doctors, nurses, midwives, and pharmacists, left the country between 1993 and 2002, leaving approximately 1.48 physicians per 100,000 people. Bleak as these figures are, they may underestimate the loss. A report on human resources by the Government of Ghana based on biannual data (table) shows significantly greater numbers of health workers lost from 1996 to 2002. The University of Ghana Medical School, the School of Medical Sciences of the Kwame Nkrumah University of Science and Technology, and the University for Development Studies Medical School train about 150 medical officers annually. But half of every graduating class leaves the country within the second year, and 80 percent leaves by the fifth year.

This exodus of medical officers is mirrored in other health professions. Of 944 pharmacists trained between 1995 and 2002, 410 had left the country by the end of 2002. The problem is most severe among nurses and midwives: of the 10,145 nurses trained during that same period, 1,996 had left Ghana by the end of 2002. And only 12 medical laboratory technologists were being produced annually as of 2002, with no guarantee of their remaining in Ghana after graduation.

Loss of trained public sector health staff in Ghana, 1996–2002

Category	1996	1998	2000	2002
Doctors	1,154	1,132	1,015	964
Nurses (including auxiliaries)	14,932	15,046	13,742	11,325
Pharmacists	n.a.	n.a.	230	200

n.a. Not available

Source: Reference 7.

underuse of facilities—cautions against jumping to the conclusion that the size of health workforce stocks alone is the major human resources problem facing the health sector in developing countries.

GEOGRAPHIC IMBALANCES IN STOCKS MATTER Another concern is the geographic imbalance of stocks across rural and urban areas, poor and less poor regions, and types of institution. Dakar, the richest and most urban region of Senegal, is home to only 24 percent of Senegal's people, yet 65 percent of the country's physicians work there: there is one physician per 5,000 people.[11] By contrast,

the peripheral region of Kolda has just one physician per 86,000 people. The problem is replicated around the world.

THE MIX OF SKILLS, NOT JUST THE SKILLS THEMSELVES, MATTER The skills of the health workforce are often woefully inadequate. Misdiagnosis is commonplace: in Burundi in 1992 only 2 percent of children with diarrhea taken to health facilities were correctly diagnosed.[12] Mistreatment is also commonplace: in the same facilities in Burundi only 13 percent of children correctly diagnosed as having diarrheal disease were correctly rehydrated.[12] Even if the correct treatment is administered, there is no assurance that it will be administered successfully: in India in the early 1990s less than 45 percent of patients in public health facilities diagnosed with tuberculosis were successfully treated.[13]

It is not just the skills that matter, it is also the skills mix. Often, unskilled labor substitutes for skilled labor. A recent study in Tanzania estimated the required full-time equivalents for service provision according to national staffing norms for unskilled and skilled labor and compared these estimates with employed unskilled and skilled staff.[5] The study found an excess of unskilled labor of 5,000 full-time equivalents and a shortage of skilled labor of 8,000 full-time equivalents. One interpretation of this finding is that every fourth task that requires a skilled health professional is performed by an unskilled worker. The results of the ongoing human resources census in Tanzania and time-and-motion studies performed in public health facilities seem to bear this interpretation out.

APPLICATION TO THE JOB IS LOW IN MANY DEVELOPING COUNTRIES One obvious indicator of low application to the job is absenteeism. Recent random surveys of primary health facilities in six developing countries found absenteeism rates between 19 percent (Papua New Guinea) and 43 percent (India).[14] Low application manifests itself in other ways, too. In Tanzania time-and-motion studies showed overall staff productivity in public facilities as low as 57 percent.[5] On average, staff was absent in 7 percent of all observations. Only 37 percent of staff time was spent on patient care. An additional 10 percent of working time was spent on irregular breaks and social contacts. Staff productivity was found to be related to the demand for services, which in turn depended on the availability of drugs in rural facilities.

Low levels of application reduce technical quality and weaken patient confidence in the health system, leading to declining demand. A recent study in five West African countries identified impoliteness, lack of attention to patient needs, verbal and physical violence, corruption and nepotism, and informal fees as key causes for the poor reputation of public health services.[15]

Tackling health workforce issues—stocks and flows

The stock of human resources in health in a country at a particular time reflects the previous period's stock and the inflows and outflows that took place during the previous period (figure 7.3). The outflow includes migration abroad (see box 7.1 on the brain drain in Ghana), deaths of medical staff (see box 7.2 on the impact of HIV/AIDS on medical staff), exit from the medical profession for other occupations (ask a taxi driver in Havana about his or her former profession and chances are it will be medicine), and retirement (many countries in which the health workforce has been aging rapidly use early retirement inducements as a policy lever). For the public sector, outflows to the private sector are a major factor. Inflows reflect the numbers of newly trained staff being produced, the number of foreigners entering the health sector, and the number of health care workers returning from abroad or re-entering the profession.

While hard data are virtually nonexistent, many developing countries appear to face the double burden of low inflows and high outflows.[1,16–19] The Philippines loses three times more licensed nurses each year than it produces.[20–22] In The Gambia, the number of newly trained nurses and midwives is insufficient even to fill vacancies in the nation's main hospital.[6] A United Nations Conference on Trade and Development study estimated that 56 percent of all migrating physicians move from developing to industrial countries, while only 11 percent move in the opposite direction. The imbalance is even greater for nurses.[23]

TACKLING COMPENSATION Differentials in compensation—both wages and benefits such as housing—have repercussions for inflows and outflows of human resources in the health sector (box 7.3). Low wages in the medical professions relative to wages in other professions discourage

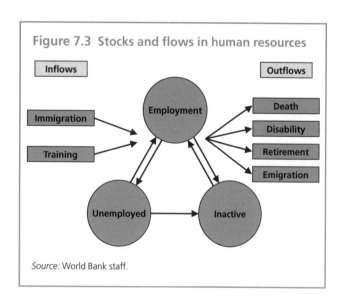

Figure 7.3 Stocks and flows in human resources

Source: World Bank staff.

Box 7.2 The devastating impact of HIV/AIDS on the health workforce

The HIV/AIDS epidemic is having a devastating impact on the stock of health workers, particularly in Africa. It has been estimated that HIV/AIDS accounts for 19–53 percent of all deaths among government staff in a typical African country. In several countries in Africa 25 percent of nurses are HIV positive. Studies of HIV prevalence among African healthcare workers suggest that doctors and nurses are at least as likely to become infected as other people. Health workers in Africa are significantly more likely to become infected with HIV than their peers in the industrial world: the HIV seroconversion risk among surgeons in Sub-Saharan Africa may be 15 times higher than in industrial countries.

Several country-specific examples confirm this bleak picture. In Botswana the share of health workers with AIDS rose from 0.3 percent in 1991 to 4 percent in 2003. By 2005 it is projected that 5 percent of healthcare workers will have HIV/AIDS and that 16 percent of healthcare workers will have died between 2003 and 2005. In Malawi deaths among nurses are equivalent to 40 percent of the annual output from nursing schools. In Mozambique the death rate of nurses tripled during the 1990s. In 2000, 20 percent of student nurses died from AIDS. In Zambia a study in two hospitals found that mortality rates among nurses rose from 2 per 1,000 deaths in 1980 to almost 27 per 1,000, largely as a result of AIDS.

Source: References 3, 24, and 25.

people from entering training institutions, from completing their studies, and from joining the profession if they graduate. They encourage people to think about leaving—by exiting the labor force, joining another profession, or leaving for another country where compensation is better.[26] Low levels of compensation encourage absenteeism, as health workers seek other earnings to supplement the earnings in their regular health sector job. This creates heavier workloads for those left behind and reduces motivation, prompting further absenteeism and exodus.

Compensation differentials across specialties influence specialization decisions during and after training.[27] Low rates of compensation in rural settings help explain rural-urban imbalances. And compensation differentials between the public and private sectors influence transitions from the public sector to the private sector—and occasionally back again.

Narrowing and even reversing compensation differentials is an important policy tool. Narrowing these differences—between healthcare and other professions, between the public and private sectors, between urban and rural areas, across countries—provides an opportunity to shift to a virtuous circle, by encouraging inflows and reducing outflows, absenteeism, and shirking. Thailand has attracted back med-

Box 7.3 Competing with the private sector in Bolivia

In Bolivia the basic pay of general physicians working in the public health system is $440 a month. Over the years, their salary increases by a maximum of $65 a month. Working in a deprived border area add another $85 to the monthly paycheck. At the same time, a single medical consultation in the private sector typically costs $10–$15 in major cities. With limited competition among private providers and the low costs of running a medical office, the large private-public salary differentials attract physicians into private practice, nullifying the monetary incentive to work in deprived border areas.

Source: Reference 35.

ical professionals through a reverse brain drain program offering generous research funding and monetary incentives.[28,29] In Zambia nursing salaries were more than doubled through the support of 16 development partners, including the European Union and the Danish and Swedish international development agencies. Several countries have experimented with bonus schemes for health workers in rural areas, some successfully.[29,30] Other countries allow public providers in rural areas to supplement their income through private practice during official working hours.[31,32] This can have disadvantages, as it is in the financial interest of public providers to lengthen waiting times and advise patients who are able to pay fees to seek private services.

Industrial countries can also help. They can raise wages at home to encourage the recruitment and retention of non-immigrant personnel, and they can provide development assistance to help developing countries raise wages to attract and retain staff. There are some signs that industrial countries are taking such steps. With growing evidence that low compensation makes recruitment and retention difficult,[26,33] the British government recently awarded nurses pay increases that were much greater than the rate of inflation.[34]

There are limits to what can be achieved through changes in compensation alone, however. Raising salaries in the developing world to the levels in industrial countries (even at purchasing power parity exchange rates) is simply unfeasible. Neither is using compensating wage differentials to keep staff in the public sector from moving to the private sector (box 7.3).

LOOKING BEYOND COMPENSATION Research suggests that nonpecuniary aspects of jobs matter to people. A recent study in India shows what health workers hope to get from their job and what they actually get (box 7.4). In Andhra Pradesh's public and private sectors, less than 40 percent of respondents felt that their current jobs provided a

good income. But having a good income was not what health workers said they aspired to most—especially workers in the private sector. Training opportunities; challenging work; relations with colleagues; a desirable location (including proximity to a good school, for example); and good physical working conditions all ranked higher than pay in both the public and private sectors. And many workers felt that their jobs did not meet expectations, especially for training opportunities.

People's job decisions do appear to reflect nonpecuniary factors.[26,27] A recent study in Uganda found that medical staff in religious nonprofit institutions are hired at below-market wages.[36] The authors suggested that this was probably due to the fact that these institutions provide more services to the poor than do other providers and more services with a public good element—dimensions of the job that presumably give health workers some satisfaction.

Pay, in short, isn't everything—what people can do in their jobs also matters. Countries could gain from better understanding the expectations that health workers have of their jobs and the degree to which these expectations are met. A recent six-country World Health Organization (WHO) study of factors that influence migration is a good example of a move in this direction.[38]

There are also encouraging signs that building policies around a better understanding of nonpecuniary motivations may work. A major reason why health professionals leave rural areas is the perceived unmet need for continuing education.[39] Retraining nurse practitioners turned out not to be very successful in Thailand, while on-the-job training in basic medical care for district hospital nurses proved to be both effective and sustainable.[28,29]

WHO YOU RECRUIT MATTERS People raised in rural areas are more likely to practice in rural locations and to choose family medicine.[40] Changing the admission criteria of training institutions can have a powerful impact on the number of physicians practicing in rural and underserved areas. Programs that targeted students based on their rural background and commitment to practice rural family medicine were able to successfully increase the physician workforce in rural areas. Family physicians seem more likely to practice in small and isolated areas.[41] Rural recruitment and training yielded some success in Thailand. Evidence suggests that the rural service of graduates lengthened, with two-thirds of graduates continuing to work in rural areas after their compulsory years of service.[28,29]

TRAINING HEALTHCARE WORKERS IN THE RIGHT SKILLS CAN HELP RETAIN THEM IN THE PUBLIC SECTOR Training opportunities are clearly valued by health workers. Training increases skills and

Box 7.4 What do health workers in India want most?

A recent study of motivation among health workers in the Indian state of Andhra Pradesh sheds light on the issue of staff morale (see figure).[37] What health workers in both the public and private sectors value most is a good working relationship with colleagues. And in both public and private sectors and in both states, a very high percentage (80 percent or so) of health workers feel that their current job provides this. Number two and three on the list of most valued job attributes are good working conditions and train-

ing opportunities to improve or learn new skills. On these issues, Indian health workers are less satisfied with their current jobs, especially with training. Although health workers in both states and in both sectors report earning less than they would like, a high income is not considered one of the most valued job attributes. Frustration over the discrepancy between actual and desired income is felt equally in both the public and private sectors.

What health workers in Andhra Pradesh want from their job—and whether they are getting it

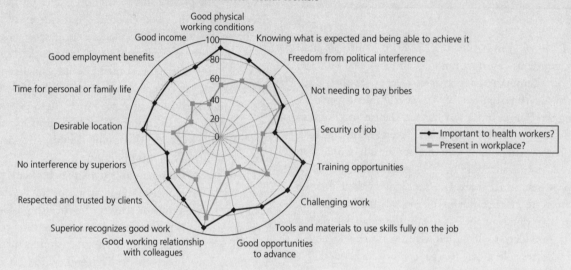

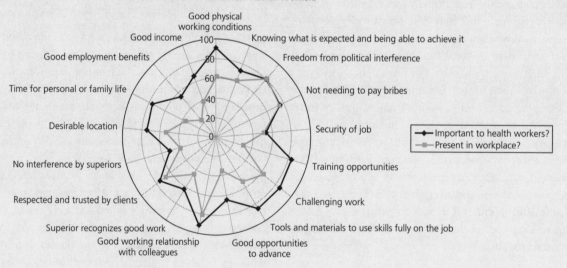

Source: Reference 37.

motivation. It is, however, a double-edged sword—training makes health workers more marketable and more likely to leave the public sector for the private sector or for other countries. This is an old problem in economics.[42] The standard way around it is to focus government spending on developing specific skills and to let health workers themselves pay—in the form of lower wages—for any general training. Such a policy seems sensible in the light of the emerging evidence on poaching and international migration of health workers. The countries that have emulated the training standards of industrial countries (such as Ghana) have been most vulnerable to poaching by them.[14] In Ethiopia and The Gambia community nurses and health officers who lack internationally recognized qualifications are less likely to migrate than those who have them.[14]

Training in areas of relevance to the Millennium Development Goals is a good example of specialized training that is unlikely to be especially valued in industrial countries. The competent training of the Integrated Management of Childhood Illness (IMCI) initiative is a case in point. It seeks to improve provider skills in the management of childhood illness, notably in the treatment of the major killers of children under five; in the delivery of preventive measures, such as immunization; and in imparting advice and counseling on feeding practices and protective behaviors.[43,44] The treatment guidelines and training methodology were developed and refined through research and field testing in numerous countries, including Bangladesh, The Gambia, Ethiopia, Kenya, Tanzania, and Uganda.[45–48] The quality of care provided by health workers trained in this methodology has been found to be significantly better than that provided by nontrained health workers in several settings. In Tanzania trained providers were twice as likely to prescribe antibiotics appropriately. In Bolivia trained providers were 10 times more likely to recognize the danger signs of a sick child. And in Niger health workers' performance (tested against the IMCI algorithm) increased 34–85 percent after training.[49–51]

REALIGNING THE SKILLS MIX CAN ALSO HELP Many Millennium Development Goal interventions can be delivered by lower-skill providers. Community health workers, for example, are providing more maternal and child health and nutrition services. (Box 6.8 on Céara describes an example of successful skill mix realignment.) A recent study estimates that at high levels of coverage, some 90 percent of full-time equivalent staff required to provide interventions related to childhood diseases in Tanzania fall into the categories of nursing and midwifery skills and unskilled labor.[52] An additional attraction of lower-skill health workers is that they are more likely to be willing to work in rural areas and less likely to be lured away by the private sector, urban provider organizations, and foreign health sectors.

Medicines and other health supplies

Medicines and other health commodities are key elements of effective interventions against child and maternal mortality and deaths from communicable diseases (see figures 3.2 and 3.3). Increased use in the developing world of good-quality vaccines, vitamin and mineral supplements, antibiotics, antimalarials, and tuberculosis and HIV/AIDS drugs would substantially reduce mortality if used rationally. So would use of insecticide-treated bednets, condoms, and other health supplies. The successful release and widespread use of medicines still under development could reduce mortality rates still further. Given this potential contribution to human health, it would be surprising if medicines were not the subject of an important array of policy issues.

What are the policy and implementation issues?

DRUGS AND OTHER SUPPLIES ARE ABSENT IN MANY FRONTLINE FACILITIES It is not just health workers who are often absent from facilities. So are drugs and other supplies (box 7.5). This is problematic—studies have shown repeatedly that when drugs are available, patients have more confidence in the public health system

---

Box 7.5 Lack of drugs threatens the Millennium Development Goals

Acute respiratory infections are one of the leading killers of children under five, accounting for about one in five deaths among children in this age group.[53] The survival of children with acute respiratory infections depends to a large extent on the availability and appropriate use of effective antibiotics. Data from health facility surveys conducted in 21 countries during 1992–97 showed that in some countries less than 30 percent of health facilities had first-line antibiotics for acute respiratory infections. The median for all 21 countries was 79 percent.[12]

In Côte d'Ivoire in 1987–88, 24 percent of rural facilities surveyed did not have antibiotics in stock, and 42 percent did not have vaccines in stock.[10] A report for the Burkina Faso Poverty Reduction Strategy Paper found that nearly 20 percent of facilities had run out of essential vaccines and that 24 percent of centers had refrigerators for storing the vaccines that did not function. In Tanzania, with its donor-funded vertically organized essential drugs program, the picture looks fairly good: 89 percent of facilities had measles vaccines in stock, 88 percent had tetanus toxoid vaccines, 86 percent had BCG vaccines for tuberculosis, and 84 percent had diphtheria, pertussis, and tetanus vaccines.[54]

---

and in government. The availability of pharmaceuticals has also been shown to motivate health professionals.

INFORMATION ASYMMETRIES LEAVE PATIENTS VULNERABLE Providers and drug vendors have a huge information advantage over patients, who are vulnerable to prescriptions of inappropriate, substandard, and counterfeit drugs (boxes 7.6 and 7.7). This asymmetry makes reliance on financial incentives to get drugs into facilities highly problematic. Informational asymmetries pose multiple challenges and suggest the need for regulation (of providers, retailers, distributors, and manufacturers) and behavior change (for patients but also for providers and retailers).

HIGH DRUG COSTS DETER EFFECTIVE USE OF DRUGS The cost of medicines can be a large part of the overall costs of treatment. As with other medical expenses, the uncertainty surrounding the need to incur drug expenses makes insurance coverage attractive. The high out-of-pocket spending on drugs in many developing countries reflects a lack of effective insurance arrangements or the lack of coverage of drugs in insurance schemes that are operating.

The high cost of drugs creates another problem as well. The medicines used to prevent and treat communicable diseases are associated with positive externalities—their

---

Box 7.6 Inappropriate or "irrational" drug use

A potentially large—and perhaps increasing—share of household spending on drugs is likely to be at best wasteful and at worst hazardous to health. Studies have indicated that 30–60 percent of patients in primary healthcare centers receive antibiotics—perhaps twice what is clinically needed. Fifteen billion injections are administered each year. Half of them are not sterile, and a large share are unnecessary.[55] It has been estimated that if Integrated Management of Childhood Illness guidelines were followed in Uganda, the number of drugs prescribed per consultation would fall sharply and the cost per consultation would drop from $0.82 to $0.17.

The consequences of inappropriate drug use are not just economic. They include increased drug resistance. A recent study reported significant increases in penicillin-resistant *Streptococcus pneumonia*, one of the most important pathogens associated with acute respiratory infections. Rates of resistance range from zero to 60 percent in developing countries, with the highest rates in South America, Sub-Saharan Africa, and parts of Asia, such as Hong Kong (China), China, and the Republic of Korea.[56]

Box 7.7 The problem of counterfeit drugs

Counterfeit drugs are a widespread global problem and a serious threat to health in developing countries. The spread of counterfeit drugs is facilitated by weak institutional regulatory structures in many developing countries and the ease of copying many drugs. According to the International Federation of Pharmaceutical Manufacturers Association (IFPMA), 7 percent of drugs sold globally are counterfeit. Counterfeiting drugs can involve changes in the active ingredients, dosage, package inserts, packaging, manufacturers' names, batch numbers, expiration dates, and documentation related to quality controls. Counterfeit drugs are associated with a spectrum of medical risks (table).

A recent editorial in the *British Medical Journal*[57] reviewed the evidence on counterfeit drugs in developing countries. A bleak picture emerged. A recent survey in the Philippines showed that 8 percent of drugs were fake.[57] In Cambodia a study found that 60 percent of drug vendors sold antimalarial tablets from stock that should have been destroyed or fakes with no active ingredient. A recent survey of mainland Southeast Asia reported that 38 percent of tablets sold as the new antimalarial drug artesunate were fakes.[57] And the list goes on.

Medical risks associated with counterfeit drugs

Type of counterfeit drug	Associated medical risk
Perfect imitation—the same active ingredients and packaging as the real drug	Limited, assuming that the quality is good
Inadequate imitation—the same active ingredient but of insufficient quality and quantity	Reduced efficacy and, in the case of antibiotics, development of pathogen resistance
"Placebo"—looks like a real drug, but contains no active ingredient	Lack of efficacy
Poisonous—contains harmful or poisonous substances	Physical injury or death

Source: Reference 57.

---

consumption by one person benefits other people as well, by reducing their risk of infection. This makes subsidization appropriate, since the price set by the market would be too high and use rates of externality-generating medicines too low.

Beyond insurance and externality arguments is an equity argument. Universal access to medicines—especially life-saving ones—is a principle that commands much support (it was endorsed in the 2001 Doha

Declaration on Trade-Related Aspects of Intellectual Property Rights, or TRIPS, and Public Health). Universal access might be interpreted to mean that poor and near-poor households ought to pay a low price even for medicines that involve no externality, so that the cost does not deter them from getting necessary medicines or push them into (or further into) poverty (boxes 7.8 and 7.9). This provides a rationale for governments seeking to influence—at least for poor and near-poor households—the retail price of all drugs, not just those used to prevent and treat communicable diseases. They have a variety of instruments at their disposal.

Because governments end up footing a sizable share of a country's drug bill, they have an interest in the price they pay for drugs, as well as in the quality and quantity of drugs dispensed. Through strategic purchasing, governments can exert a substantial influence on the price they pay for drugs. Governments also have several means to influence prescribing behavior and use patterns.

PATENTS AND THE PAUCITY OF R&D ON DISEASES AFFECTING PEOPLE IN DEVELOPING COUNTRIES LIMIT TREATMENT OPTIONS The use of patents to provide incentives for research and devel-

Box 7.8 Do we know how affordable drugs really are?

Despite the importance of drug prices, little is known about the prices people pay for medicines in developing counties. A new approach to measuring drug prices focuses on a range of 30 key medicines that address the global disease burden, particularly for low- and middle-income countries.[58] Several of these drugs—including antibacterial medicines, such as co-trimoxazole pediatric suspension for treatment of acute respiratory infection in children under five, and antimalarials, such as artesunate and pyrimethamine with sulfadoxine—are relevant to the Millennium Development Goals.

The preliminary results of surveys based on this new approach show that in South Africa the price that the lowest-paid government worker needs to pay to afford a course of treatment with amoxicillin (an antibacterial drug) in the private sector is between half a day's and a day and a half's wages, depending on the type of amoxicillin used.[59] In Armenia the lowest-paid government worker had to work for 148 days to pay for a course of treatment with branded aciclovir, an antiviral drug. The same money would be enough to pay for enough rice or sugar for 10 years. The use of a generic drug reduced the price by 40 percent but still left it unaffordable for most people. In Kazakhstan surveys found that the prices of only 4 of 85 drugs were lower than the international median.[60]

Box 7.9 High drug costs in Vietnam deter use and cause impoverishment

In Vietnam in 1993 a single visit to a public hospital by a member of a household in the poorest fifth of the population resulted in outlays on medicines equivalent to 40 percent of the household's annual nonfood consumption (discretionary income) (see figure). A single visit to a commune health center resulted in a bill for drugs equal to 11 percent of the household's annual nonfood consumption.

Not surprisingly, a large number of Vietnamese—3 million people according to one estimate[61]—were pushed into poverty as a result of high out-of-pocket payments for healthcare, much of it attributable to drug expenditures. Households in Vietnam appear to have been deterred from using health services because of high drug costs: having insurance coverage for drugs and inpatient care has a substantial positive effect on the use of hospital care.[62,63]

The high cost of drugs in Vietnam, by source, 1993 and 1998

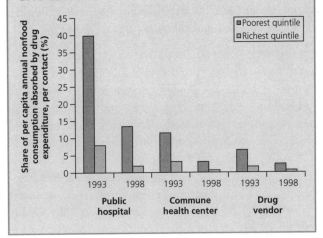

opment (R&D) leaves many key drugs beyond the financial reach of poor countries. The extension of the patent period to 20 years under the TRIPS agreement (even the United States, with its robust patent system, previously had only a 17-year period) made this problem worse. These concerns have led to heated debate, brinkmanship by some developing country governments, and exemptions for public health crises.

The concerns, it should be noted, currently apply to relatively few drugs, since most drugs on WHO's Essential Drug List (the most cost-effective therapies for a broad list of diseases) are off-patent in all countries. But as resistance to some essential medicines increases, replacements are being developed. These new treatments will be unaffordable to developing countries. In 2002, for example, the cost for the antimalarial drug chloroquine was $0.10 per treatment.

But resistance to chloroquine is growing in many parts of the world, and alternative treatments are far more expensive—30 times more for coartem and 400 times for malarone. Similarly the six-month treatment under the directly observed treatment, short-course (DOTS) regimen for people with tuberculosis is $20, while the newer multidrug therapy treatment is $400.[64]

Another concern is the low levels of R&D for drug treatment of "neglected" diseases—diseases that disproportionately or exclusively affect poor countries, with effective demand that is too limited to make R&D profitable. The facts are striking. Global expenditure on health R&D has risen significantly and continues to rise. Yet of the 1,393 new drugs approved between 1975 and 1999, only 16 (just over 1 percent) were specifically developed for tropical diseases and tuberculosis—diseases that account for 11.4 percent of the global disease burden but which are disproportionately concentrated among poorer populations.[65] By contrast, 179 new drugs were developed for cardiovascular diseases.[65]

What are the options for getting drugs and other supplies to the frontline and enhancing treatment practices?

CHANGING BEHAVIOR AMONG CONSUMERS AND PROVIDERS Providing health education (information on dosage and mode of administration) to patients and building trust between patients (and their caregivers) and prescribers (particularly as part of DOTS) have proved successful in addressing low patient compliance as well as high levels of self-medication.[66] Group discussions with mothers, training seminars for providers at the community level, and districtwide monitoring have reduced the use of "irrational" injections in children.[67] Treatment guidelines and training and continuing education for health providers on the use of drugs are also potentially useful tools.

IMPROVING THE MANAGEMENT CHAIN TO GET THE DRUGS TO THE FRONT LINE In the retail sector in the industrial world, supply-chain costs are as low as 3–6 percent of the cost of goods sold in the grocery sector and 6–8 percent in the retail sector. In healthcare, supply-chain costs are as high as 38 percent of the cost of goods. Some of this reflects a lack of continued investment in healthcare supply chains, resulting in manually controlled logistics systems with considerable paper shuffling, lengthy order and delivery cycle times, excessive inventory, multiple product handling activities, lack of information sharing among trading partners, and an operational rather than a customer focus.[68] Few of these problems are limited to the logistics sector. One study estimates that because of waste and inefficiencies in drug selection and procurement, only

12 percent of government spending allocated to the purchase of drugs in Africa is used effectively.[69]

The management chain can be improved, however. Key measures include:

- moving the logistics functions from the backroom to the boardroom, recognizing that it is a core function that needs to be strategically managed and invested

- putting computerized information management systems in place that gather timely consumption and stock data and using information to drive the system

- preparing annual forecasts and revising them semiannually

- negotiating better purchase prices through group purchasing organizations

- strategically managing distribution by reducing intermediate distribution points and outsourcing the distribution

- establishing key performance measures to continually assess the performance of the system

- focusing on driving down the total delivered cost, rather than the unit cost[70]

All of this is doable. In Ghana, as part of the Strategies for Enhancing Access to Medicines (SEAM) initiative funded by the Bill and Melinda Gates Foundation, a portion of the drug distribution system was extensively reformed to improve the use of medicines by mission hospitals. The effort has included dovetailing pharmaceutical distribution with other proven logistics systems (such as social marketing).

CREATING INCENTIVES TO ENCOURAGE RESPONSIBLE PRESCRIBING Behavior change programs for providers and retailers will have only limited effects if there are strong economic incentives not to be responsible in prescribing drugs. An extreme example is that of doctors in Georgia, who contributed to the spread of drug-resistant tuberculosis (box 7.10). Prescribing DOTS drugs to tuberculosis patients offers the doctors, who are paid just $50 a month, no additional income, since the drugs are provided free by the German government. Instead, the doctors prescribe a cocktail of other drugs, at a cost of $300–400 a month, causing patients to develop multidrug-resistant tuberculosis. This is a classic example of a well-intentioned policy—to protect the poor from drug costs—that has not been thought through. If irresponsible prescribing is to be deterred, providers have to have a financial incentive to prescribe responsibly. This can be done through a voucher scheme in which patients present the provider with a voucher (usable only for

Twenty-three-year-old Gia is thin, and his eyes shine with fever. "Please tell me, isn't there anything to get rid of this heat?" he asks, sitting hunched on a bench in a damp hall in the Abastumani hospital, 1,500 meters high in Georgia's forested mountains. "A thousand paracetamol won't get rid of this temperature."

Gia and his fellow patients are hoping to be cured of tuberculosis, but they are at the center of a public health disaster that threatens Europe with a deadly form of tuberculosis resistant to standard drug regimens, the so-called multidrug-resistant tuberculosis. To blame is the treatment these patients receive in places like Abastumani, 125 miles west of the capital Tbilisi.

Gia had to sell his apartment, leaving his wife and two-year-old son homeless, to pay for a cure at the hospital after more than three years of treatment elsewhere failed to rid him of his cough, night sweats, and crushing fatigue. He now rests in a wing of the run-down hospital. The myth of fresh, mountain air as a cure for tuberculosis still holds among Georgia's 4 million people. The Soviet system once supported a large network of such hospitals, which allowed patients to convalesce for two years or more. The system was rich in time but poor in medication, giving only a small fraction of patients the antituberculosis drugs with proven efficacy.

In the chaos that followed Georgia's independence and the conflicts that racked the country between 1991 and 1994, the tuberculosis notification rate tripled, from 29 new cases for every 100,000 people in 1988 to 89 in 2001. To combat the disease, in 1995 Georgia adopted the World Health Organization's standard strategy—the directly observed treatment, short-course (DOTS).

Widely promoted in the developing world, DOTS is a simple regimen of four to five drugs taken three times a week for at least six months under the observation of trained staff who make sure that the medicine is taken properly. Finishing the course is essential, as patients often feel better after a month or so, stop taking their drugs, and promptly relapse with a tougher strain of tuberculosis that is resistant to standard DOTS medicines.

The hospital's director, Tariel Endeladze, is an enthusiastic convert to the DOTS regimen. But the collapse of Georgia's healthcare system means that the misuse of antituberculosis drugs is widespread. The government has no money to pay its nurses and doctors, it cannot afford health education, and the market in pharmaceuticals is unregulated.

Recognizing tuberculosis as a disease of poverty, the DOTS strategy requires the treatment to be free. The German government has been donating antituberculosis drugs to Georgia since 1995. Dr. Endeladze said patients did not pay for their treatment at Abastumani, but nearly all the patients interviewed said they were paying far more than the $50 it costs to treat a patient with a standard course of DOTS. Gia and others said they paid $300–$400 a month for treatment, a small fortune in a country where a doctor's monthly salary—if it is paid—is $50.

With cash rather than cure on many impoverished doctors' minds, the uncontrolled distribution of antituberculosis drugs has created the perfect breeding ground for multidrug-resistant tuberculosis, dubbed "ebola with wings" by a Harvard medical school study. Annabel Baddeley, manager in Georgia of the British aid agency Merlin, which is working to adapt DOTS to Georgia's rural areas, said that unpaid doctors were one of the greatest threats to health there. "Doctors will charge tuberculosis patients who come to them without referring them to the specialized tuberculosis facilities and treat them for 'pneumonia' or 'bronchitis' with one or two tuberculosis drugs when they should be using four or five. The patients will then eventually find their way to the tuberculosis facilities with advanced tuberculosis, having developed drug resistance as part of the unnecessarily expensive package they've paid for."

Patients like Gia are also being treated incorrectly at Abastumani with drugs usually reserved for treatment of multidrug-resistant tuberculosis, worsening the resistance problem and condemning those infected with tuberculosis to years of debilitating illness or death as second-line drugs such as kanamycin lose their potency. Treatment for multidrug-resistant tuberculosis is about 100 times more expensive than standard DOTS. The World Health Organization will not sanction the use of second-line drugs until the standard strategy is up and running, leaving patients like Gia without treatment. They could go on to infect 15 people in a year.

Reliable statistics are hard to come by in Georgia, but tuberculosis specialists estimate that as many as 10 percent of new patients with tuberculosis and up to 25 percent of patients being retreated for the disease could have multidrug-resistant tuberculosis. The structural health problems that created this crisis in Georgia are repeated in almost all the former Soviet states.

Source: Reference 74.

approved drugs), which the provider takes to a payer (possibly a donor) to convert into cash.

OTHER INCENTIVES MATTER, TOO Better prescription and management are important. But without institutional arrangements that give the right incentives to all parties involved in drug distribution and prescription, availability will improve only marginally. Part of the reason—sometimes a major part—why facilities lack drugs is that providers have little incentive to have drugs there. Sometimes drugs are

absent because they have been "borrowed" by providers: surveys in Uganda suggest that an average of 70 percent of medical supplies and drugs in public facilities were appropriated by staff for use in their private work.[71–73] Where providers have an incentive to have drugs available, they often are. In China, where providers and retailers make much of their income from selling drugs, drugs are readily available—the public policy challenges are to reduce the prescription of inappropriate and unsafe drugs and to make drugs more affordable. The same story emerges in Georgia (box 7.10).

The drawback to creating incentives to prescribe drugs, of course, is that inappropriate or poor-quality drugs will be prescribed. Creating regulation and behavior change programs to limit this response is not impossible, but it is not easy. It is almost certainly unwise to try to solve the drug availability problem by providing financial incentives to prescribe drugs. There may, however, be scope for changing the incentive arrangements in the distribution of drugs. Some countries have contracted out the distribution of medicines to the private sector. Doing so may yield efficiency gains (evaluations do not appear to have been undertaken).

REGULATING DRUGS According to the WHO, an effective drug regulatory system ought to include a full drug registration process, unbiased drug information, oversight of promotional activities, post-approval drug safety monitoring, quality-control testing, pharmaceutical inspection services, and certified compliance with good manufacturing practices.[75] Just one in three drug regulatory agencies works effectively in developing countries, as became clear in a recent WHO study of pharmaceutical regulation in Australia, Cuba, Cyprus, Estonia, Malaysia, the Netherlands, Tunisia, Uganda, Venezuela, and Zimbabwe.[76]

Some countries, such as the Lao People's Democratic Republic, have no formal drug regulatory agency. Others require only a notification from the manufacturer or importer in order to market the product, not authorization from a regulatory agency. On paper Nigeria has an appropriate formal system: market authorization requires evidence of safety and efficacy, and samples of the product must be regularly analyzed. But implementation is usually weak because of lack of human and financial resources. Guyana applies a reasonable, pragmatic approach, making authorization dependent on proof of registration by a drug regulatory agency in Australia, Canada, the United States, or the United Kingdom.

Developing countries will not be able to set up a drug regulatory agency with the resources and capacity of the U.S. Food and Drug Administration or the European Medicines Agency. But almost all countries should be able to set up a drug regulatory agency that can handle the most essential functions in an efficient, transparent, and affordable way. One important policy issue is whether the agency should be a department of the ministry of health or an independent agency. An independent status is assumed to allow the drug regulatory agency to perform its functions without political interference. There can, however, be disadvantages in having an autonomous drug regulatory agency. Badan POM, Indonesia's drug regulatory agency, once a department of the Ministry of Health, is now directly accountable to the President's Office. But lines of authority are not clear, resulting in dysfunctional competi-

tion between the two organizations. An autonomous entity might not be an efficient option for small and very poor countries. In such cases, countries could rely on international or regional mechanisms, such as the WHO Certification Scheme, created in 1975 to help small importing countries gain access to relevant information and establish minimum safeguards. More recently the WHO, supported by several UN organizations and the World Bank, launched a pilot procurement initiative to prequalify manufacturers of HIV-AIDS drugs.

INSURANCE POLICIES ON DRUG PRICES AND DRUG SPENDING Drug costs are often not covered or only partly covered by insurance (box 7.11). Whether the exclusion of outpatient drug costs makes sense is debatable. It makes sense for insurance to focus on high-cost, low-frequency costs, such as expensive inpatient drug treatment. But not covering outpatient drug costs may deter people from taking preventive measures and seeking care from a low-level provider as soon as they fall ill. They may well get even sicker later and end up in a hospital, incurring large bills against which they are fully insured. The result may be higher costs for the entire insurance scheme. The fact that private insurers in countries like the United States cover drug expenses likely reflects a belief that covering certain preventive measures and outpatient-administered medicines lowers overall costs.

DRUG PRICES AND THE ROLE OF GOVERNMENT Governments have ways of influencing drug prices—both the prices they (and ultimately taxpayers) pay when they subsidize the cost of drugs and the prices consumers pay out of pocket. Governments can exert a direct influence by regulating retail prices through fixed prices, risk-sharing agreements, and reference-based pricing schemes. In China, where the majority of drugs are purchased from retailers, a sizable fraction of drugs are sold at a regulated price.

Governments can influence retail prices indirectly through policies affecting the domestic pharmaceutical industry (antitrust regulation, profit controls, incentives to encourage market entry by new competitors) and foreign trade. The large increase in affordability of drugs in Vietnam between 1993 and 1998 (see box 7.9) was due largely to deregulating the pharmaceutical industry and opening the sector to international trade. These two measures resulted in a 33 percent decline in real terms in the medical price index.[63] Governments can also influence retail prices indirectly by making large bulk purchases from manufacturers and then selling drugs at wholesale prices to the private nonprofit sector, as the governments of Ethiopia, Ghana, Malawi, Tanzania, Uganda, Zambia, and Zimbabwe do.[81]

In Hungary drugs are free of charge or reimbursed at 50 percent, 70 percent, or 90 percent, depending on patient characteristics. Generic products on the pharmaceutical benefits list are reimbursed at 90 percent of the price. People on public assistance and those with chronic diseases receive free drugs, or they are reimbursed at 90 percent.[77]

Estonia has had a drug reimbursement system since 1993 for pharmaceuticals purchased from outpatient pharmacies. There is a mandatory patient copayment for each purchase of drugs. All prescription drugs exceeding the patient's copayment are covered by at least a 50 percent reimbursement. The reimbursement rate increases up to 90 percent or 100 percent for medicines on a list of more serious diseases, in which case the copayment is also lower.[77]

Since July 1997 in Albania only children under the age of one, war veterans, and people with disabilities receive a full subsidy for essential drugs.[77]

In Lithuania drug costs are fully covered for inpatient care but are not covered for the majority of the population for outpatient care.[77]

In Azerbaijan drugs are free of charge for inpatient care but not for outpatient care, except for people with cancer and some psychiatric diseases.

In Indonesia drugs are provided free of charge to specific groups—poor families, schoolchildren, people with disabilities, the elderly, government officials, and public enterprise employees and their families—through primary health centers and public hospitals.[78] People not included in any medical insurance system have to pay for drugs obtained from public or private facilities.[79]

In Nepal drugs are distributed free of charge in public health facilities. Large hospitals, managed by semi-autonomous hospital management committees, can sell drugs at either subsidized or full price.

In Myanmar cost-sharing drug shops have opened in hospitals, with 43 drug items supplied by the Central Medical Stores Depot (CMSD). Drugs are sold at a maximum 15 percent profit margin over the CMSD price. The CMSD cost of drugs has to be returned to the government budget from the proceeds of sales.[79]

In Guatemala the Ministry of Health provides drugs free of charge in primary or secondary health centers and hospitals. In 2001 almost 70 percent of the population had access to essential drugs.[80]

Ghana is currently scaling up for a national health insurance scheme that will include limited coverage for pharmaceuticals.

Source: World Bank staff.

Whether governments sell such drugs to the private sector or keep them for use or sale in their own facilities, they can exert a major influence over drug prices by engaging in strategic purchasing. One issue is whom to purchase from. In the past many governments relied heavily on their own domestic industry. Considerations of economies of scale, however, point to purchasing from multinational companies—or at least from domestic affiliates of multinational companies. Today developing countries seem to be relying less and less on domestic manufacturers, whose share of world pharmaceutical production decreased from 11 percent in 1985 to 7 percent in 1999. A few cases buck this trend. Cuba's industry has been highly innovative, bringing $100 million a year in export earnings. And Brazil recently fell back successfully on its domestic industry to make credible a threat to invoke a compulsory license to produce its own antiretrovirals unless significant price concessions were made by the research-based global pharmaceutical industry (they were). But there are also plenty of failures, with governments wasting scarce revenues supporting uncompetitive domestic industries.[82]

The second issue is whom to purchase with. Governments can increase their monopsony (single buyer) power by getting donors to engage in pooled procurement with the government (box 7.12). Governments can increase their bargaining power still further by joining forces with other governments to set up a multinational purchasing pool. The scope for putting downward pressure on drug prices is very large.

The third issue is what governments should purchase. A major choice is between brand name drugs and generics. Since generics are sold under an international nonproprietary name, there is limited scope for product differentiation and much greater scope for competition. This puts downward pressure on the prices not only of generic drugs but also of brand drugs. If the generic and the brand drug are therapeutically equivalent, quality should not need to be compromised. Drugs not subject to any exclusive marketing rights, patents or otherwise, such as most of the drugs on the WHO's Essential Drug List, are the obvious target of a generics policy.

SUBSIDIZING DRUGS Many drugs—even those for communicable diseases—are not subsidized, in part because of budget constraints in developing countries. According to the WHO, a regular supply of "essential" drugs would cost at least $5 per capita per year.[79] This is beyond the means of many developing countries—many spend this much on all healthcare costs. Donors can help

Box 7.12 The attractions of pooled procurement

In Mozambique drug imports are financed largely by donor assistance. In the past a lack of coordination in drug procurement resulted in huge inefficiencies.[83] The government determined which types and quantities of drugs to purchase only after a donor had allocated a specific amount of finance. This resulted in unpredictable funding, erratic purchasing cycles, difficulties with long-term planning, and tied donations that resulted in frequent stockouts and expiring drugs. Decisions on what and how much to buy were offer driven, and drug imports expanded or shrank according to donor financing. After several agencies pushed for restructuring based on the Ministry of Health's specification of needs, in 1997/98 donors pooled their funds and responded to the government's priority. Currently, seven donors are making multiyear commitments to a common pool for drugs.

The benefits of pooled purchasing are also illustrated by the use of multinational purchasing pools for HIV drugs in the Americas. Almost 2 million people in Latin America and the Caribbean are living with HIV/AIDS, according to Joint United Nations Program on HIV/AIDS (UNAIDS) figures.[84] The Caribbean, where about 500,000 people are living with HIV/AIDS, has the second-highest HIV prevalence rate in the world after Sub-Saharan Africa. The high cost of antiretroviral drugs to treat HIV/AIDS makes it difficult for patients to pay for the drugs and for public and private insurance to make treatment affordable. Negotiated agreements between ministries of health and pharmaceutical companies reduced the prices of antiretroviral drugs in Latin America and the Caribbean,[85] but the prices were still high compared with generic prices in countries like India. There were also wide differences between countries, with some countries paying up to 10 times more for the same treatment.

Analysis of the negotiations for HIV/AIDS drugs suggests that regional pooling procurement benefits not only countries with small markets, high need, lack of private insurance, and lack of a pharmaceutical industry, such as countries in Central America and the Caribbean, but also countries with large markets and an established pharmaceutical industry, such as Argentina, Colombia, and Mexico. The use of generic manufacturers prequalified by the WHO allowed for greater price competition and further reduction of prices.

The Rockefeller Foundation, Management Sciences for Health, and the South Center recently identified lessons from pooled procurement initiatives in Latin America and the Caribbean, the Middle East and North Africa, and Sub-Saharan Africa.[86] The analysis identified several success factors: political will and organizational commitment, adherence to a single purchasing agreement, secure and trustworthy finance and payment mechanisms, a permanent and autonomous procurement secretariat, harmonization and standardization, good pharmaceutical procurement practices, and effective quality assurance.

Pooled procurement is more likely to succeed if pool members share similar economic, regulatory, and cultural backgrounds. Currency, language, and a harmonized drug registration procedure seem to be key factors of success. Two regional groups were identified with significant potential for expansion: the Association Africaine des Centrals d'Achats de Médicaments Essentiels and the Commonwealth Regional Health Community and Southern African Development Community. Each organization has 16 member countries, with 12 countries belonging to both organizations. The expected next steps are to agree and formally request assistance for funding proposal development.

Source: World Bank staff.

---

governments meet the cost of providing free or subsidized drugs. Between 1999 and 2002, $400 million in World Bank loans was spent on pharmaceuticals and other medical goods. In Tajikistan external donations accounted for more than 40 percent of pharmaceutical expenditures in 1998.[77] This level of support is clearly not sustainable (see chapter 4 on financing issues).

The long-term solution is to set priorities for government health spending so that sufficient funds are available to subsidize activities that genuinely warrant a subsidy (such as medicines against communicable diseases) and to scale back spending on programs of lower priority or programs for which government spending is not indicated or is poorly targeted. Donor finance to cover recurrent drug costs should be time limited, tied to policies that support the development of a robust and sustainable pharmaceutical system, and linked to support for the reallocation of government spending. The World Bank's recent Kyrgyzstan

Health Sector Reform project set out to do precisely this: accompanying the $6.9 million four-year loan were a series of promised policy reforms, including strengthening the government's drug regulatory capabilities and improving the cost-effectiveness of public financing.[77]

PATENTS, TRIPS, AND THE AFFORDABILITY OF NEW DRUGS The strengthening of patent rights under TRIPS led to concerns that new drugs would become even less affordable to developing countries. In November 2001 WTO ministers announced the Doha Declaration on TRIPS and Public Health, stating, "We affirm that the Agreement can and should be interpreted and implemented in a manner supportive of a WTO member's right to protect public health and, in particular, to promote access to medicines for all." Under this interpretation of article 31(f) of the TRIPS Agreement, countries with a public health crisis can forgo patent law and issue a compulsory license to a local manufacturer. But since most developing countries lack the domestic capacity and technical expertise to manufacture on-patent pharmaceuticals, interpretation of what this meant became the subject of a global pharmaceutical policy debate. In August 2003 it was agreed that countries without the capacity to manufacture medicines could still use compulsory licensing by contracting-out agreements with firms in other countries. So far the provision has been invoked only to increase the supply of antiretroviral therapy globally.

The August 2003 provision should encourage competition and make antiretrovirals more affordable to the developing world, but the administrative intricacies of implementing the compulsory licensing provision are likely to prove cumbersome for most developing countries. An additional route to making antiretrovirals affordable is the Accelerating Access Initiative (box 7.13).

PUSH AND PULL FOR R&D TO DEAL WITH NEGLECTED DISEASES One way out of this impasse is to separate R&D from drug manufacturing and sales.[89] Industrial countries, donors, or foundations would commit to purchase—for a sizable fee—any patents resulting from the development of a major new vaccine or drug and to make the patent freely available to drug manufacturers. This would increase the incentive to engage in R&D on diseases for which effective demand for drugs is limited (push), while allowing the drug to be sold at marginal cost immediately after approval (pull). Another approach is the global public-private partnership known as the International AIDS Vaccine Initiative (box 7.14). And Médecins sans Frontières is leading a global initiative that would encourage research and development of drug therapies for most neglected diseases by developing countries themselves.

Box 7.13 The Accelerating Access Initiative for antiretroviral drugs

The Accelerating Access Initiative, launched in May 2000 by five UN agencies and five pharmaceutical companies,[87] aims to address the high cost of antiretroviral drugs and to increase access to HIV/AIDS care and treatment. The initiative was structured into working groups for country support, communications, and procurement. UN agencies offered technical support on planning for the care and support of people living with HIV/AIDS, particularly on how to increase access to antiretroviral drugs. The countries then negotiated with pharmaceutical companies in discussions facilitated by the UN agencies.

By May 2002, 80 countries had expressed an interest in the initiative, and 39 countries had developed or were developing national plans to improve the care of people living with HIV/AIDS. Also by May 2002, 19 countries had reached agreements with the pharmaceutical companies to supply their antiretroviral drugs at significantly reduced cost. The countries agreed to waive import taxes and duties on the drugs. Some countries have also introduced generic antiretroviral drugs at competitive prices.

By December 2002 the cost of the drugs offered by the pharmaceutical companies in the Accelerating Access Initiative had decreased substantially, in some cases to 10–20 percent of their price in industrial countries. In the 19 countries that reached agreements with the pharmaceutical companies, 27,000 people had gained access to antiretroviral treatment, almost 10 times the number of patients treated before the agreements. Despite these efforts, however, less than 6 percent of people in developing countries who could benefit from antiretroviral treatment are receiving it.[88]

Source: World Bank staff.

References

1. Upadhyay, A. 2003. "Nursing Exodus Weakens Developing World." Inter Press Service News Agency. www.Ipsnews.Net/Migration/Stories/Exodus.Html.

2. Lindelow, M., P. Serneels, and T. Lemma. 2003. "Synthesis of Focus Group Discussions with Health Workers in Ethiopia." World Bank, Washington, DC.

3. U.S. Agency for International Development. 2003. *The Health Sector Human Resource Crisis in Africa: An Issue Paper.* Washington, DC.

4. World Health Organization. 2003. *Global TB Control. 2003 Report.* Geneva.

5. Kurowski, C., S. Abdulla, and A. Mills. 2003. *Human Resources for Health: Requirements and Availability in the Context of Scaling-Up Priority Interventions. A Case Study from Tanzania.* London School of Hygiene & Tropical Medicine.

6. World Bank. 2002. *The Gambia: A Country Status Report on Health and Poverty.* Washington, DC.

7. Blanchet, N., G. Dussault, and B. Liese. 2003. "The Human Resource Crisis in Health Services." Background Paper to the 2004 *World Development Report: Making Services Work for Poor People.* World Bank, Washington, DC.

8. Hammer, J., I. Bnabi, and J. Cercone. 1995. "Distributional Effects of Social Sector Expenditures in Malaysia 1974–89." In *Public Spending and the Poor: Theory and Evidence,* ed. K. Nead. Baltimore: Johns Hopkins University Press.

9. Lavy, V., J. Strauss, D. Thomas, and P. De Vreyer. 1996. "Quality of Care, Survival and Health Outcomes in Ghana." *Journal of Health Economics* 15 (3): 333–357.

10. Thomas, D., V. Lavy, and D. Strauss. 1996. "Public Policy and Anthropometric Outcomes in the Côte d'Ivoire." *Journal of Public Economics* 61 (2): 155–192.

11. Diop, F., A. Soucat, A. Wagstaff, and F. Zhao. 2002. "Health and the Poor in Senegal." Draft chapter for Senegal Country Economic Memorandum. World Bank, Washington, DC.

12. World Health Organization. 1998. *CHD 1996–97 Report.* Geneva.

13. Ministry of Health and Social Welfare. 2002. *RNTCP Performance Report, India, 3rd Quarter.* Central TB Division, Delhi.

A company's decision to invest in developing and commercializing a vaccine is based largely on an evaluation of economic factors: costs, risks, and timing of investments, and expected returns. To influence these economic factors, governments are seeking new ways to assess and share risk and accelerate the development and introduction of priority vaccines. They are using "push" mechanisms to reduce the risks and costs of investments and "pull" mechanisms to ensure future returns. The benefits and constraints of each mechanism, and examples of how they have been used, are shown in the table.

The role of partnerships

It is unlikely that adequate resources can be raised to finance all the costs of vaccine development and production (100 percent push) or to purchase vaccines at prices equivalent to those paid in the United States or Europe (100 percent pull). So the public sector must leverage its resources by targeting as directly as possible the obstacles inhibiting a vaccine's progress. If the risks are linked to scientific uncertainty, as for an HIV/AIDS vaccine, push mechanisms may prove more valuable than pull mechanisms. If the risks stem from the market, as for the meningococcal A conjugate vaccine, pull mechanisms become more important.

Public-private partnerships allow for sharing the risks and costs of developing and introducing priority vaccines in novel ways. Several public-private partnerships are accelerating the development of specific vaccines (HIV/AIDS, malaria, acute respiratory infection, and diarrheal disease). To move forward with credible partnerships, both partners must understand the costs, risks, and benefits in order to identify the costs and risks that are sensitive to public sector support. And both public and private partners must be confident that the agreements defining the partnership protect both of their interests—more rapid development, expanded capacity, and lower prices on one side and real financial commitments that cover investments on the other.

The impact of partnerships

Public-private partnerships are expanding the number and quality of vaccine candidates in the pipeline and accelerating late-stage development activities (ensuring clinical trials in developing countries, influencing production capacity decisions, working with governments to collect data for national decisionmaking). The International AIDS Vaccine Initiative (IAVI) and the Malaria Vaccine Initiative (MVI) have supported these efforts. More than 75 percent of IAVI's resources are slotted for vaccine development and a number of vaccines are targeted for trials in 2003 in such countries as China, India, Kenya, South Africa, and Uganda. The MVI currently has nine vaccine development projects in its portfolio, with clinical trials under way in Africa for two of those projects.

Source: References 90–95.

Push and pull mechanisms to accelerate the introduction of new vaccines

Mechanism	Benefits	Constraints	Examples
Push	• Reduces risk and cost of investment and thus may spur or accelerate product development • Well-known policy tool with proven track record • Credible to industry since money is offered upfront	• Requires "picking a horse" early in the process • Difficult to estimate value and negotiate some return from industry • No promise of a successful outcome	• Direct financing: provides funds to implement activities critical to vaccine development (clinical trials) • Facilitating environment builds clinical trial capacity and helps gain government support • Tax credits on R&D
Pull	• Reduces risk to manufacturer, thus creating incentives for private investment • Public sector not forced to select one product; instead, competition encouraged • Public funds not committed unless a vaccine is developed • If structured correctly, highly credible to industry	• Locked in even if results are unfavorable (if commitments are made early, the public sector may be locked in to a suboptimal outcome) • Mechanisms untested and risky • Promised return may be too distant and risky to spur investment	• Increased uptake of existing vaccines (Global Alliance for Vaccines and Immunization and the Vaccine Fund): provides five-year commitments to governments for purchase of vaccines • Copayments: fixed copayment (less than price) guaranteed • Market guarantee: commits to purchase a vaccine if it is developed

14. World Bank. 2003. *World Development Report 2004: Making Services Work for Poor People.* Washington, DC: World Bank.

15. World Bank. 2003. "Briefing Note: A Global Trust for Health: Revitalizing the Workforce." Health, Nutrition, and Population Department, Washington, DC.

16. Raufu, A. 2002. "Nigeria Concerned over Exodus of Doctors and Nurses." *British Medical Journal* 325: 65.

17. Federation for American Immigration Reform. 2002. "Brain Drain." www.Fairus.Org/Immigrationissuecenters/ Immigrationissuecenters.Cfm?ID=1242&C=17.

18. Marcelo, R. 2003. "Hospital 'Angels' Look for Heaven Elsewhere." *Indian Financial Times,* October 13.

19. Padarath, A., C. Chamberlain, D. Mccoy, A. Ntuli, M. Rowson, and R. Loewenson. 2003. "Health Personnel in Southern Africa: Confronting Maldistribution and Brain Drain." EQUINET Discussion Paper 3.

20. Adversario, P. 2003. "Philippines Suffer from Hemorrhage of Nurses." *Manila Times,* April 21.

21. Adversario, P. 2003. "Quality of Nursing Education Deteriorating." *Manila Times,* April 22.

22. Adversario, P. 2003. "Confusing Policies Worsen Outflow of Nurses." *Manila Times,* April 23.

23. Zarilli, S., and C. Kinnon. 1998. *International Trade in Health Services: A Development Perspective.* Geneva: United Nations Conference on Trade and Development/World Health Organization.

24. Buve, A., S.D. Foaster, C. Mbwili, E. Mungo, N. Tollenare, and M. Zeko. 1994. "Mortality among Female Nurses in the Face of the AIDS Epidemic: A Pilot Study in Zambia." *AIDS* 8 (3): 396.

25. Tawfik, L., and S. Kinoti. 2001. *The Impact of HIV/AIDS on the Health Sector in Sub-Saharan Africa: The Issue of Human Resources. The HRM Response to the Impact of HIV/AIDS on the Health Sector.* USAID, Washington, DC.

26. Holmas, T.H. 2002. "Keeping Nurses at Work: A Duration Analysis." *Health Economics* 11 (6): 493–503.

27. Thornton, J., and F. Esposto. 2003. "How Important Are Economic Factors in Choice of Medical Specialty?" *Health Economics* 12 (1): 67–73.

28. Wilbulpolprasert, S. 1999. "Inequitable Distribution of Doctors: Can It Be Solved?" *Human Resources Development Journal* 3 (1): 2–22.

29. Wilbulpolprasert, S. 2002. "Integrated Strategies to Tackle Inequitable Distribution of Doctors in Thailand: Four Decades of Experience."

30. Organisation for Economic Co-operation and Development. 2002. *Geographical Imbalances of HRHC: Size, Determinants, and Policy Responses.* Working Party on Social Policy, Human Resources for Health Care Systems, Paris.

31. Setiadi, G. 1999. Discussion of S. Wibulpolprasert, "Inequitable Distribution of Doctors: Can It Be Solved?" *Human Resources for Health Development Journal* 3 (1): 2–22.

32. Zurn, P. 2002. "Imbalances in the Health Workforce: Briefing Paper." World Health Organization, Geneva.

33. "Nursing Nursing Back to Health," *Lancet* 352, no. 9124 (1998): 249.

34. Carvel, J. 2001. "Inflation: Busting Rise for GPs and Nurses." *Guardian,* December 18.

35. World Bank. 2003. "Bolivia: Health Sector Reforms in the Context of Decentralization." 26140–BO. Washington, DC.

36. Reinikka, S. 2003. "Working for God? Evaluating Service Delivery of Religious Not-for-Profit Health Care Providers in Uganda." Policy Research Working Paper 3058, World Bank, Washington, DC.

37. Peters, D.H., A.S. Yazbeck, R. Sharma, G. Ramana, L.H. Pritchett, and A. Wagstaff. 2002. *Better Health Systems for India's Poor: Findings, Analysis and Options.* Washington, DC: World Bank.

38. Awases, M., A. Gbary, and R. Chagtora. 2003. *Migration of Health Professionals in Six Countries: A Synthesis Report.* Geneva: World Health Organization.

39. Srinavichakron, S. 1998. "Conditions, Constraints, and Strategies Increased Contribution of General Practitioners to the Health System in Thailand." *Human Resources for Health Journal* 2 (1) 48–59.

40. Rabinowitz, R. 1999. "A Program to Increase the Number of Family Physicians in Rural and Underserved Areas: Impact after 22 Years." *Journal of the American Medical Association* 281 (3): 255–260.

41. Rosenblatt, R.A., M.E. Whitcomb, T.J. Cullen, D.M. Lishner, and L.G. Hart. 1992. "Which Medical Schools Produce Rural Physicians?" *Journal of the American Medical Association* 268 (12): 1559–1565.

42. Becker, G.S. 1993. *Human Capital: A Theoretical and Empirical Analysis, with Special Reference to Education.* 3rd ed. Chicago: University of Chicago Press.

43. Tulloch, J. 1999. "Integrated Approach to Child Health in Developing Countries." *Lancet* 354 (Suppl. 2): SII16– SII20.

44. Gove, S. 1997. *Integrated Management of Childhood Illness by Outpatient Health Workers: Technical Basis and Overview.* WHO Working Group on Guidelines for Integrated Management of the Sick Child. *Bulletin of the World Health Organization* 75 (Suppl. 1): 7–24.

45. Weber, M.W., E.K. Mulholland, S. Jaffar, H. Troedsson, S. Gove, and B.M. Greenwood. 1997. "Evaluation of an Algorithm for the Integrated Management of Childhood Illness in an Area with Seasonal Malaria in The Gambia." *Bulletin of the World Health Organization* 75 (Suppl. 1): 25–32.

46. Perkins B.A., J.R. Zucker, J. Otieno, H.S. Jafari, L. Paxton, S.C. Redd, B.L. Nahlen, B. Schwartz, A.J. Oloo, C. Olango, S. Gove, and C.C. Campbell. 1997. "Evaluation of an Algorithm for Integrated Management of Childhood Illness in an Area of Kenya with High Malaria Transmission." *Bulletin of the World Health Organization* 75 (Suppl. 1): 33–42.

47. Simoes, E.A., T. Desta, T. Tessema, T. Gerbresellassie, M. Dagnew, and S. Gove. 1997. "Performance of Health Workers after Training in Integrated Management of Childhood Illness in Gondar, Ethiopia." *Bulletin of the World Health Organization* 75 (Suppl. 1): 43–53.

48. World Health Organization, Division of Child Health and Development and Regional Office for Africa. 1997. "Integrated Management of Childhood Illness: Field Test of the WHO/UNICEF Training Course in Arusha, United Republic of Tanzania." *Bulletin of the World Health Organization* 75 (Suppl. 1): 55–64.

49. Schellenberg J., and the MCE Tanzania Working Group on the 2001 Health Facility Survey. 2001. *Report of the Health Facility Survey Submitted to the Department of Child and Adolescent Health and Development.* World Health Organization, Geneva.

50. Ministry of Health, Bolivia, World Health Organization, BASICS/USAID, and Sociedad Boliviana De Pediatria. 1999. *Report of the Health Facility Survey in Bolivia.* Geneva.

51. Kelley E., C. Geslin, S. Djibrina, and M. Boucar. 2001. "Improving Performance with Clinical Standards: The Impact of Feedback on Compliance with the Integrated Management of Childhood Illness Algorithm in Niger, West Africa." *International Journal of Health Planning and Management* 16 (3): 195–205.

52. Oliveira-Cruz, V., C. Kurowski, and A. Mills. 2003. "Delivery of Priority Health Services: Searching for Synergies within the Vertical versus Horizontal Debate." *Journal of International Development* 15 (1): 67–86.

53. Black, R.E., S.S. Morris, and J. Bryce. 2003. "Where and Why Are 10 Million Children Dying Every Year?" *Lancet* 361 (9376): 2226–2234.

54. World Bank. 2002. *Tanzania: A Country Status Report on Health and Poverty.* Washington, DC.

55. Quick, J. 2002. "Essential Medicines: Twenty-Five Years on Closing the Access Gap." *Bulletin of the World Health Organization* 80 (11): 913–914.

56. Schrag, S., B. Beall, SF. D. 2001. "*Resistant Pneumococcal Infections: The Burden of Disease and Challenges in Monitoring and Controlling Antimicrobial Resistance.* WHO/CDS/CSR/DRS/2001.6. ed. World Health Organization, Geneva.

57. Newton, P.N., N.J. White, J.A. Rozendaal, and M.D. Green. 2002. "Murder by Fake Drugs." *British Medical Journal* 324 (7341): 800–801.

58. World Health Organization and Health Action International. 2003. *Medicine Prices: A New Approach to Measurement.* Geneva: WHO.

59. Kishuna, A. 2003. "Drug Pricing Survey in Kwazulu-Natal." *Essential Drugs Monitor* (32): 4–7.

60. World Health Organization. 2003. *Essential Drugs Monitor.* Geneva: WHO.

61. Wagstaff, A., and E. Van Doorslaer. 2003. "Catastrophe and Impoverishment in Paying for Health Care: With Applications to Vietnam 1993–98." *Health Economics* 12 (11): 921–933.

62. Wagstaff, A., and M. Pradhan. 2003. "Evaluating the Impacts of Health Insurance: Looking beyond the Negative." World Bank, Washington, DC.

63. World Bank, SIDA, AusAID, Royal Netherlands Embassy, and Ministry of Health of Vietnam. 2001. *Vietnam. Growing Healthy: A Review of Vietnam's Health Sector.* Hanoi: World Bank.

64. Hogerzeil, H. 2002. "WHO Department of Essential Drugs and Medicines Policy: The Concept of Essential Drugs and the WHO Model List of Essential Medicines." Presentation to the Expert Committee on the Use of Essential Drugs, April, World Health Organization, Geneva.

65. Médecins Sans Frontières. 2001. *Fatal Imbalance: The Crisis in Research and Development for Drugs for Neglected Diseases.*

66. Olivera-Cruz, V., K. Hanson, and A. Mills. 2001. "Approaches to Overcoming Health Systems Constraints at the Peripheral Level: A Review of the Evidence." WG5 15. CMH Working Paper Series, Geneva.

67. Santoso, B., S. Suryawati, and J.E. 1996. "Prawaitasari Small Group Intervention vs. Formal Seminar for Improving Appropriate Drug Use." *Social Science Medicine* 42 (8): 1163–1168.

68. Brumburgh, S., and S. Raja. 2001. *Ghana: Process Mapping: First Step to Reengineering the Health Supply Chain of the Public Sector System.* Arlington, VA: Deliver/John Snow, Inc. for USAID.

69. World Bank. 1994. *Better Health in Africa : Experience and Lessons Learned.* Washington, DC: World Bank.

70. John Snow, Inc. 2000. *Programs that Deliver: Contribution to Better Health in Developing Countries.* Arlington, VA: Family Planning Logistics Management/John Snow, Inc. for USAID.

71. Reinikka, R. 1999. "Using Surveys for Public Sector Reform." *PREM Notes.* World Bank, Washington, DC.

72. Mcpake, B., D. Asiimwe, F. Mwesigye, M. Ofumbi, L. Orthenblad, P. Streefland, and A. Turinde. 1999. "Informal Economic Activities of Public Health Workers in Uganda: Implications for Quality and Accessibility of Care." *Social Science and Medicine* 49 (7): 849–865.

73. Ablo, E., and R. Reinikka. 1998. " Do Budgets Really Matter? Evidence from Public Spending on Education and Health in Uganda." Policy Research Working Paper 1926, World Bank, Washington, DC.

74. Bird, C. 2003. "Impoverished Georgia Harbours Fatal Form of TB." *Guardian* August 9.

75. World Health Organization. 2001. *The Impact of Implementation of ICH Guidelines in Non–ICH Countries.* Geneva.

76. Ratanawijitrasin, S., and E. Wondemagegnehu. 2002. *Effective Drug Regulation: A Multicountry Study.* Malta. Geneva: World Health Organization.

77. World Health Organization. 2004. *Country Profiles.* WHO Regional Office for Europe (Hungary). www.Euro.Who.Int/Pharmaceuticals/Topics/20020226_1.

78. Andajaningsih. 1997. "Implementation of Essential Drug Concept and Drug Financing Strategies." World Health Organization, Geneva.

79. Santoso, B., H. Shein, and S. Suryati. 1997. "Financing Drugs in South East Asia." *Health Economics and Drugs* DAP Series(8).

80. Government of Guatemala. 2002. *Evaluación del sector farmacéutico en Guatemala.* Ministerio de Salud Pública y Asistencia Social, Dirección de Regulación y Control de Programas de la Salud. Report is in Spanish.

81. Bennett, K., and E. Ngalande-Banda. 1994. "Public and Private Roles in Health: A Review and Analysis of Experience in Sub-Saharan Africa." SHS Paper 6. World Health Organization, Division of Strengthening Health Systems, Geneva.

82. Kaplan, W. 2003. "Local Production: Industrial Policy and Access to Medicine: An Overview of Key Concepts, Issues, and Opportunities for Future Research." Prepared for World Bank meeting on the role of generics and local industry in attaining the MDGs in pharmaceuticals and vaccines (June 24, 2003).

83. Pavignani, D. 1999. "Managing External Resources in Mozambique: Building New Relationships on Shifting Sands?" *Health Policy and Planning* 14 (3): 243–253.

84. UNAIDS and World Health Organization. 2002. *AIDS Epidemic Update 2003.* Geneva. www.unaids.org/en/default.asp/.

85. Pan American Health Organization. 2002. "AIDS Dugs Prices Drop 54 Percent in Latin America." www.Paho.Org/English/DPI/Pr020718.Htm.

86. Rockefeller Foundation, Center for Pharmaceutical Management, and Management Sciences for Health. 2002. *Regional Pooled Procurement of Drugs: Evaluation of Programs.* Arlington, VA..

87. World Health Organization and UNAIDS. 2002. *Accelerating Access Initiative: Widening Access to Care and Support for People Living with HIV/AIDS.* Progress Report, June. Geneva.

88. UNAIDS. 2003. "Access to HIV Treatment and Care Fact Sheet." Geneva.

89. Weisbrod, B. 2003. "Solving the Drug Dilemma." *Washington Post,* August 22.

90. International AIDS Vaccine Initiative. 2003. *Improving and Accelerating the Clinical Pipeline of AIDS Vaccine Candidates for Use Worldwide: The IAVI Research and Development Agenda 2002–2004.* New York.

91. Malaria Vaccine Initiative. 2003. *MVI Vaccine Development Projects.* http://www.malariavaccine.org/ab-current_projects.htm.

92. Kremer, M. 2000. *Creating Markets for Vaccines. Part II: Design Issues.* Cambridge, MA: National Bureau of Economic Research.

93. Madrid, Y. 2001. *A New Access Paradigm: Public Access to Assure Swift Global Access to AIDS Vaccines.* New York: International AIDS Vaccine Initiative.

94. Performance Innovation Unit, UK Cabinet. 2001. *Tackling the Disease of Poverty.* London. www.pm.gov.uk/output/page4162.asp.

95. Batson, A., and M. Ainsworth M. 2001. "Obstacles and Solutions: Understanding Private Investments in HIV/AIDS Vaccine Development." *Bulletin of the World Health Organization* 79 (8): 721–728.

96. World Bank. 2003. *World Development Indicators 2003.* Washington, DC.

CHAPTER 8

Strengthening Core Public Health Functions

Chang Sun's wife is HIV positive. So is his mother. So is his aunt. So are his cousin and his cousin's wife. So is the woman next door and, probably, so is her husband. In fact, it is quite possible that almost every adult and many of the children in his small, remote village are infected. Among them is Chang's father, who died of AIDS last year, and his three-year-old daughter, who succumbed the year before that. His first wife is there too—she threw herself down the village well in 2000 after a doctor told her she was no longer worth treating because she had the virus.

This is Xiongqiao village in Henan Province, the ground zero of arguably the world's worst HIV/AIDS epidemic, with up to a million people infected in this single province through a vast, largely unregulated blood-selling operation. The situation is already a catastrophe, but the risks are growing.

It was almost inevitable that the outbreak occurred in Henan. Here in the most populous and impoverished of China's provinces, life is cheaper than almost anywhere else in the world. The average Henan farmer survives on 80¢ per day. Henan's officials turned to almost their only untapped resource: the blood of the province's 90 million population. Vans were converted into mini-clinics and driven out into the countryside. Ambitious peasants established themselves as "bloodheads" (brokers) to meet the demand among both buyers and sellers. For an 800 cc donation, villagers were paid 45 renminbi (about $5.50), enough to feed a family for a week. Realizing that they could get far more for milking their veins than for tending the land, they lined up day in and day out for years to make dona-

tions. By the peak—around 1995—Henan had become the nation's blood farm. The system had been adapted so that villagers could give such huge amounts of blood without suffering anemia. After extracting plasma from each 800 cc donation, the collectors would pump 400 cc back into the arms of the donors. It is believed that people's blood often got mixed up in this way, spreading HIV to almost everyone involved.

"Almost everybody did it," said Chang's cousin, Ming. "We would sell extra if there was a marriage ceremony coming up or if we wanted to build a house. The most I ever did was four donations in a single day."

The consequences for China will be devastating as many infected villagers are migrating to work in Beijing and other big cities.

GUARDIAN, *October 25, 2003*

The Chinese government has started providing free treatment for poor people with HIV and AIDS and plans to expand the program next year until every poor person who has tested positive is receiving medical help, a top health ministry official said in a speech this week.

NEW YORK TIMES, *November 8, 2003*

This account from ground zero of one of the world's major AIDS epidemics and the 2002 outbreak in China of severe acute respiratory syndrome (SARS) serves as a forceful reminder of the importance of strong public health systems. Vulnerable populations need to be empowered, protected from risks, informed and educated, and encouraged to participate in health activities. Public health regulations need to be established and enforced. Infrastructure needs to be in place to reduce the health impact of emergencies and disasters. All of this needs to be done through a public health system that is transparent and accountable.

Thus governments have responsibilities that go beyond providing and financing health services in attaining the Millennium Development Goals. Strengthening core public health functions such as policy formulation, monitoring and evaluation, disease surveillance, provider and insurance regulation, social mobilization, and cross-sectoral actions are government responsibilities that must be discharged as part of the Millennium Development Goal effort. Good practices in these areas need to be carefully analyzed and multiplied. It is important for national leaders and donor agencies to appreciate the necessity of investing in these core public health functions, which are often overlooked as politicians and funders focus exclusively on service delivery. It will not be possible to go to scale with basic services for HIV/AIDS, tuberculosis, malaria, or maternal and child health with faltering or absent public health infrastructure and weak public health functions.

What is public health?

The previous chapters emphasize the importance of governments building strong policies and institutions across the health sector. Without such improvements, increases in government health budgets in most countries will have little impact on Millennium Development Goal outcomes. Governments play a role in developing and implementing policies to lower the barriers that households—especially poor ones—face. Households, as users of health services and producers of health, are key actors in the health system. Governments also play a role in improving the quality and efficiency of service providers, which are also key actors. They can do so through a combination of measures to improve management in provider organizations and improve the accountability of provider organizations to the public, whether directly to patients and community organizations or indirectly through interactions with policymakers. Because provider organizations rely on inputs—human resources and medicines—government policies aimed at increasing stocks of human resources and improving their distribution and quality are crucial. Policies to get medicines to providers and ensure that providers face the right incentives for prescribing medicines are also important, as are global policies to ensure appropriate levels of research and development in "neglected" diseases and affordable medicines for poor countries.

These responsibilities are vital elements of the government's stewardship role in the health sector. But beyond them lies another set of essential responsibilities of the public sector: those in public health (table 8.1).[1,2] Many of these responsibilities are examined in other chapters of the report, including financing health services (chapter 9), managing health services (chapter 6), pharmaceutical policy (chapter 7), and health promotion and behavior change (chapter 5). Several others are discussed in this chapter.

Market failure and public health

In each of these areas of public health is at least one element of "market failure." This means that without some form of government involvement, a free market would produce an outcome that is inefficient. In many of these areas are elements of "externalities" and "public goods." Immunizations, for example, benefit not only the immunized person but also whole communities, by reducing the risk of others getting infected. The same is true of the use of insecticide-treated nets (ITNs) and antimalarials. Externalities also provide an important rationale for the public health agenda to concern itself with intersectoral issues. For example, investments in water and sanitation infrastructure enable households to improve their hygiene, reducing their risk of contracting communicable diseases and also the risk to others.

Communicable disease programs—surveillance, prevention, treatment and control—are classic examples of public goods: benefits to some do not diminish the benefits to others, and it is typically not feasible to exclude specific people from benefiting from such programs. Data collection and analysis and monitoring and evaluation are other examples of public goods. In some cases the rationale for government involvements stems from informational asymmetries: the patient, having less knowledge than the provider, can be vulnerable to exploitation by unscrupulous providers (chapter 7). This asymmetry goes beyond medicines. It arises, for example, in blood contamination, as in Henan Province.

Government involvement is required to deal with these market failures. Externalities call for government subsidies,

Table 8.1 Public health responsibilities and functions

Policy development	Collection and dissemination of evidence for public health policies, strategies, and actions	Prevention and control of disease	Intersectoral action for better health	Human resource development and capacity building for public health
Public health regulation and enforcement[a]	Health situation monitoring and analysis[a]	Surveillance and control of risks and damages in public health[a]	Environmental protection and health, including road safety, indoor air pollution, water and sanitation and disease vector control in infrastructure, management of medical wastes, tobacco legislation, school health, and education	Development of policy, planning, and managerial capacity[a]
Evaluation and promotion of equitable access to necessary health services[a]	Research, development, and implementation of innovative public health solutions[a]	Management of communicable and noncommunicable diseases		Human resources development and training in public health[a]
Assurance of the quality of personal and population-based health services[a]	Provision of information to consumers, providers, policymakers, and financiers	Health promotion[a]		Community capacity building
Health policy formulation and planning	Development of health information and management systems	Behavior change interventions for disease prevention and control		
Financing and management of health services	Research and evaluation	Social participation and empowerment of citizens in health[a]		
Pharmaceutical policy, regulation, and enforcement		Reducing the impact of emergencies and disasters on health[a]		

a. Pan American Health Organization, World Health Organization, and the U.S. Centers for Disease Control "essential" public health function.[2]

Source: Reference 1.

since without them, caregivers fail to take into account the external benefits (the benefits to others) of their actions. Too few people would be immunized. Surveillance activities, research and development, and monitoring and evaluation would be inadequate. Indeed, in some cases, without government intervention none would be produced at all. For activities involving externalities and public goods, governments need not undertake the activities themselves, but at a minimum they need to provide some financing and close oversight, to ensure an acceptable level of performance, given the information asymmetries. Monitoring a nongovernment supplier can be difficult, so governments often undertake these activities themselves in the belief—sometimes mistaken—that government officials are less likely to exploit their informational advantages over patients.

Obstacles to performing public health functions

Developing country governments generally recognize that these public health functions are important—for making progress toward the health- and nutrition-related Millennium Development Goals and for health policy in general—but they often lack the capacity and financial resources to implement them. Indeed, few low-income countries invest in these public health functions. Because these functions deal with broad health system issues rather than specific diseases,

they lack the immediate urgency and concrete appeal of disease-specific programs and thus tend to be neglected. That their influence on health outcomes is difficult to measure also contributes to their frequent neglect by governments and donors.* It is difficult, for example, to say just how much a strong disease surveillance and reporting system contributes to reducing the incidence of tuberculosis, whereas the benefits of distributing and consistently using drugs for treating tuberculosis are obvious. Still, where these core functions are well performed, countries tend to have greater success in achieving their health targets.

Why do core public health functions matter for the Millennium Development Goals?

The core public health functions complement vertical programs for achieving disease-specific goals (see table 8.3 at the end of this chapter). Investing in these functions helps build capacity across all of the Millennium Development Goals, whether the challenge is HIV/AIDS, malaria, tuberculosis, or communicable diseases in childhood.

---

*It has also been difficult to define and estimate the cost of implementing core public health functions, although the Bank and its partners (the Pan American Health Organization, the U.S. Centers for Disease Control and Prevention) are trying to do so as part of national health accounts and public expenditure reviews.

Of the many potential public health functions, four are key:

- establishing national strategies for disease prevention, treatment, and control;

- installing government-led monitoring and evaluation systems through integrated disease surveillance, program assessment, and collection and analysis of demographic and vital registration data;

- establishing and strengthening national institutions and local capacities; and

- taking intersectoral actions that go beyond the remit of ministries of health.

Establishing national strategies for disease prevention, treatment, and control

By employing skilled public health professionals, governments can effectively monitor the health of communities and broader populations, develop and enforce standards, and emphasize health education, public information, health promotion, and disease prevention. Public action can improve consumers' knowledge and change attitudes so that private markets can operate effectively to meet the needs of the poor. Examples are social marketing of ITNs to reduce malaria transmission (box 8.1) and social marketing of condoms for protection against HIV/AIDS.

Installing government-led monitoring and evaluation systems

Integrated disease surveillance, program assessment, and collection and analysis of demographic and vital registration data are essential if governments and donors are to determine whether policies and programs are having an impact on the health Millennium Development Goals. Box 2.1 in chapter 2 lists intermediate indicators and proxy indicators for the Millennium Development Goals that can help monitor progress, assess the impact of policies, and adjust programs going forward. Much greater investments are needed in systems to monitor these intermediate indicators. Disease surveillance helps determine whether health outcomes are improving. Some good practices in surveillance are being developed (box 8.2).

Not all developing countries can afford to invest in the infrastructure required for strong surveillance systems. Most rely on alternative short- to medium-term solutions for data gathering, such as intermittent household surveys, health facility surveys, and simplified facility-based routine reporting systems. In a few cases countries have made special efforts to improve surveillance for specific interventions, such as tuberculosis treatment or immunization, while others attempt to monitor progress toward a specific Millennium

---

Box 8.1 Increasing the supply of and demand for insecticide-treated nets

Several large-scale efficacy trials have demonstrated that the regular use of insecticide-treated bednets reduces child deaths by some 25 percent. The Roll Back Malaria Global Partnership has adopted the widespread use of insecticide-treated nets (ITNs) by children and pregnant women as a core strategy for reaching its goal of halving malaria illness and death by 2010.

In many countries, insecticide-treated nets are available only in a small number of commercial outlets in major cities. The nets are often of poor quality, and the cost is high ($5–$15 each). Insecticide retreatment kits are rarely available. Even where activities to boost demand have been successful, commercial markets have not always responded by scaling up supply.

Governments and their partners have used several approaches to increase demand and supply. The most common have been social marketing and public-private partnerships. In both, governments and donors have supported demand-creation activities and provided subsidies for the purchase of nets, through voucher schemes or sales of subsidized products. Eighteen countries have also waived or significantly reduced taxes and tariffs on nets, insecticides, and treated bednets.

These approaches have increased the accessibility and use of ITNs. In Tanzania a social marketing scheme stimulated local textile manufacturers to produce high-quality bednets, while the government drastically reduced taxes and tariffs on these products. The resulting competition in the marketplace caused the price of treated bednets to drop from almost $15 to $2, making the treated bednets accessible to a much larger segment of the population. Use of ITNs has increased in some districts from less than 2 percent to more than 25 percent.

Source: World Bank staff.

Development Goal. Cuba has made the Millennium Development Goal for reducing child mortality a national priority and established a surveillance system to monitor and follow up each child death. Some governments, including the Dominican Republican, are developing or modifying their monitoring and evaluation framework to focus on the Millennium Development Goals (box 8.3).

Establishing and strengthening national institutions and local capacities

Ideally, national institutions that implement core public health functions include a national center for disease surveillance, associations of health professionals with a strong licensing arm, associations of health providers with strong licensing and accreditation arms, a drug safety and regulatory agency, a health insurance regulatory body, interagency task forces for such multisectoral issues as road safety and tobacco control, and others. These institutions and capacities are entirely lacking or in short supply in many low-income countries.

With these institutions and capacities in place, a country can more readily adapt to changes in its health profile and deal with new challenges as they arise, including the range of health challenges related to the Millennium Development Goals. The recent rapid response to severe acute respiratory syndrome (SARS) in Vietnam demonstrates the critical role of a strong public health system. Successful management of the disease outbreak in Vietnam was due not only to high-level political commitment but also to strong surveillance, enforcement of regulations to isolate infected individuals and protect the public from further exposure to the SARS virus, and cross-sector collaboration with officials responsible for water and sanitation, education, and local government services. Drawing on this experience, China's strategy following the SARS epidemic will be to improve SARS–related diagnosis, clinical management, and infection control. It also aims to strengthen the capacity of the public health system to prevent and control infectious disease—improving surveillance and case-reporting systems and setting up alert and response

mechanisms to address public health crises and lower the fatality rate should the disease reemerge.

Additional lessons on how countries can strengthen the institutions responsible for core public health functions can be drawn from a review of public management of these functions. Box 8.4 identifies some of the key lessons.

One of the best examples of institutional changes resulting in improved health outcomes is the often mentioned

A recent review of the main themes of public management literature drew lessons on how public management relates to the core public health functions. Some of the key lessons include the following:

- Curative services, preventive services, and core public health functions have distinct properties requiring different policy prescriptions.

- Because core public health functions have characteristics of public goods, user fees are not appropriate.

- Promoting competition among agencies responsible for public health functions does not improve efficiency. On the contrary, it may hamper collaboration and technical assistance, compromising the effectiveness of such activities as surveillance and health promotion.

- Contracting works for some services but not for others. For preventive services that are measurable and discrete, such as immunization or campaign-based programs, contracting can be effective. But since measurement of core public health functions is complex, expensive, and requires strong information systems, contracting imposes transactions and monitoring costs that make efficiency gains unlikely and can reduce effectiveness.

- If introduced cautiously and with instruments to ensure consistency across units and jurisdictions, managerial autonomy can be an important way of promoting adaptation and innovation in the core public health functions.

- Decentralizing the core public health functions can be a risky strategy, because of the importance of central coordination, oversight, and technical assistance for these functions

and because local governments have little incentive to invest in public goods and may neglect them. Core public health functions should either remain under central control—with managerial autonomy or other strategies to permit local adaptation and responsiveness—or if already decentralized should be subject to alternative forms of central oversight and control, such as grants-in-aid or earmarking.

- Since core public health functions are heavily influenced by rules and norms in the broader institutional environment that cannot be addressed through training alone, efforts to build management capacity should include components in addition to training. Public sector norms and rules that impede effective administration should be changed whenever possible.

- Provider incentives are difficult to design for core public health functions. For incentives to be useful, measurement indicators should be chosen carefully. Incentives should be team based or network based rather than individualized and should include nonfinancial benefits. Performance improvement can also be achieved in more traditional ways—say, by implementing merit-based selection and promotion criteria and clear job descriptions.

- Increasing hierarchical accountability within the public health system is critical for strengthening core public health functions. Doing so requires changes in the capacity, autonomy, and behavior of service managers, and it requires monitoring systems and instruments. Monitoring instruments need to strike the right balance between simplicity and complexity and should be designed for operational rather than research use.

Source: Reference 4.

---

case of Céara, Brazil (see box 6.5). Several government actions there were important. Substantial investment in public information about public health services led communities to hold elected mayors accountable for these services in their area. Careful control over selected human resource issues reduced patronage at the local level. A phased approach to implementing programs allowed early adopters to be nurtured to success and news about "success stories" to spread widely, influencing nonadopting areas. And there was strong state government involvement in motivating frontline health workers.

Taking intersectoral actions—going beyond the remit of ministries of health

A review of the evidence for key determinants of the health and nutrition Millennium Development Goals identifies significant potential for intersectoral synergies (table 8.2).

Roads and transport, water, hygiene, and sanitation, indoor air pollution, and agriculture require multisectoral activities with the potential to contribute to the Millennium Development Goals for health and nutrition.

ROADS AND TRANSPORT Improving transport of intermediate services reduces poverty not by directly increasing consumption of transport but by improving the quality and security of access to work, markets, and services, according to a recent World Bank report.[5] Better transport and roads can reduce delays that contribute to maternal deaths. In Tanzania 63 percent of women who died after reaching a hospital had traveled 10 kilometers or more for treatment.[6] In India a study found that half of maternal deaths occurred before the women reached a treatment facility.[7]

Several developing countries have improved access to health services using locally available resources for emer-

Table 8.2 Potential for intersectoral synergies to achieve the Millennium Development Goals for health and nutrition

Millennium Development Goal	Target	Multisectoral inputs	Country examples	Key sectors
Reduce maternal mortality	Improve access to emergency obstetric care	Availability of transport, roads, and referral facilities	Bangladesh, Tanzania, Vietnam,	Transport, road infrastructure, health
	Reduce indoor air pollution	Improved cooking practices, fuel, and ventilation	China, Guatemala, India, Kenya	Energy, housing, health
Reduce child mortality	Reduce diarrheal diseases in children through hand-washing, use of latrines, and proper disposal of young children's stools	Improved hand-washing practices, using soap and plenty of water	Costa Rica, El Salvador, Guatemala, Ghana, India, Nepal, Peru, Senegal	Water and sanitation, health private sector (soap manufacturers)
	Reduce indoor air pollution	Improved fuel, ventilation, and childplay practices	China, Guatemala, India, Kenya, Mongolia, Nicaragua	Energy, housing, private health, private sector (improved stove production)
Reduce hunger and improve nutrition	Regulate food prices, raise women's income, and promote dietary diversity and food security at the household level	Improved agricultural practices, tariffs, and trade; reduced women's workload; better gender relations and intrahousehold decisionmaking	Bangladesh, India, Kenya, Tanzania, Vietnam	Agriculture, rural development, gender, trade

Source: World Bank staff.

gency transport and communication. Better transportation can increase the ratio of health facilities to population.[8] Several community-driven development programs have demonstrated that women's access to health services can be improved by making arrangements with local transporters and by organizing emergency interest-free loans financed and managed by the communities.[9] Preliminary evidence from Mali, where referral funds managed by local health communities financed a system of radio calls and ambulances, shows an increase in emergency referral rates from 1 percent to 3 percent.[10]

A 10-year study in Rajasthan, India, showed that better roads and transport helped women reach referral facilities but that many women continued to die because there were no corresponding improvements at the household and facility levels.[7] This illustrates the need to improve performance in all relevant sectors to achieve results on the Millennium Development Goals.

WATER, HYGIENE, AND SANITATION Better hygiene (hand-washing) and sanitation (use of latrines, safe disposal of children's stools) are at least as important as drinking water quality to health outcomes, especially the reduction in diarrhea and associated child mortality.[11] Increased quantity of water has been shown to have greater impact than improved quality of water,[11] possibly because an adequate supply of water increases the feasibility of adopting safe hygiene behaviors and reduces the length of time that water must be stored and may become contami-

nated by handling. And constructing water supply and sanitation facilities is not enough to improve health outcomes—sustained human behavior change must accompany the infrastructure investment.

So what can the public health sector do? In collaboration with other sectors, it can develop public health promotion and education strategies. It can work with agencies that plan, develop, and manage water resources and those responsible for monitoring water quality and sanitation, and it can provide leadership for action on hygiene education. It can also provide other sectors with reliable data on water-associated diseases and the effectiveness of interventions—and advocate for water, sanitation, and hygiene interventions in poverty reduction strategies. And it can work with the private sector to manufacture, distribute, and promote affordable in-home water purification solutions and safe storage vessels.

Hand-washing is one of the most effective interventions for reducing diarrhea. Measurable reductions in diarrhea-associated child mortality have been achieved through public-private partnerships to promote hand-washing.[12] The Bank's water sector is working with a consortium to improve the water supply questions on standardized health surveys used in the developing world (such as the Demographic Health Surveys and Multiple Indicator Cluster Surveys) to gather more accurate information on the links between water and health. The Bank's health, nutrition, and population and water sectors are implementing a joint work program with the World Health Organization to update scientific evidence on water, sanitation, hygiene, and health links to inform policies at national level.

INDOOR AIR POLLUTION Most indoor air pollution in developing countries is caused by the use of low-cost, traditional energy sources, such as coal and biomass (wood, cow dung, crop residues), in primitive stoves for cooking and heating—the main source of energy for some 3.5 billion people. The health burden from indoor air pollution is greatest in high-altitude rural areas among poor families who use biomass in primitive stoves without proper ventilation. Indoor air pollution is a major risk factor for pneumonia and associated deaths in children and for lung cancer in women who are at risk of exposure during cooking.

Eventually, most developing countries will move up the energy ladder, but this move is delayed by low income and limited access to high-quality fuel. Improved biomass stoves have been effective in improving health outcomes in India and elsewhere.[13] Large community-based intervention trials are documenting the affordability, cost-effectiveness, feasibility, and sustainability of multisectoral interventions. Studies in China, Guatemala, and India are under way to improve access to efficient and affordable energy sources through local design, manufacturing, and dissemination of low-cost technologies, modern fuel alternatives, and renewable energy solutions.[14] In China the health sector initiated a large community-based project to reduce indoor air pollution in rural areas, after policymakers became troubled by the leveling off in child mortality rates among the rural poor. Having already achieved high immunization rates and other child health interventions, China is now seeking ways to reduce risk factors beyond the health sector. The health sector is generating the data, assessing the impact of interventions, and promoting behavior change that will reduce exposure to indoor air pollution and complement the provision of hardware, such as improved stoves and ventilation.

AGRICULTURAL POLICIES AND PRACTICES Agricultural policies and practices that affect food prices, farm incomes, diet diversity and quality, and household food security also require government leadership to achieve better Millennium Development Goal outcomes. Agricultural policies that focus on women's access to resources (land, training, agricultural inputs); their role in production; and their income from agriculture are likely to have a greater impact on nutrition than policies that do not focus on women, particularly if combined with other strategies, such as strategies for improving women's education and effecting behavior change communication.[15,16]

Box 8.5 Strengthening the health system and core public health functions to combat HIV/AIDS

To achieve the Millennium Development Target for HIV/AIDS, massive efforts are needed to strengthen health systems. In the most severely affected countries, the health sector suffers from severe shortages of human and financial resources. Many health sector services are struggling to cope with the growing impact of HIV/AIDS. In Sub-Saharan Africa, people with HIV–related illnesses occupy more than half the hospital beds, overwhelming health services and other organizations providing care and support. And just as demand for health services increases, more and more healthcare personnel are becoming infected with HIV/AIDS and unable to work. Added to this is the ongoing attrition of healthcare workers for other reasons and weakened infrastructure.

In many African countries healthcare systems also suffer from chronic shortages of drugs, infrequent equipment maintenance, inadequate logistical support, and weak supervision. Also lacking are procedures or systems to monitor and evaluate the quality of healthcare and to ensure that providers are accountable to clients. All this needs to change, not only to meet the HIV/AIDS treatment target but to achieve the health Millennium Development Goals.

Because of the high cost of antiretroviral drugs, the complexity of the regimens, and the need for careful monitoring, specific services and facilities must be in place in order to introduce antiretroviral therapy:

- ensured access to voluntary counseling and testing

- capacity to recognize and manage common HIV–related illnesses and opportunistic infections

- reliable laboratory monitoring services, including routine hematological and biochemical tests for the detection of drug toxicity as well as access to facilities for monitoring the immunologic and virologic parameters of HIV infection

- ensured supply of good-quality drugs

- sufficient resources to pay for treatment on a long-term basis

- information and training on safe and effective use of antiretroviral drugs for health professionals in a position to prescribe antiretroviral therapy

- establishment of reliable regulatory mechanisms to prevent misuse and misappropriation of antiretroviral drugs

Only through investments in strengthening of health systems and core public health functions will these conditions be met.

Source: References 17–19.

What do governments and donors need to do next to improve public health?

To accelerate progress toward the Millennium Development Goals, most countries need to significantly increase investments in the core public health functions, in addition to providing and financing health services. Strengthening these functions should be included in the Poverty Reduction Strategy Paper process and public expenditure framework exercises. Many existing health partnerships and initiatives could contribute more to strengthening public health functions by helping build surveillance capacity. In India a World Bank–supported $146 million immunization project was instrumental in strengthening disease surveillance over the succeeding two years and beyond. The project spurred development of a new national surveillance strengthening program, now being implemented with additional World Bank financing.

Unless low-income countries strengthen such core public health functions as surveillance, policy formulation, and program monitoring and evaluation, they will find it difficult to deliver the basic health interventions to fight diseases and achieve the Millennium Development Goals for health and nutrition. The key constraints to progress on HIV/AIDS, for example, are weak government systems for policy analysis, disease surveillance, and monitoring and ineffective policies for human resources in health. To achieve their goals, national HIV/AIDS programs need to strengthen these core public health functions rather than focus exclusively on prevention, condoms, testing and counseling services, and treatment for HIV and opportunistic infections (box 8.5).

References

1. World Bank. 2002. *Public Health and World Bank Operations.* Human Development Network, Washington, DC.

2. Pan American Health Organization. 2000. *National Level Instruments for Measuring Essential Public Health Functions. Public Health in the Americas.* PAHO/Centers for Disease Control/Centro Latino Americano de Investigaciones en Sistemas de Salud, Washington, DC.

3. Khaleghian, Peyvand, and Monica Das Gupta. 2004. "Public Management and Essential Public Health Functions." Policy Research Working Paper 3220, World Bank Development, Research Group, Washington, DC. econ.worldbank.org/working_papers/33192/.

4. Khaleghian, P., and M. Das Gupta. 2004. "Public Management and the Essential Public Health Functions." World Bank Policy Research Working Paper, Washington, DC.

5. World Bank. 2002. "Transport." In *A Sourcebook for Poverty Reduction Strategies,* 325–362. Washington, DC.

6. Biego, G., ed. 1995. *Survey on Adult and Childhood Mortality, Tanzania.* Calverton, MD: Macro International.

7. Pendse, V. 1999. "Maternal Deaths in an Indian Hospital: A Decade of (No) Change?" *Reproductive Health Matters* (Special Issue on Safe Motherhood Initiatives).

8. Samai, O., and P. Sengeh. 1997. "Facilitating Emergency Obstetric Care through Transport and Communication, Bo, Sierra Leone." *International Journal of Gynecology and Obstetrics* 59 (Suppl. 2): 157–64.

9. Eissen, E., D. Efenne, and K. Sabitu. 1997. "Community Loan Funds and Transport Services for Obstetric Emergencies in Northern Nigeria." *International Journal of Gynecology and Obstetrics* 59 (Suppl. 2): S37–S46.

10. Debrouwere, V., R. Tonglett, and V. W. Lerbergh. 1998. "Strategies for Reducing Maternal Mortality in Developing Countries: What Can We Learn from the History of the Industrialized West?" *Tropical Medicine and Hygiene* 100: 771–782.

11. Esry, S., J. Potash, and L. Roberts, and C. Schiff. 1991 "Effects of Improved Water Supply and Sanitation on Ascariasis, Diarrhea, Dracunculiasis, Hookworm Infection, Schistosomiasis, and Trachoma." *Bulletin of the World Health Organization* 69 (5): 609–621.

12. Saade, C., M. Batemen, and D.B. Bendahmane. 2001. "The Story of a Successful Public-Private Partnership in Central America." Arlington, VA: BASICS II, EHP, UNICEF, USAID, and World Bank.

13. Hughes, G., K. Lvovsky, and M. Dunleavy. 2000. "Environmental Health in India: Priorities in Andhra Pradesh." World Bank, Environment and Social Development Unit, Washington DC.

14. World Bank. 2003. "Public Health at a Glance Fact Sheet: Indoor Air Pollution." Health, Nutrition, and Population Department, Washington, DC.

15. Quisumbing, A.R. 1995. "Gender Differences in Agricultural Productivity: A Survey of Empirical Evidence." *FCND Discussion Paper-IFPRI* 15.

16. Johnson-Welch, C. 1999. "Focusing on Women Works: Research on Improving Micronutrient Status through Food Based Interventions." International Center for Research on Women (ICRW)/Opportunities for Micronutrient Interventions (OMNI), Washington, DC.

17. World Health Organization. 2000. *Use of Antiretroviral Treatments in Adults with Particular Reference to Resource Limited Settings.* Geneva: WHO.

18. World Health Organization. 2003. *Global Health Sector Strategy for HIV/AIDS 2003–2007: Providing a Framework for Partnership and Action.* Geneva: WHO.

19. World Bank. 1994. *Better Health in Africa: Experience and Lessons Learned.* Washington, DC: World Bank.

Table 8.3 Examples of public health functions and infrastructure requirements for preventing and controlling communicable diseases

Public health function	HIV/AIDS	Tuberculosis	Malaria	Acute respiratory infection, diarrhea, and measles
Developing policy and strategy				
Adopting and reinforcing legislation	Providing HIV testing, ensuring confidentiality, and protecting the rights of people living with HIV/AIDS	Controlling drug quality and the monitoring of private sales of drugs Notifying people with tuberculosis when their cases are detected	Removing taxes and tariffs on essential commodities (ITNs, insecticides, drugs)	Regulating antidiarrheal drugs use
Promoting equitable access to health services	Targeting vulnerable groups (often poor or marginalized) with HIV/AIDS services Addressing gender barriers Contracting NGOs and community-based organizations (which are often more effective in reaching high-risk groups)	Providing free diagnosis and treatment Increasing community-based treatment options Addressing gender barriers	Authorizing mid-level and community workers to provide effective treatment in the community Adjusting or removing user fees for people at high risk (such as children under five)	Encouraging community-based prevention and treatment Monitoring the cost of services and establishing protective mechanisms for poor families
Developing quality standards and norms	Implementing protocols in voluntary counseling and testing, treating opportunistic infections, reducing mother to child transmission, and providing antiretrovirals Providing training and incentives to service providers Strengthening supervision and monitoring and evaluation	Ensuring adequate supervision and accountability based on monitoring and evaluation and performance-based contracting	Balancing the needs of the health sector in discussions on civil service reform Contracting out health services Crafting malaria treatment policies	Establishing guidelines and standards for clinical care for pneumonia and diarrhea Evaluating clinical performance
Developing national strategies for disease control	Developing strategies that take into account the specifics of the situation (stage of the epidemic, high-risk groups, capacity, resources)	Establishing disease control within sector programs	Incorporating malaria control policies in strategic plans for the health sector	Adopting integrated control of acute respiratory infections, diarrhea, and measles and incorporating it into the overall child health policy and plan (Integrated Management of Childhood Illness)
Providing finance and resource management	Calculating the cost of a package of key HIV/AIDS interventions and ensuring its financing	Ensuring financing for drug supplies; accountability of health personnel; strong central normative, surveillance; and a monitoring and evaluation unit	Including malaria control in sector budgets Expanding allocation for nonsalary recurrent expenditures commensurate with need	Including child health preventive and curative services in the overall sector budget
Developing policies for rapid approval of drugs and monitoring the quality of drugs	Adopting a policy on antiretrovirals	Developing efficient planning, procurement, and supply of quality-assured drugs and monitoring private sales, where feasible	Monitoring the availability of insecticides and effective antimalaria drugs in the marketplace	Monitoring drug resistance, particularly for pneumonia and dysentery

Table 8.3 Examples of public health functions and infrastructure requirements for preventing and controlling communicable diseases *(continued)*

Public health function	HIV/AIDS	Tuberculosis	Malaria	Acute respiratory infection, diarrhea, and measles
Measuring results: Collecting and disseminating evidence for policies, strategies, and actions Conducting health situation monitoring and analysis, including surveillance	Implementing second-generation surveillance	Applying a standardized quarterly system of recording and reporting on case detection and outcomes Conducting periodic surveys, where feasible	Using existing survey tools (such as the Demographic and Health Survey and the Multiple Indicator Cluster Survey) to monitor outcomes and impacts Conducting population-based surveillance Making decisions based on data	Conducting routine monitoring of health facility data Conducting periodic household surveys of immunization coverage, oral rehydration therapy coverage, and acute respiratory therapy treatment Conducting disease surveillance
Conducting research and development of innovative solutions	Fostering partnerships to conduct operational research on AIDS vaccines, new drugs, and new preventive tools	Fostering partnerships to pursue operational research and extending access to new technologies and strategies	Strengthening partnerships with research and technical partners to conduct operational research on efficacy and effectiveness of new drugs, insecticides, and preventive tools	Conducting operational research on new delivery mechanisms, such as community management of acute respiratory infections Strengthening partnerships for new pneumonia vaccine development and distribution
Providing information to consumers, providers, policymakers, and financiers	Providing information to policymakers on the socioeconomic costs of HIV/AIDS, the costs of scaling up interventions, and the cost-effectiveness of different interventions	Expanding information, education, and communication programs and social mobilization efforts to increase case detection and demand for services within communities and using key stakeholders	Disseminating best practices Providing information, education, and communication that promote behavior change	Using information, education, and communication programs and social marketing techniques to promote appropriate behaviors, such as handwashing
Strengthening health information and management systems	Strengthening health information systems, surveillance, HIV/AIDS program monitoring and evaluation, and their linkages	Integrating standard TB reporting into regular health systems without losing required depth of data for decision making	Using health information systems data to monitor performance of health workers and facilities	Providing health workers at the most peripheral level with feedback of results of health information systems
Conducting research and evaluation	Evaluating HIV/AIDS programs and conducting intervention research on interrupting modes of transmission, epidemiological risk and burden research, and health systems and operational research	Ensuring periodic evaluation at the local and national levels that increases accountability and motivation to perform	Conducting operations research on innovative methods to improve treatment and prevention practices at the community level Monitoring and evaluating programs using standardized indicators	Developing standardized indicators for program monitoring and evaluation

Table 8.3 Examples of public health functions and infrastructure requirements for preventing and controlling communicable diseases (continued)

Public health function	HIV/AIDS	Tuberculosis	Malaria	Acute respiratory infection, diarrhea, and measles
Preventing and controlling diseases Managing communicable diseases	Implementing effective interventions with adequate coverage to make an impact Strengthening links between HIV/AIDS and other diseases control programs (sexually transmitted diseases, tuberculosis, maternal and child health) Ensuring a reliable supply of good-quality condoms and drugs for treating sexually transmitted infections and opportunistic infections	Adapting design of case detection, diagnostic, and treatment delivery schemes to local conditions and resources	Collaborating with public health centers on implementing Integrated Management of Childhood Illness Establishing good-quality community-based treatment capacity through NGOs and the private sector Supervising and monitoring public and private sector health workers	Managing supervision, supply chain, immunization and other child health programs at the central, regional, and district levels
Providing health promotion information, education, and communication	Providing information, education, and communication programs for high-risk groups as well as the general population	Expanding information, education, and communication programs and social mobilization efforts to expand case detection and demand for services within communities using key stakeholders	Promoting use of insecticide-treated nets and improving home treatment practices by sponsoring behavior change campaigns	Promoting key family and community practices for child health
Promoting social participation and empowerment of citizens	Adopting a multisectoral approach to HIV/AIDS Involving people living with HIV/AIDS and high-risk groups in HIV/AIDS activities	Expanding information, education, and communication programs and social mobilization efforts to expand case detection and demand for services within communities using key stakeholders	Promoting use of insecticide-treated nets and improving home treatment practices by sponsoring behavior change campaigns	Promoting social mobilization for national immunization days and community-based child health and nutrition interventions
Reducing the impact of emergencies and disasters	Establishing social support networks for people living with HIV/AIDS and AIDS orphans Establishing social safety nets for poor households affected by HIV/AIDS and AIDS orphans (if possible)	Undertaking routine reporting and conducting periodic surveys to identify special risks (emergence of multidrug-resistant disease or outbreaks in prisons or health facilities)	Rapidly providing preventive tools (insecticide-treated nets) Establishing readily accessible treatment capacity	Establishing effective surveillance for detection of outbreaks of measles or diarrheal diseases common in population displacement Establishing effective, rapid access to immunization and treatment
Undertaking intersectoral action to improve health Improving environmental health	Treating medical waste generated by HIV/AIDS services	Encouraging improvement in conditions (ventilation, space) of households, worksites, prisons, and refugee camps in order to reduce exposure	Using proven, safe, and cost-effective environmental management techniques	Reducing indoor air pollution Forging public-private partnerships to improve water and sanitation (hand-washing) and other hygiene behaviors
Improving school health	Supporting school-based HIV/AIDS education programs	Increasing awareness to improve case detection and youth participation in treatment supervision	Facilitating rapid treatment and access to preventive strategies through schools	Promoting water and sanitation and life skills through Focusing Resource(s) on Effective School Health (FRESH)

Table 8.3 Examples of public health functions and infrastructure requirements for preventing and controlling communicable diseases *(continued)*

Public health function	HIV/AIDS	Tuberculosis	Malaria	Acute respiratory infection, diarrhea, and measles
Taking intersectoral actions	Supporting HIV/AIDS activities in other sectors: tourism, transport, labor, education	Supporting public-private collaboration on drug supply and drug quality control and stimulating research and development	Institutionalizing health impact assessment for new initiatives and projects in other sectors Using appropriate environmental management and vector control strategies in agricultural, water, and infrastructure projects	Collaborating with education, water and sanitation, and other sectors on key family practices
Developing human resources and building capacity for public health Developing policy, planning, and managerial capacity	Sharing the experience of success stories Maximizing the role of in-country HIV/AIDS Theme Groups in capacity building for policymakers and planners	Ensuring that policymakers and donors understand the impact improved distribution, retention, and quality of primary healthcare workers has on outcomes	Establishing capacity for short-, medium-, and long-term planning and budgeting to support malaria control programs Integrating planning for malaria control in health sector planning activities	Establishing a comprehensive human resources development plan with capacity building, follow-up, retention, and incentives to work in rural areas
Providing human resource development and training	Training health professionals, social workers, counselors, peer educators, program managers, and epidemiologists	Integrating technical and managerial training needs within larger preservice and in-service training and supervision efforts	Ensuring adequate numbers of trained health workers at facilities and in communities, including through use of contracting with NGOs and private sector	Training epidemiologists, and program managers Providing preservice and in-service Integrated Management of Childhood Illness skills-based training
Building capacity in communities	Training and funding NGOs and community-based organizations in HIV/AIDS programming and management, prevention, care, and support	Ensuring that the benefits to the community of engagement in disease control efforts are known and barriers to participation overcome	Engaging NGOs and private sector in community-based prevention and treatment activities	Engaging and training NGO staff and other private sector actors in delivering services and preventive messages at the community level

Financing Additional Spending for the Millennium Development Goals—In a Sustainable Way

Nha's family has 12 members. They used to be one of the richest families in the village (in Lao Cai Province, Vietnam). Now they are one of the poorest. They have suffered two shocks in recent years. First Nha's father died two years ago. So there are now only two main laborers in the family—Nha, 26, and his mother, 40. Nha has two young children. Two years ago, his daughter Lu Seo Pao also had a serious illness and had to be operated on in the district and province hospital. Nha's family had to sell four buffaloes, one horse, and two pigs to cover the expenses of treatment. The operation cost several million VND, but Lu Seo Pao is still not cured. All the people in Nha's community helped, but no one can contribute more than 20,000 VND (a little over $1). Nha's younger brother, Lu Seo Seng, who was studying in grade 6, had to leave school to help his family. If Lu Seo Pao was not ill, says Nha, his family would still have many buffaloes, he could have a house for his younger brother, and Seng could stay in school.[1]

Additional health spending is necessary in at least some countries. How should the extra spending be financed? How should the cost be divided between governments and donors? Many developing countries spend less than they appear to be able to afford. Other countries with similar per capita incomes devote larger shares of their GDP to health spending. Countries that spend less do so either because they place a lower priority on health in their public expenditure allocations or because they raise smaller shares of GDP in tax and nontax revenues.

Mobilizing additional domestic resources—by raising the share of government spending on the health sector or raising the share of GDP that is taxed—is worth exploring. But raising additional domestic resources for government health spending takes time. Even on optimistic assumptions about the growth of the health share of government spending, the tax share of GDP, and economic growth, health spending per capita might easily take 10 years to double in real terms.

Official development assistance for health can play a temporary role in financing additional expenditures. It increased in the 1990s, but overall development assistance did not, so development assistance for health probably will not increase indefinitely. Development assistance also entails difficulties, including its volatility. That volatility makes it an unreliable source of funding for permanent increases in recurrent expenditures. And increased expenditures financed through development assistance eventually have to be accommodated within each country's budget. The sustainability of increased expenditures therefore requires efforts on both domestic and external fronts.

Private health spending, whether out-of-pocket or from private insurance, is another source of funding for health. The importance of private spending as a share of GDP varies across country income groups, but it is higher in low-income countries (figure 9.1).

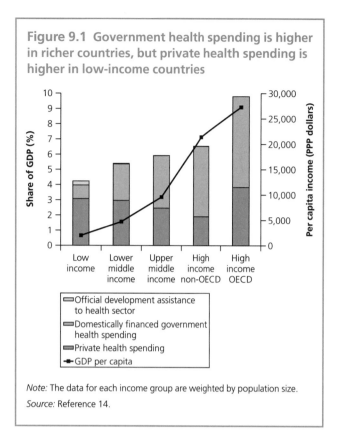

Figure 9.1 Government health spending is higher in richer countries, but private health spending is higher in low-income countries

Legend:
- Official development assistance to health sector
- Domestically financed government health spending
- Private health spending
- GDP per capita

Note: The data for each income group are weighted by population size.

Source: Reference 14.

Health spending—government isn't the only player

Private spending absorbs a larger share of income in poorer countries. In fact, in low-income countries, private health spending absorbs a larger share of GDP, on average, than domestically financed public spending. If private spending were private insurance, this might not matter. But in low-income and lower middle-income countries, private spending almost invariably means out-of-pocket expenditures, not private insurance.[2] In Cambodia, where the private health spending share of GDP is 6 percent, or in India and Vietnam, where the share is 4 percent, private health spending is almost entirely out-of-pocket. The same is true of many lower middle-income countries, such as China.

The large share of private spending leaves many near-poor households heavily exposed to the risk of impoverishing health expenses. In China evidence suggests that exposure to the risk of medical expenses[3] causes rural households to hold more wealth—and to hold more of it in liquid form.[4] This self-insurance is only partly successful at smoothing consumption when income shocks occur (due to a variety of factors, including illness). The problem is most pronounced for the poor: for the poorest 20 percent, 40 percent of an income shock is passed on to current consumption, while the richest 20 percent is protected from almost 90 percent of an income shock.[5]

In India a study estimated that nearly a quarter of people admitted to the hospital were above the poverty line when they went in and below it when they came out.[6] In Vietnam health expenses are estimated to have pushed about 3.5 percent of the population into absolute poverty in both 1993 and 1998.[7] In Cambodia a single hospital stay is estimated to have absorbed 88 percent of an average household's non-food consumption in 1997; for a household in the poorest 20 percent, the cost was greater than its entire annual non-food consumption.[8] The risk of large-scale impoverishment is clearly greater the poorer the country, since poorer countries tend to have larger shares of poor people.[9] A country's private share of health spending in GDP may not in practice be related to its per capita income. But on poverty-reduction grounds, there are good reasons to wish that it were.

Government has a clear role. It must not end up paying the medical bills of people who can afford to spend their own resources. Instead, it needs to concentrate financing on essential public goods and other areas where private spending is inefficient, target its limited resources on the poor, and use its stewardship capacity and resources to leverage private spending at lower levels of care to protect against catastrophic risks through some type of pooling mechanism. Vietnam—a country with one of the highest private spending shares in the world—has recently started doing just this, by providing central government support to the provinces to allow them to enroll poor and other disadvantaged groups in the national social insurance scheme.

Government spending—what's affordable?

Government spending is an important part of the picture, but how much can governments afford to spend? In contrast to private spending, government spending as a share of GDP is higher in richer countries (figure 9.1). But at any given per capita income, there is a surprising amount of variation across countries in the share of GDP allocated to government health programs. Countries that appear able to spend similar shares of GDP on government health programs end up spending quite different amounts.

A regression of the share of GDP absorbed by government health spending on per capita income provides some indication of what a country could afford to spend on government health programs (see figure 9.2). Bolivia, whose domestically financed government health spending accounts for 4.2 percent of its GDP, is considerably above the 2 percent predicted by the regression line. By contrast, Uganda's domestically financed government health spending accounts for barely 0.5 percent of GDP, well below its predicted share of 1.4 percent.

Countries above the regression line have a stronger case for additional development assistance than countries below it. For countries below the regression line, the focus

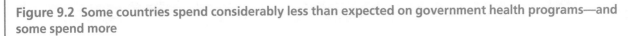

Figure 9.2 Some countries spend considerably less than expected on government health programs—and some spend more

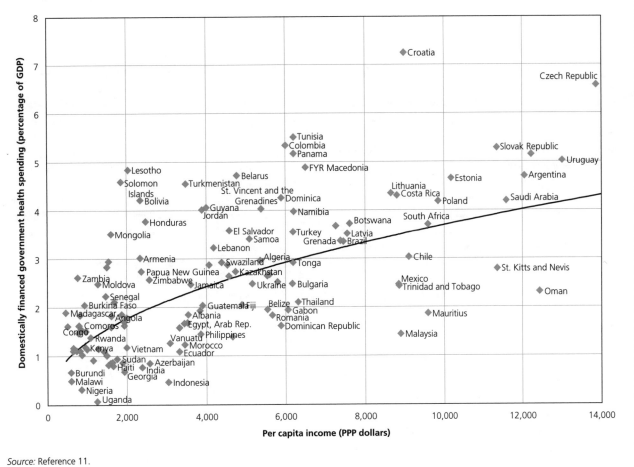

Source: Reference 11.

of the health financing debate should initially be on why health spending appears to be less than what the country could afford and on finding ways of remedying the situation. External assistance in such a setting is not precluded, however. Indeed, countries in that setting could benefit from technical assistance and are likely to require financial assistance to meet the adjustment costs of mobilizing additional resources to move to affordable spending (box 9.1).

Reasons for underspending

Domestically financed government health spending comes from general revenues and social insurance contributions. The amount of general revenues flowing into the health sector depends on both the amount of general (tax and nontax★)

★ Some countries with large public sector companies, especially in the Middle East and North Africa, South Asia, and Sub-Saharan Africa, have important nontax revenues, which can represent as much as 9 percent of GDP. Increasing revenues from this source would require consideration of the competitive environment in which the companies operate and the need for reinvestment in the companies.

revenues collected by the government (the general revenue share) and the share of general revenues allocated to the health sector (the health share of government spending).[10] Low government health spending could be due to either or both being low. In poorer countries, both shares are typically lower than they are in richer countries (figure 9.3). But there are differences across countries that cannot be explained by per capita income alone.

Figure 9.4 divides low-income countries into those below the regression line in figure 9.2 (those spending less than appears affordable by international standards) and those above the regression line. Countries in quadrant I have above-average values of both government health spending as a share of total government spending and total government spending as a share of GDP. Not surprisingly, these countries are well above the regression line in figure 9.2. Countries in quadrant I place a strong emphasis on the health sector in government spending allocations, along with a strong emphasis on government finance in the economy in general. By contrast, countries in quadrant III have

Box 9.1 Raising tax levels in the developing world—hard but doable

Direct taxes include taxes on personal income, corporate profits, payrolls, property, and wealth. Indirect taxes (taxes on transactions and commodities) include general sales taxes, value-added taxes, excise taxes, turnover taxes, import duties, and export taxes. The ratio of tax revenues to GDP increases with GDP. Low-income countries raise an average of 14 percent of their GDP through taxation, while lower middle-income countries raise 19 percent (see table). These averages conceal large variations: a low-income country may raise as little as 4 percent of GDP in taxation (Myanmar) or as much as 36 percent (Lesotho), while a lower middle-income group may raise as little as 9 percent of GDP (Guatemala) or as much as 30 percent (Ecuador).

The small size of the formal economy is a major constraint to the use of payroll taxes to collect personal income taxes. In Bolivia, for example, 45 percent of the population lives in rural areas, and a large part of the urban population works in the informal economy. As a consequence, only about 30 percent of household income is paid through payroll taxes. Increasing personal income taxes would be a burden only for civil servants and employees of a few companies and would increase the incentives for transferring activities to the informal sector.

Increasing tax revenues by raising corporate income taxes may also be difficult when there are only a handful of companies reporting income, as is the case when extractive and service sectors are in the hands of the government. A high concentration of the tax burden on a few firms makes raising taxes difficult, especially if the owners are politically influential. If extractive and service sectors have been privatized, international corporations are likely to be involved (especially in petroleum and mineral industries), and a high corporate income tax rate risks driving them away.

Import taxes, especially on luxury goods (tobacco, alcohol, cars), are a politically attractive option. But import taxes can create significant economic distortions, especially if imports have a high capital content. Such taxes may also be hard to collect. Bolivia has more than 6,000 kilometers of borders with its five neighbors, making it impossible to control illegal imports. Thousands of people carry all types of products—from alcoholic beverages to flour and rice—on their backs through the borders each day, depending on the relative prices on each side of the border.

Increasing revenues through tax reforms requires political commitment and administrative will, but it is possible. Bolivia raised tax revenues from 3 percent of GDP in 1983 to 17 percent by the end of 1987. Facing hyperinflation of 25,000 percent in 1985, Bolivia, with World Bank technical assistance and financing for adjustment costs, undertook major structural reforms, including tax reform. It replaced a complex tax system of more than 100 tax rates (differential import tariffs, earmarked taxes, progressive personal income taxes, and corporate taxes with

Taxes as a percentage of GDP, by income group

Country income group	Total tax revenue	Taxes on international trade	Excise duties	General sales tax	Social security
Low-income (less than $760 per capita)	14.0	4.5	1.6	2.7	1.1
Lower middle-income ($761–$3,030 per capita)	19.4	4.2	2.3	4.8	4.0
Upper middle-income ($3,031–$9,360 per capita)	22.3	3.7	2.0	5.7	5.6
High-income (more than $9,360 per capita)	30.9	0.3	3.1	6.2	8.8

below-average health shares in government spending and below-average general revenue shares. By international standards these countries place comparatively little emphasis on health and on public finance in the economy in general.

Countries in quadrant II attach importance to health in government spending allocations, but they tax comparatively small shares of their GDP. As a result, these countries fall below the regression line in figure 9.2. Countries in quadrant IV attach relatively little priority to the health sector in government spending allocations, but they tax relatively large shares of their GDPs. In some cases, the general revenue share is sufficiently large to offset the relatively small health share and the country spends more than is expected on the basis of its per capita income (Angola and Zimbabwe are examples). In other cases—such as Burundi and Eritrea—the relatively high general revenue share is more than offset by the relatively small health share and the country spends less than expected on the basis of its per capita income.

many exceptions and loopholes) with a simple structure of six taxes:

- a uniform import tariff rate of 20 percent, reduced to 10 percent in 1988

- a 10 percent value-added tax on a broad base, excluding only housing and financial services

- taxes on consumption of luxury goods (alcoholic beverages, perfumes, cosmetics, tobacco, and jewelry)

- a 1 percent transaction tax (a cumulative turnover tax)

- a progressive tax on vehicles (1.5–5 percent) and urban real estate (1.5–3 percent), which was shared with municipalities

- a 2 percent tax, increased to 2.5 percent in 1988, on the net worth of public and private enterprises (small informal enterprises paid a fixed lump sum instead)

All other taxes, including personal and corporate income taxes, were eliminated. At the same time, Bolivia established a strong and credible tax administrative structure.

Although far from perfect, the tax reform dramatically increased revenues and equilibrated oil prices to international standards. The reform has endured for more than 12 years, and taxes now represent 19 percent of GDP. The government is currently considering a reform that would introduce a progressive income tax.

Social expenditures must be accommodated within each country's budget constraint over a reasonable time span. Although difficult, such accommodation can take place if government commitment is strong and reforms are well planned, preferably within a Poverty Reduction Strategy Paper and medium-term expenditure framework structure.

Source: World Bank staff.

Figure 9.3 Health absorbs a higher share of government spending, and general revenues absorb a higher share of GDP in richer countries

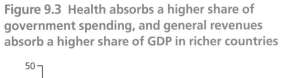

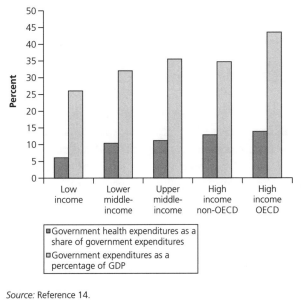

Government health expenditures as a share of government expenditures

Government expenditures as a percentage of GDP

Source: Reference 14.

Mobilizing extra domestic resources—where you push depends on where you're coming from

Countries spending less than seems affordable by international standards and wanting to mobilize additional domestic resources for government health programs face different challenges depending on whether they are in quadrants II, III, or IV.

For countries in quadrant II the challenge is to push for a higher share of general revenues in GDP rather than to raise the health share of government spending, which is already relatively high by international standards. This can be done. Some countries have achieved high average annual growth of the share of general revenue in GDP, though others have slipped backwards (figure 9.5). Bolivia increased the tax share of GDP at an annual average rate of 5 percent during the 1990s, the result of a sustained reform process that boosted the tax share of GDP from 3 percent in 1983 to 17 percent by the end of 1987 (see box 9.1). The health sector in Bolivia has benefited from this growth of tax revenues, with government health spending as a share of GDP growing at an annual rate of nearly 10 percent during the 1990s (figure 9.5). Ministries of health rarely interest themselves in tax reform. But Bolivia shows that this indifference is probably misplaced.

For countries in quadrant IV the challenge is to push for a higher share of health in government spending allocations, since general revenues already represent a relatively high share of GDP by international standards. Several countries raised their government health spending share in the 1990s, often considerably (figure 9.6). A challenge is to demonstrate to an often skeptical ministry of finance that additional resources in the government health budget are warranted.

One cause of skepticism may be a misplaced perception that the health sector is necessarily an "unproductive" sector. The perception is misplaced because—as emphasized in chapter 1 and as the recent SARS episodes in Canada, China, and Vietnam illustrate—better health outcomes are closely linked to economic growth and poverty reduction.

Figure 9.4 Small health shares and low government revenues cause some low-income countries to spend less than they can afford on health

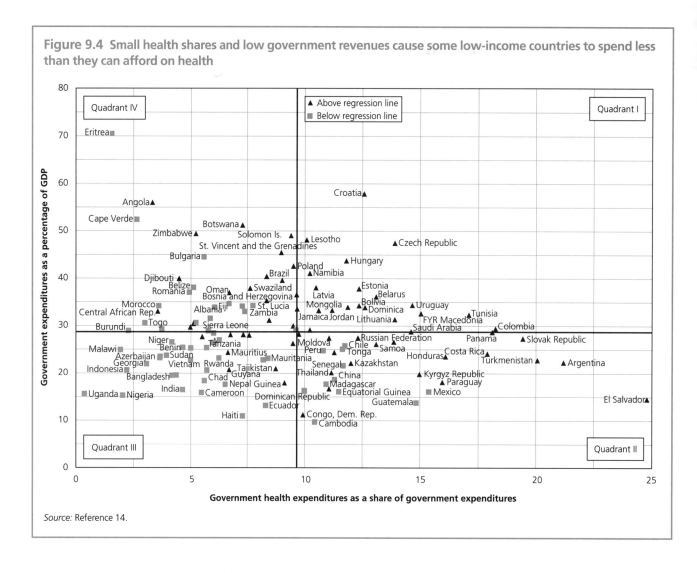

Source: Reference 14.

Insofar as more health spending leads to better health outcomes, the health sector may be as "productive" as, say, the education sector. The issue is not whether better health carries economic benefits, which is indisputable—it is whether more spending will lead to better health outcomes. Both issues tend to get overlooked by ministries of health, which often view the importance of their mission of improving health outcomes as self-evident and take for granted that government programs are achieving their intended health outcomes.

Some uncomfortable arithmetic: Raising domestic resources takes time

There are, then, two ways to mobilize additional domestic resources for tax-financed health spending—increase the share of government spending going to health and increase the share of GDP that is taxed. Pursuing these two avenues, how quickly could a country reach the regression line? And what level of spending would it reach?

Table 9.1 shows the implications for trends in government health spending as a share of GDP and in dollar terms per capita of different assumptions about the growth of government health spending as a share of total government spending, government revenues as a share of GDP, and GDP per capita. The figures in table 9.1 are hypothetical but realistic enough to be worrying. In the pessimistic scenario A, the share of government health spending grows at 2 percent a year, government tax revenues at 0.5 percent, and GDP per capita at 1 percent. These figures are achievable, though many countries have failed to sustain them in the past. A country spending 1 percent of its GDP on health in 2000 would end up spending 1.45 percent in 2015; if its 2000 level of spending per capita were $10 (about that of Mauritania or Zambia), its 2015 level would be $16.84. Scenarios B, C, and D are progressively more optimistic about how quickly growth would proceed. But even in the most optimistic scenario, government health spending in 2015 is only 2.8 percent of GDP, or $32 per

Figure 9.5 General revenues as a share of GDP rose significantly during the 1990s in some countries and fell in others

Annual percentage change in share of GDP absorbed by taxes and general revenues

Turkey
Dominican Republic
Argentina
Maldives
Peru
Bolivia
Paraguay
Nepal
Namibia
St. Vincent & the Grenadines
Uruguay
Iran, Islamic Rep.
Bhutan
Chile
South Africa
Madagascar
India
Panama
Mexico
Jordan
Philippines
Tunisia
Mauritius
Costa Rica
Pakistan
Venezuela, RB
Thailand
Romania
Swaziland
Sri Lanka
Côte d'Ivoire
Bulgaria
Hungary
Oman
Myanmar

Source: Reference 14.

Figure 9.6 The share of GDP going to government health spending during the 1990s rose significantly in some countries and fell in others

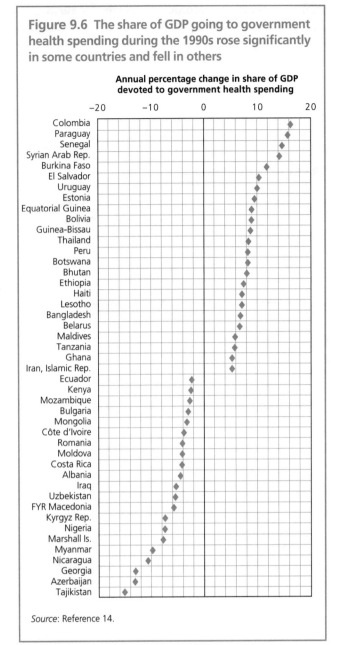

Annual percentage change in share of GDP devoted to government health spending

Colombia
Paraguay
Senegal
Syrian Arab Rep.
Burkina Faso
El Salvador
Uruguay
Estonia
Equatorial Guinea
Bolivia
Guinea-Bissau
Thailand
Peru
Botswana
Bhutan
Ethiopia
Haiti
Lesotho
Bangladesh
Belarus
Maldives
Tanzania
Ghana
Iran, Islamic Rep.
Ecuador
Kenya
Mozambique
Bulgaria
Mongolia
Côte d'Ivoire
Romania
Moldova
Costa Rica
Albania
Iraq
Uzbekistan
FYR Macedonia
Kyrgyz Rep.
Nigeria
Marshall Is.
Myanmar
Nicaragua
Georgia
Azerbaijan
Tajikistan

Source: Reference 14.

capita. That 2.8 percent could still be below what appears to be affordable by international standards. And $32 would probably be too little to fund a basic health program.

That the share of GDP flowing into the health sector cannot be raised overnight[10] does not mean that countries that can apparently afford to spend more out of their own resources should not be encouraged to start. Development agencies have a role in helping them do so—through technical support of tax reform, assistance in developing government commitment to health in public expenditure allocations, and financial assistance to ease the adjustment costs and provide support while the gap between current and affordable spending is being closed.

Development assistance—a mixed blessing

Development assistance tends to account for a larger share of government health spending in poorer countries (see figure 9.1). Development assistance for health is especially important in Sub-Saharan Africa: all 12 countries with external funding exceeding 35 percent of total health expenditures in 2000 were in Africa.[11]

Development assistance is not, however, without drawbacks. Although development assistance for health increased in the 1990s, total development assistance did not, and there is no assurance that development assistance for health will continue to grow. Industrial countries show no signs of closing the gap between current levels of development assistance and the proposed 0.5 percent of GDP. Judging by the past, relying on continually increasing levels of development assistance for health would not be wise. Furthermore, donor financing depends on donor budgets, which are subject to

Table 9.1 Some uncomfortable arithmetic—how long to raise domestic resources for health?

Item	Scenario			
	A	B	C	D
Assumed annual growth (percent)				
Government health expenditure as a percentage of government expenditure	2.00	3.00	4.00	5.00
Government expenditure as a percentage of GDP	0.50	1.00	1.50	2.00
GDP per capita	1.00	1.50	2.00	2.50
Implied annual growth (percent)				
Government health expenditure as a percentage of GDP	2.51	4.03	5.56	7.10
Government health expenditure per capita	3.54	5.59	7.67	9.78
Trend in government health expenditure (percent of GDP)				
2000	1.00	1.00	1.00	1.00
2005	1.13	1.22	1.31	1.41
2010	1.28	1.48	1.72	1.99
2015	1.45	1.81	2.25	2.80
Trend in government health expenditure per capita (U.S. dollars)				
2000	0.00	10.00	10.00	10.00
2005	11.90	13.13	14.47	15.94
2010	14.15	16.40	18.98	21.93
2015	16.84	21.00	26.14	32.48

Source: World Bank staff.

the usual business and political cycles and may go up or down each year.

From a country perspective, development assistance is a very volatile source of funding for health. The ratio of external financing to total health expenditures increased or decreased yearly in selected countries in South and East Africa that showed improvements in child mortality between 1995 and 2000—in some cases sharply, as it did in Somalia (figure 9.7). Obviously, then, it is not prudent for countries to commit to permanent expenditures for such items as salaries for nurses and doctors on the basis of uncertain financing flows from development assistance funds.

Donors often require that assistance be kept in parallel budgets outside the ministry of finance, which precludes appropriate planning and targeting of expenditures. In 2000 off-budget spending was estimated to represent more than 46 percent of health spending in Tanzania and more than 50 percent in Uganda.[12,13] Although some off-budget spending, such as the resources collected from user fees, is domestically funded, most is funded by donors, who encourage this practice in order to facilitate accounting for the direct impact of their resources.

But because money is fungible, once external financing becomes available for health, ministries of finance may substitute donor funds for regular treasury financing of expenditures, resulting in only marginal increases in overall health expenditures (chapter 10). This is especially so in countries

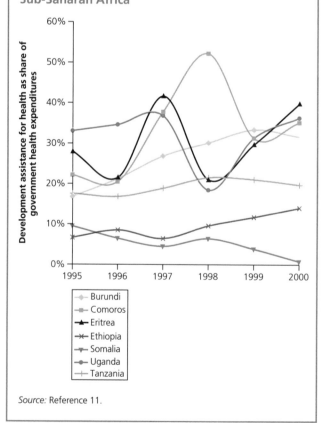

Figure 9.7 Importance of external financing in total health expenditures in selected countries in Sub-Saharan Africa

Source: Reference 11.

operating under strict budget constraints, where increased expenditures in many sectors have been suppressed for some time. As resources from abroad become available for health, political pressures are likely to divert resources previously available to health to other uses. So a simple assessment of the impact of external resources on outputs or the purchase of additional inputs does not take into account the impact of reduced resources from regular budgets.

Off-budget expenditures in health may partly explain the low government expenditures in some countries, such as Uganda. Moreover, off-budget expenditures make it impossible to properly target resources to particular interventions, geographic locations, or population groups. Such targeting may be essential for improving the impact of expenditures on outcomes and for reaching the health Millennium Development Goals, as explained in chapter 4.

Most important, spending commitments in the health sector must be permanent. This means that any external financing must eventually be replaced by additional domestic revenues or by reallocating expenditures from other sectors. Because both these policy measures are difficult to implement, countries must carefully analyze the commitments they make to their populations on the basis of temporary external financing.

Sustainability of health expenditures—a dim picture?

A dim picture of the sustainability of additional health expenditures can emerge from some of the main messages of this chapter and chapter 4:

- Health outcomes are influenced by multiple factors, many of them outside the health sector, such as access to roads and clean water, and requiring additional investment.

- Not all the Millennium Development Goals are for health, and countries have many other priorities.

- Raising additional domestic revenues requires increased capacity and takes time.

- Development assistance has not increased to expected levels and may be volatile at the country level, so expenditures financed with such funding must eventually be accommodated within each country's budget constraints.

In discussing resource mobilization—whether domestic or external—a sense of realism needs to be maintained. All countries face budget constraints. They are more difficult to live with in low-income countries with limited capacity to increase tax revenues and relatively inflexible expenditures. The possibility of accommodating increased expenditures in health diminishes when economies are in a downturn and facing decreased tax revenues (as many countries in Latin America and the Caribbean are) or when they have to reduce the overall nonfinancial public sector deficit in order to be fiscally prudent, meet regional commitments (such as joining the European Union), meet commitments to International Monetary Fund programs, or maintain international credit ratings. Commitments outside the health sector also need to be kept in mind. Expenditures that improve health outcomes—such as infrastructure projects crucial for enabling people to get to health facilities—may even have to be increased. All expenditures must be considered to avoid excessive leveraging at the country level that would threaten fiscal sustainability (maintaining a country's debt-to-GDP ratios and liquidity requirements for debt service).

While difficult, the prospects for achieving sustainable health expenditures are not necessarily bleak. Fiscal sustainability implies working on all fronts of the fiscal deficit: raising tax revenues, reallocating expenditures across the budget, and increasing donor funding in the form of grants or other forms that may be registered as part of the revenue stream. The issues point to a range of tasks that require a joint effort by developing countries and donors.

What needs to be done domestically

Low spenders need to increase resources for health by raising taxes, raising allocations to health, or both. All countries need to strive for good-quality Poverty Reduction Strategy Papers and medium-term expenditure frameworks. They need to align targets and goals with resources. They need to manage resources through improved public expenditure management systems, focus resources at the margin on programs that will have the largest impact on outcomes, and improve the impact of expenditures on outcomes through appropriate targeting of interventions and population groups. As indicated in chapter 4, policies and institutions in the health sector need improving. Countries need to find mechanisms for pooling out-of-pocket expenditures and expand the financial envelope beyond fiscal efforts.

What donors need to do

Donors need to make good on the promise of increased financing. Development assistance needs to be timely and predictable, so that it can be used to finance carefully planned recurrent expenditures that may eventually be covered by domestic financing. Donors need to improve coordination among themselves, eliminating off-budget financing, for example, which inhibits appropriate country budgeting and targeting.

References

1. Vietnam-Sweden Mountain Rural Development Programme, ActionAid, Save the Children Fund, and Oxfam. 1999. *A Synthesis of Participatory Poverty Assessments from Four Sites in Vietnam.* Hanoi.

2. Musgrove, P., R. Zeramdini, and G. Carrin. 2002. "Basic Patterns in National Health Expenditure." *Bulletin of the World Health Organization* 80 (2): 134–142.

3. Akin, J.S., W.H. Dow, and P.M. Lance. 2004. "Did the Distribution of Health Insurance in China Continue to Grow Less Equitable in the Nineties? Results from a Longitudinal Survey." *Social Science and Medicine* 58 (2): 293–304.

4. Jalan, J., and M. Ravallion. 2001. "Behavioral Responses to Risk in Rural China." *Journal of Development Economics* 66 (1): 23–49.

5. Jalan, J., and M. Ravallion. 1999. "Are the Poor Less Well Insured? Evidence on Vulnerability to Income Risk in Rural China." *Journal of Development Economics* 58 (1): 61–81.

6. Peters, D.H., A.S. Yazbeck, R. Sharma, G. Ramana, L.H. Pritchett, and A. Wagstaff. 2002. *Better Health Systems for India's Poor: Findings, Analysis, and Options.* Washington, DC: World Bank.

7. Wagstaff, A., and E. van Doorslaer. 2003. "Catastrophe and Impoverishment in Paying for Health Care: With Applications to Vietnam 1993–98." *Health Economics* 12 (11): 921–933.

8. World Bank, SIDA, AusAID, Royal Netherlands Embassy, Ministry of Health of Vietnam. *Vietnam. Growing Healthy: A Review of Vietnam's Health Sector.* Hanoi: World Bank.

9. World Bank. 2000. *World Development Report 2000/2001: Attacking Poverty.* Washington, DC: World Bank.

10. Hay, R. 2003. "The 'Fiscal Space' for Publicly Financed Health Care." Oxford Policy Institute Policy Brief.

11. World Health Organization. 2002. *The World Health Report 2002: Reducing Risks, Promoting Healthy Life.* Geneva.

12. World Bank. 2003. "Health Sector Public Expenditure Review Update FY 03." Washington, DC.

13. Republic of Uganda. 2002. "Public Expenditure Review: Report on the Progress and Challenges of Budget Reform." Republic of Uganda.

14. World Bank. 2003. *World Development Indicators 2003.* Washington, DC: World Bank.

CHAPTER 10

Applying the Lessons of Development Assistance for Health

Development assistance to the health sector has been increasing, both in real terms and as a proportion of official development assistance. It can be effective in countries with sound policies and institutions. But in countries with weak policies and institutions, it has little impact on health outcomes. Recent work on development effectiveness yields other important lessons, too. Conditionality can work—but only if governments are committed to the conditions they agree to. Donors cannot force policies on governments, but they can help design them. And aid is at least partially fungible, with governments shifting their spending patterns in response to donor allocations.

These and other lessons have spurred interest at the World Bank and among other donors in broader development assistance mechanisms, such as sectorwide programs and poverty reduction support credits, which aim to have countries leading donor coordination, with strategic coherence ensured through a Poverty Reduction Strategy Paper. To be effective, the strategy should contain a careful analysis of the Millennium Development Goals and be linked firmly to outcomes. The related financial coherence then needs to be expressed in the medium-term expenditure framework. A practical lesson for donors is to work more closely with each other and with governments to ensure that the number of country coordination bodies for health is limited, that resources are pooled, and that aid is untied to

procurement only from the country of origin of the funding. Also needed is a common framework for reporting and assessing progress, with a commitment to learn from it and make appropriate policy adjustments.

Are the lessons of development assistance being learned and applied in practice? They appear to be. In the World Bank's analytical work, policy dialogue, and financial operations over the past 18 months are many positive signs of change.

The previous chapters point to the many actions developing country governments can take to accelerate the pace of progress on the Millennium Development Goals for health while ensuring that much of the benefit accrues to the poorest and most disadvantaged households. At the same time, the many international partners to health and nutrition—bilateral and multilateral agencies, philanthropic organizations, and transnational companies—have a heavy responsibility to assist. This chapter assesses the track record of development assistance to health, outlines the lessons learned, and reviews some recent attempts to improve the effectiveness of development assistance to health and its contribution to meeting the health goals. It also reviews the Bank's responses to the Millennium Development Goal challenge—how the Bank's commitment to the goals has influenced its analytical work, its dialogue with and technical assistance to countries, its country assistance strategies, its lending activities, and its work on monitoring and evaluation.

The review highlights breakthroughs and promising new approaches and identifies continuing constraints to better performance.

At the High-Level Forum on the Millennium Development Goals for health held in Geneva in January 2004, a wide variety of actors—donors, international technical agencies, philanthropists, and developing countries—agreed broadly on a number of points. They agreed that the Millennium Development Goals for health indeed pose formidable challenges and that it is vital for all to rise to those challenges. They agreed that a greater sense of urgency is required if 2015 is not to pass by with a large number of countries having missed the targets. And they agreed on actions to mobilize resources for health, to enhance aid effectiveness and harmonization, to increase human resources, and to monitor performance.

Development assistance to health— what have we learned?

Despite a decline in overall official development assistance, development assistance to health rose in real terms and as a proportion of official development assistance in the 1990s (figure 10.1).[1] With new funding sources for health in 2000–02—including the Bill and Melinda Gates Foundation; the Global Fund to Fight AIDS, Tuberculosis and Malaria; the special U.S. financing for HIV/AIDS; and World Bank International Development Association (IDA) grants—commitments from all external sources including foundations rose from an average of $6.4 billion in 1997–99 to about $8.1 billion in 2002.* And funding can be expected to continue to rise in the coming years.[2]

What has development assistance to health achieved in recent years? Can this money be spent in a way that will have a greater impact on health outcomes? What are some of the lessons of experience that can be carried forward as the external financing envelope expands?

Development assistance to health works— in a good policy environment

Development assistance to health supports a vast array of activities and services, some focused on specific diseases (polio, tuberculosis, HIV/AIDS); some on strengthening health systems (disease surveillance, training nurses and midwives); and some on particular services (reproductive and child health services). Did this assistance actually change health outcomes? Recent work from the World Bank suggests that it did.[3,4] But development assistance to health does not improve health outcomes in countries where the policy environment is poor.[4] With "good" policies and institutions (strong property rights, little corruption, an efficient bureaucracy), an extra 1 percent of GDP in aid is estimated to have lead to a decline in infant mortality of 0.9 percent. By contrast, where policies were only average, the decline was only 0.4 percent. And where policies were poor, aid is estimated to have had no significant effect on infant mortality.

Corroborating the finding that aid has little or no effect if policies and institutions are poor is the World Bank's experience with projects. Numerous evaluation studies, development effectiveness reports, implementation completion reports, and quality reviews demonstrate that the major weaknesses in the use of development assistance to health arise from institutional issues. Projects are more likely to have a development impact if adequate institutional analysis is undertaken before a health sector operation is approved, if clear institutional lines of responsibility are established, and if implementation is entrusted to a strong team.

This finding is influencing IDA allocations, which are no longer based only on per capita income but also on Bank staff assessments of countries' policies and institutions. A similar approach is being followed at the subnational level. The Bank's country assistance strategy for India over the past five years has focused on a few states, such as Andra Pradesh and Karnataka. These states have

---

* The International Development Association provides "credits" to the world's poorest countries—loans at zero interest with a 10 year grace period and maturities of 35–40 years.

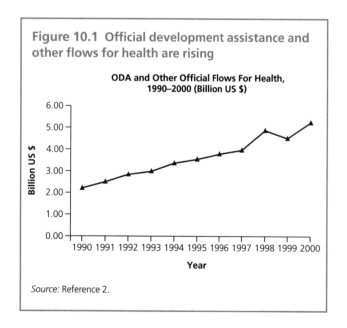

Figure 10.1 Official development assistance and other flows for health are rising

ODA and Other Official Flows For Health, 1990–2000 (Billion US $)

Source: Reference 2.

put fiscal reform, governance issues, and sectoral strategy at the top of the development agenda—and been rewarded by development partners with new financing for health and other sectors.

But the productivity of aid is not a black-and-white issue. There are graduations of good policy, and as policy gets better the productivity of aid increases. Improving governance can enable countries to get more out of health spending. In Bangladesh, for example, an additional dollar of government health spending spent after improvements in governance are made is estimated to reduce under-five mortality by 14 percent; without such improvements, under-five mortality would fall just 9 percent. Bangladesh has made large strides in reducing child mortality in recent years, relying on nongovernmental organizations to deliver many services. Raising the quality of governance from below average to above average (based on the internationally agreed governance index) would allow it to reap gains more quickly at given levels of public spending.[5]

There may be a tradeoff between targeting assistance on the neediest countries and achieving the greatest impact from development assistance to health. But if there is, it is not an all-or-nothing decision: countries need not move from "bad" policies to "excellent" policies in order for aid to be justified. And in countries with weak policies, a focus by donors on policy dialogue and technical assistance to improve the environment for development assistance to health can set the stage for a larger infusion of financial support.

Aid can help improve health policies—under certain conditions

Conditionality can work—if country commitment is in place. Tying aid to policy changes is a common practice, but recent studies have cast doubt on the ability of conditions to bring about reform.[6] If governments are committed to reform, conditions can help—by enabling governments to commit publicly to certain reforms and persuade private investors of their seriousness. But if governments are not committed to reform, conditions will not make them reform, often because disbursements continue anyway.

Donors cannot force policies on governments—but they can help design policy. Donors can alert governments to the reasons for reform and help nurture commitment. But at the end of the day, it is governments that have to sustain it (box 10.1). Analytical work, training and technical assistance, disseminating ideas about policy reform and development, and stimulating debate in civil society can all be valuable activities for donors to support while the government's commitment to reform is growing.

Vietnam in the late 1980s and early 1990s is a good example. At a landmark meeting in 1986, the ruling communist party decided to break with the past and introduce sweeping economic reforms. In the health sector this included introducing user fees at public facilities, legalizing private medicine, deregulating the pharmaceutical industry, and opening the pharmaceuticals and medical equipment industries to

---

Box 10.1 The importance of country commitment: How Bangladesh and Thailand have fared in reducing malnutrition

Nutrition has not made it to the national political agenda in most countries, because nutrition advocates have not succeeded in linking improved nutrition with political and economic goals or creating popular demand to eliminate malnutrition. Can donors help? In Bangladesh, UNICEF and the Bank partnered with the government to present the case that the country could not achieve its economic goals without reducing malnutrition. They persuaded policymakers that funding a national nutrition program was a good investment, and a new nutrition project was approved in 1995. But commitment is often fragile, and careful and continuing efforts are needed to sustain the initial commitment through changes in political scenarios.

The issue is not just how to build initial commitment, but how to broaden and maintain commitment and complement it with systematic investments in institutional capacity development. The first nutrition investment in Bangladesh was wound up in 2001. Child care and health-seeking behaviors improved substantially in project areas, and malnutrition rates in the country declined. A new follow-on nutrition investment was approved, but is struggling in the challenging policy environment for social sectors. Contradictory messages from donors and other partners, and frequent changes in governmental portfolios, have added to the challenge.

In Thailand, commitment-building for nutrition was achieved and nurtured with little external support. It generated commitment for nutrition by building a wide consensus (among the government, nongovernmental organizations—NGOs—and the private sector) around the benefits of nutrition—not as a welfare issue but as a human development issue. This initial commitment was sustained by ensuring that policy statements were closely linked to national investment plans, building strong technical and managerial capacity for nutrition in the country (often through external aid), and linking these actions with a strong buy-in and demand from communities. Malnutrition rates in Thailand declined from 51 percent in the early 1980s to 18 percent in 1990.

Source: World Bank staff.

international trade. Initially, Vietnam saw no increase in aid. But institutions such as the United Nations Development Programme and the World Bank helped facilitate the reform process by organizing international workshops for the Vietnamese to exchange ideas on policy with their neighbors. This set the stage for a large inflow of donor financing, starting about 1995 and continuing to the present.

Donors can support innovative financing mechanisms to improve performance by linking disbursements to specific performance measures, including better policies. This is the tack taken by the Global Fund for AIDS, Tuberculosis and Malaria. And it is one way the Global Alliance for Vaccines and Immunization disburses its funds to countries, using a per capita payment for each additional child fully vaccinated against a target schedule. Recent programmatic social adjustment loans to Peru and Brazil by the World Bank link disbursement of large single tranches of funding to policy changes targeting public health spending toward the poor. Performance-based lending is also at the heart of the new scheme for IDA credit buy-downs for polio (box 10.2).

Box 10.2 Helping eradicate polio through IDA credit buy-downs

To ensure financing for the Millennium Development Goals, governments, foundations, agencies, and development banks are all exploring new financing approaches that have the potential to increase resource flows, adjust the concessionality of funding where appropriate, and help focus more attention on impact.

The IDA credit buy-down mechanism was recently piloted in several projects supporting polio eradication, clearly a global public good. The mechanism enhances the concessionality of IDA's assistance in priority areas, mobilizes additional resources from external partners, and focuses the attention of governments, partners, and Bank staff on clearly defined performance objectives.

Two projects—in Nigeria and Pakistan—were implemented in fiscal 2003, in partnership with the Bill and Melinda Gates Foundation, Rotary International, and the United Nations Foundation. The partnerships will buy down a country's IDA loans on successful completion of the country's polio eradication program. Because of the generous loan terms, each grant dollar unlocks roughly $2.50 for countries to fight polio. To fund the buy-downs, the partnership has established a trust fund with $25 million from the Gates Foundation and $25 million from Rotary International and the United Nations Foundation. This $50 million investment has the potential to buy down roughly $125 million in World Bank IDA loans. In this way, developing countries can mobilize what ultimately becomes grant funding to eradicate polio—and contribute beyond their borders to the global campaign to eliminate polio.

Source: World Bank staff.

The fungibility in development assistance to health is substantial

Much aid is earmarked—both across sectors and within them. One part of a development agency gives a grant to the ministry of health for a health sector reform while another does the same for a primary education project. One agency makes a loan to the ministry of health for a tuberculosis project while another makes a loan for a malaria control project. The intention of donors is that these activities remain tightly sealed—the health sector reform funds are to be kept separate from the primary education project funds, and the tuberculosis project funds are to be kept separate from the malaria control project funds. The idea is to ensure that the government makes a certain spending choice that it would not have made had it been handed a check for the same amount.

One view of aid is what-you-see-is-what-you-get: a government receives $1 million for a water project, and the net impact is $1 million worth of extra spending on the water sector. This view has recently been challenged, on the grounds that aid is fungible—at least partially. Where aid is not fungible, the recipient government increases spending on the health sector by an amount equal to the aid. For each dollar of aid to the health sector, government health spending rises by a dollar. The other extreme is where aid is fully fungible. The recipient government treats the extra dollar of aid as if it represented an extra dollar of government revenue, and it increases its spending in the health sector by whatever amount it increases its health spending when its own revenues rise by a dollar. The intermediate position is incomplete fungibility—government spending on health rises by less than a dollar but by more than it would if the government received an extra dollar in its overall budget.

Assessing whether aid is indeed fungible is not straightforward. The difficulty is knowing how the government would have responded if its own resources had increased by the amount of the aid, or equivalently if it had received a check for the same amount. Recent research suggests that while an extra dollar of development assistance does result in an extra dollar of government spending in some countries, in many it does not.[6] Where it does, only 29 cents of the additional dollar of aid goes into government development programs—the rest leaks out into nondevelopment programs, though not apparently into reduced tax effort. So official development assistance at the level of overall government spending is fungible—the average government spends an additional dollar in exactly the same way, irrespective of whether it comes from domestic resources or from a donor.

Research also suggests that aid in many countries is fungible across sectors within the government's development program—aid intended for the health sector gets spent on other development sectors, and aid intended for other development sectors gets spent on health. Fungibility implies, for example, that when development assistance to health is earmarked for primary health services and excludes tertiary care, governments simply focus their resources on health services for the population served by public hospitals—a wealthier, urban population in many poor countries.

One important implication is that donors should not spend time and effort trying to channel their external funding to specific programs for certain priority diseases and populations, without engaging in a dialogue with the government on basic changes in the overall patterns of public spending for health—the total allocation and the amounts allocated to, say, child health and communicable disease control services or improving community and primary level health delivery systems. If these basic changes were enacted, donors would then transfer their financial assistance to the health sector as a whole, knowing that they are likely to have a positive impact on Millennium Development Goal outcomes.

The transactions costs of aid are still too high

In a single low-income country, more than 20 donors—including bilaterals, multilaterals, global programs, foundations, and large NGOs—can be involved in health. The demands placed on recipient countries can be huge, as donors are starting to acknowledge. They are recognizing that their individual procedures for reporting, accounting, and managing funds—often encompassing different budget structures, ways of measuring progress toward objectives, regulations for the procurement of goods, services and works, and approaches and cycles to disbursing funds—place heavy and unreasonable demands on recipient countries. This is particularly so in poor countries forced to allocate limited human resources away from managing service delivery to managing donors.

Donors have also learned that individual project management units have not made sustainable contributions. They have sometimes run parallel to local structures. They have also fostered a sense that the project staff are more accountable to the financier than the government. And they have redirected the most qualified human resources away from government employment toward employment in development assistance agencies.

There is a need to enhance coordination, explicitly pool aid, and put countries in the driver's seat

There is a growing view that if aid is indeed fungible and earmarking imposes transactions costs on recipient countries, donors should dispense with the fiction that donors can

identify what their money buys. This recognition has encouraged donors to search for broader development assistance mechanisms that recognize the importance of the entire expenditure program. These mechanisms range from the Multi-Country AIDS Program in Africa, which supports national HIV/AIDS strategies, to sectorwide approaches in health to poverty reduction support credits, which back a broad public spending agenda. In several countries, including Ethiopia, Ghana, Mozambique, Senegal, Tanzania and Uganda, these principles have improved country-level coordination of development assistance to health. Some key elements include the following:

- ensuring that countries, not donors, drive the coordination

- ensuring strategic coherence, as expressed in the poverty reduction strategy and the health, nutrition, and population analysis that feeds into it

- ensuring financial coherence through a medium-term expenditure framework and an agreement that all donor funding will respect the overall spending plans and limits of the government

- pooling donor funds in a single account and untying aid to procurement only from the country of origin of the funding

- limiting the number of country coordination bodies that can bring together national and international actors involved in health

- establishing a common framework for reporting and assessing progress, with a strong focus on countries conducting the monitoring and evaluation, learning from it, and using the information to make their programs more effective

Some of the experiments in country-level coordination of development assistance to health reveal the difficulties in implementing the principles of better donor harmonization. In some instances, it has been hard to persuade donors to pool their funds and break the tie between funding and procurement. Monitoring and evaluation systems have sometimes not been strong enough to yield timely and meaningful data on progress, a critically important feature if disbursements are linked to performance. Multiple national coordination bodies for government, donors, and NGOs for different diseases and services also persist in many settings.

Global partnerships add value but involve risks

Chapter 1 provided a long list of diverse global initiatives and partnerships (box 1.2). Each responds to priorities in public health in developing countries and to health problems that represent global threats.

Are these efforts competing to garner attention on an already overwhelmed global development agenda? Are they fragmenting the complex health challenges facing societies? Possibly both. But they reflect genuine collective attempts to solve large common problems, after long periods of moribund, parallel, or conflicting efforts. The partnerships speak different technical languages, have vastly different resource bases, and target different risk groups. But they all seek to add value through a common array of functions, including the following:

- *National and global coordination.* Committees, forums, communication channels, and Web sites make resource or knowledge flows more efficient, identify where cross-national efforts are best merited, and reduce burdens on those on the "frontlines" at the country or local levels.

- *Strategy development and evaluation.* Partnerships such as the Roll Back Malaria core strategies, the Global Plan to Stop TB, and the current search for a common position on antiretroviral drug resistance strive for consensus on effective intervention packages, monitoring indicators, and replicable solutions to specific implementation obstacles or opportunities.

- *Global financing and delivery mechanisms and new tools.* Partnerships such as the Global Fund to Fight AIDS, Tuberculosis and Malaria; the Global TB Drug Facility; the Vaccine Fund; and the Global Alliance for Improved Nutrition, as well as public-private partnerships for developing new diagnostics, drugs, and vaccines provide global public goods and respond to common externalities or market failures.

- *Resource mobilization, social mobilization, and advocacy.* Nearly all partnerships grapple with resource mobilization, advocacy, and community mobilization.

Recent external evaluations of some of the major health partnerships, such as Stop TB and the Global Alliance for Vaccines and Immunization, suggest that these collaborations are indeed adding substantial value. But some partnerships lack strategic focus and try to do too much. Others committed to stimulating a scaling-up of disease control and other interventions fail to engage enough with country-level processes to make things happen on the ground.

The global partnerships can also have cumbersome and costly governance and management arrangements, with large governing boards that fail to make strategic decisions or micromanage the full-time staff of the partnership secretariats. And some ignore, or exacerbate, the problems afflicting the entire health system, such as the lack of human resources for service delivery and weaknesses in integrated monitoring and evaluation. The challenge is for

countries and donors to learn how to capitalize on these global partnerships at the country level to throw light on health system issues and ultimately strengthen the underlying human and physical infrastructure.

So far there has been little cross-fertilization across the major health partnerships, although efforts are under way—through the High-Level Forum for the Millennium Development Goals for health and through development of a global partnership for child survival—to bring together different partners around a common goal or around all the Millennium Development Goals for health. It may be useful for countries active in multiple partnerships to initiate cross-partnership learning and collaboration. The small Initiative for Public-Private Partnerships for Health, based in Geneva, is one example of a modest effort to share the lessons of the roughly 70 active programs involving industry and public institutions in research and development and new product development to solve the health problems of developing countries.

Getting funds to the frontline

Central government funds can easily leak as they move through the system to the periphery of the country. And in the absence of local initiative and the right incentives, service provision can fail to reflect the views of local people. Effective development assistance to health needs to address these impediments. It needs to channel technologies, ideas, finance, and technical assistance closer to households and health providers and supervisory officials in ways consistent with national policies and amenable to monitoring and reporting.

Development assistance to health is likely to be more successful with four things in place:

- a decentralized system of fiduciary and technical management in the public sector (financial procedures, competent officials, open reporting)

- strong financial capacity of NGOs and private providers

- a government body equipped and charged with regulating the quality of public and private providers

- a balanced approach to community-driven development in health, to ensure that social fund–type financing for community health initiatives is sustainable

Examples of development assistance to health reaching frontline workers in an expeditious and sustainable way include block grants for districts in Uganda, social funds in Central America, contracting with urban and rural NGOs in the Reproductive and Child Health Program in India, and support to community-led initiatives in the Multi-Country AIDS Program (MAP). MAP is supporting thousands of community-led initiatives, including 2,500 subprojects in Ghana, 1,200 community-based activities in Kenya, and support to more than 4,600 villages in Ethiopia.

Development assistance to health is still unpredictable

Donor financing for health has not been as reliable or sustained as is often claimed or hoped for, even under new "long-term" arrangements. In some countries the cuts in development assistance to health have been sharp. Donor budgets are subject to the usual business and political cycles—and may go up or down yearly during budgetary processes. For countries such as Comoros and Eritrea, where the year-to-year changes in external funding can amount to as much as a fifth of all public spending for health, the fluctuations are so great that they make it nearly impossible to plan and implement a coherent national program (see figure 9.7).

Further work is needed in designing mechanisms for development assistance to health that provide greater assurance of sustained financial support. The challenges are to overcome the factors that result in interruptions in long-term development assistance to health, including changes in political leadership and aid agency management that lead to reneging on earlier agreements.

Applying the lessons in World Bank programs

What are governments and development agencies actually doing to align their efforts with the Millennium Development Goals? What new approaches are they taking to improve their contributions? Are they applying the lessons from experience with development assistance for health?

Within the World Bank, a review of recent trends and changes in the Bank's principal instruments—country analyses, policy dialogue with government, and financing of country-based projects and programs—suggests some important and encouraging developments in the way the institution is responding to the Millennium Development Goal challenge. While much more needs to be done in the coming years, there are some positive signs. What follows is a brief description of activities in the following areas:

- conducting country analyses of Millennium Development Goal trends, prospects, and challenges to inform Poverty Reduction Strategies

- incorporating the Millennium Development Goals in government policies and budgets, including medium-term expenditure frameworks

- strengthening the Millennium Development Goal focus in Bank assistance strategies

- integrating the Millennium Development Goals in Bank sectorwide and programmatic instruments

- reorienting lending and grants toward Millennium Development Goal outcome objectives

- using the Millennium Development Goals to build monitoring and evaluation capacity

Conducting country analyses of Millennium Development Goal trends, prospects, and challenges

The worldwide focus on the health, nutrition, and population goals has led to the production of several innovative analyses of Millennium Development Goal performance, trends, and determinants. In India the Bank recently completed a multivariate analysis of the large disparities in Millennium Development Goal performance across states and an assessment of the impact of public expenditures and other policies on Millennium Development Goal outcomes.[7] The study concludes that the impact of additional public spending for improved child health and nutrition would be greatest in the poorer Indian states. The study recommends steps to improve the efficiency of public expenditures, by targeting certain services (such as immunization and community-based nutrition activities) and villages and districts in the poorer states in which health and nutrition indicators are the worst. A similar approach to geographical targeting has been proposed by the Hunger Task Force under the Millennium Project, which has identified 75 nutrition "hot spots" in Africa where more than 40 percent of the continent's malnourished children live.

In Egypt a recent Millennium Development Goal analysis found that targeting publicly financed services and involving civil society in implementing programs and monitoring progress for the health, nutrition, and population goals are critical for success.[7] In Burkina Faso an indepth review of the child mortality target identified key constraints at the household, health system, and policy levels.[8] The review also analyzed policy reforms already undertaken and recommended further actions.

The Bank has collaborated with local analysts and policymakers in several African countries over the past two years to conduct studies on health, nutrition, and population trends and services nationally and as they relate to different socioeconomic groups, with a special emphasis on the poorest households. The studies, known as country status reports, have been completed for nine countries—Burkina Faso, Chad, The Gambia, Guinea, Malawi, Mauritania, Mozambique, Niger, and Tanzania—and are ongoing for another seven (e.g., box 10.3). The reports, important inputs into the national dialogue on the Millennium Development Goals and development policy,

The country status report for Guinea shows that the outlook for reaching the Millennium Development Goals is bleak. In 1999 children born in the poorest 20 percent of the population were twice as likely to die before reaching their first birthday as children born in the richest 20 percent. Service use is particularly low for children, as evidenced by low rates of vaccination and treatment for acute respiratory infections. Despite high use rates for antenatal care, the rates of assisted deliveries are extremely low in rural areas. Cost is a major barrier to use, particularly for poor households. About 10–15 percent of households are permanently unable to pay for health services, and few exemption schemes and subsidization mechanisms are in place. As a result, many poor households frequently resort to self-medication.

The key health sector performance issues included the following:

- *Mismatch between where money is spent and epidemiological needs.* Public expenditure in the 1990s focused on services in urban areas, particularly in the capital city of Conakry.

- *Low availability of resources.* More than 60 percent of health personnel work in Conakry, serving only 20 percent of the country's population. Drugs and vaccines are not readily and consistently available. Spending on operations and maintenance at the primary level is too low.

- *Low perceived quality of services.* Shortages of vaccines and drugs continue to undermine service quality, both technical and perceived. The perceived quality of services is often low. For example, many households do not view assisted delivery services as being of good quality.

The report recommends providing a package of essential interventions to the poor, strengthening institutional capacity by developing a framework for decentralization, reallocating resources to primary and essential secondary care, and increasing the government's commitment to sustainable financing.

Source: References 9 and 10.

the Millennium Development Goals. In Mauritania the analysis shaped the Poverty Reduction Strategy Paper and resulted in salary incentives for health workers serving in remote areas and an increase in the health sector budget of nearly 70 percent over two years (box 10.4). Mauritania used "marginal budgeting of bottlenecks" tool to link the Millennium Development Goals for health outcomes with essential services and the marginal cost of providing these services on a sustainable basis. The tool enabled the Mauritanians

Mauritania's Poverty Reduction Strategy, launched in 2000, profoundly reexamined health sector strategies, assessing past successes and failures and reorienting resources toward poor regions, poor groups, and efforts on outcomes related to the Millennium Development Goals. To address demand- and supply-side constraints, the strategy focused on reorienting public spending along three main lines: addressing gaps in service delivery to the poor, developing income protection mechanisms, and strengthening the voice of poor people and communities in service design and management. The strategy identified performance parameters and key inputs, such as incentives for rural practice, training and recruitment, facility support, subsidized essential supplies, vaccination costs, emergency AIDS plan, subsidized third-party payer hospital funds, and monitoring of priority programs. The reform issues addressed include human resources, drug purchasing, logistics, autonomy of management committees, reform of budget procedures, and performance contracts with regional directorates based on coverage objectives.

The Ministry of Health developed a medium-term expenditure framework that showed explicitly how it would strengthen three approaches to service delivery: family-oriented services, population-based services, and clinical care to "purchase results" in child and maternal mortality and malnutrition with investments in health services. The Minister of Health led the budget preparation process, consulting at each step with the Minister of Finance. Budgeting was done on the basis of the service delivery bottlenecks identified during the assessment phase.

Results of the budget reform process have been impressive. The health sector budget increased by more than 50 percent in 2002 and by 13 percent in 2003. An early evaluation of the impact of the changes in the budgeting process shows an increase in immunization coverage from 32 percent in 2001 to 82 percent in 2002. The clear links in the national health budget between the new activities to be funded and the objectives of the Poverty Reduction Strategy proved essential in the subsequent discussions with the Ministry of Finance and the International Monetary Fund.

Source: Reference 11.

have, in some countries, helped in drafting poverty strategy papers, estimating the cost of policies and programs, and designing medium-term public spending proposals.

Incorporating the Millennium Development Goals in government policies and budgets

The main findings of country status reports from African nations have been fed into country-led processes—the Poverty Reduction Strategy Papers and the medium-term expenditure frameworks—changing key policies in the health sector and reallocating public spending toward health, nutrition, and population services likely to have an impact on

to estimate, for example, the cost of investments that would allow for wider immunization of children and a higher percentage of women delivering babies under good conditions.

Using the Millennium Development Goals to assess World Bank country assistance strategies

To better align its country assistance strategies to the Millennium Development Goals, the Bank has conducted informal assessments in several regions. One example is the portfolio ranking in Benin, which found that the Bank's activities were weakly related to the goals: they had only low-to-moderate relevance for maternal and child mortality reduction and mixed relevance for communicable diseases. The ranking concluded that the Bank needed to do more, through the Benin poverty reduction credit and other projects, to have a substantial impact on health outcomes. The Benin social fund was seen as a promising instrument for increasing the Bank's impact. The country assessment also highlighted the importance of tracking intermediate indicators to measure progress in the short and medium terms.[12]

In the Europe and Central Asia region of the Bank, staff drafted a Millennium Development Goal "business plan," including a country-by-country analysis showing that official data on child mortality and malnutrition were of questionable accuracy—and that many countries in the region were unlikely to meet the goals for 2015. The business plan called for special efforts to strengthen capacity for monitoring and evaluation, align Bank projects better to support achievement of the Millennium Development Goals, and expand multisectoral linkages.

Integrating the Millennium Development Goals in the Bank's sectorwide and programmatic instruments

In many cases the goals provide the strategic underpinnings of sectorwide programs in health and multisectoral budget support. The Dominican Republic health project uses Millennium Development Goal intermediate and outcome indicators to monitor progress. The health information system has been designed to capture data on these indicators, augmented by the results of periodic household surveys. In Bolivia performance indicators for the Bank-financed health project include coverage and quality of key child and maternal health and disease control services, as well as changes in the incidence of diseases and deaths. Monitoring at the municipal and national levels, with the involvement of civil society, will increase local participation and make local politicians and healthcare providers more accountable for results.

Some sectorwide operations for health in Africa embody a sharp focus on the goals. Since sectorwide approaches combine donor resources in a single budget envelope and apply common procedures to their disbursement, they provide a good vehicle for reducing transactions costs and

bringing the government and external partners together around a common set of outcome targets—tied to the goals. The Ghana sectorwide approach, now entering its second five-year phase, has led to a substantial upswing in the use of health services for better child and maternal health, with the largest increases in the poorest areas of the country. Success factors include joint appraisal by all partners, strong government leadership, and expanded capacity to manage donor funds. Some challenges to enhance the impact of the Ghana sectorwide approach on the health goals will be to address persistent inequalities across regions and households, the brain drain of Ghanaian health personnel, and the limited use of NGOs to increase coverage.

Reorienting and increasing Bank loans and grants to achieve Millennium Development Goal outcomes

To underpin national efforts to improve health outcomes, the World Bank has significantly expanded its financial commitments in health over the past four years, through projects focused on specific diseases (the tuberculosis and AIDS loan in the Russian Federation) and population groups (the Brazil Family Health Project) as well as through broader health sectorwide approaches and other multisectoral operations. This increase has been consistent with the stated goal of boosting health lending from $1 billion in fiscal 2001 to $2.2 billion in fiscal 2005. Mirroring this target, actual lending has grown from yearly commitments of $0.95 billion in fiscal 2000 to $1.7 billion in fiscal 2003. Projected lending for fiscal 2004 is expected to be more than $2 billion. And the lending target for fiscal 2005 is likely to be met.

An important feature of health lending is that more of it is being incorporated in health components in other sectors, such as transport, social protection, and water supply and sanitation. For example, of the $1.7 billion in fiscal 2003 commitments, about 44 percent of total health lending was in projects and programs outside the health sector.

These changes in the World Bank's response to the Millennium Development Goal agenda create three problems. First, the Bank's organizational structure and incentives make it difficult to bring health specialists into project teams led by staff from other disciplines, such as water supply and transport. Unless this problem is solved, inadequate attention may be devoted to the health dimensions of these multisectoral operations. To address the problem, the Bank has organized special training and coaching arrangements for multisectoral teams, and it is testing budgeting and performance assessment techniques to encourage more effective teamwork in a multisectoral environment.

Second, the new projects require effective monitoring and evaluation systems to track progress on intermediate indicators and Millennium Development Goal outcomes. Traditionally, too little effort has gone to establishing such monitoring systems at the outset of Bank-supported programs. And most governments continue to be reluctant to invest in the kind of operations research needed to evaluate the impact of these programs. Recent efforts to standardize the use of intermediate indicators for the Millennium Development Goals for health—as well as initiatives to build strong monitoring into AIDS programs in Africa, tuberculosis control projects in China and elsewhere, and child health programs in Africa and Latin America—are pointing in the direction of a solution to this problem.

Third, the Bank needs to address the in-house mix of skills needed to manage relations with countries in an environment in which the focus is on the Millennium Development Goals and on a new set of financial instruments. Required are staff with knowledge and experience of health policy, institutional reform, and the economic, financial, and regulatory dimensions of health. Existing staff will need to be retrained and additional staff with the right skill sets recruited. Over the past two years the Bank has begun to tackle this challenge by expanding its external recruitment and introducing new training programs on scaling up programs related to the Millennium Development Goals and on using new lending and financing instruments.

Using the Millennium Development Goals to build monitoring and evaluation capacity

Effective national programs to pursue the health, nutrition, and population Millennium Development Goals depend on the use of intermediate indicators to track progress—and on building national monitoring and evaluation systems with local capacity. The Bank is supporting efforts in both areas. It convened a meeting of technical experts in November 2001 to review and agree on a framework of intermediate determinants. Those determinants were later published in a booklet now used in setting Millennium Development Goal targets in Poverty Reduction Strategy Papers and other national strategies and in developing monitoring and evaluation systems.[13]

Strengthening monitoring and evaluation capacity is taking different forms. In Albania, as part of a recent Bank-financed poverty reduction credit, a monitoring and evaluation template was prepared to help four ministries (including health) develop their own monitoring and evaluation systems, and a specialized advisory body on monitoring was established. In Mali a health card has been developed to give government officials and the public a snapshot of policy actions, health service indicators, and health outcomes for the entire country and for different income groups.

One of the most important global and national efforts to improve monitoring and evaluation of progress toward the Millennium Development Goals is for HIV/AIDS, where the Bank has been asked to take the lead role in coordinating partners (box 10.5)

Toward coordinated donor actions to accelerate country level progress

To pull together the lessons of effective development assistance for the health goals, the donor community, in concert with leaders from developing countries, has begun to

---

Box 10.5 Harmonizing, monitoring, and evaluating HIV/AIDS programs

The success of the Multi-Country AIDS Program (MAP) and other investments in HIV/AIDS will be determined by the degree to which implementing partners, countries, and the donor community can learn by doing. This requires better information on program reach and effectiveness. Yet few countries have adequate capacity to collect and use basic coverage data. Managerial and budgeting structures in most countries lack performance incentives, and motivation is undermined by lack of feedback on whether programs are succeeding or failing.

Recognizing this, and fueled by the intense demand for results at all levels, UNAIDS decided to form the Global HIV/AIDS Monitoring and Evaluation Support Team (GAMET) at the World Bank.

GAMET made considerable progress in its first year of operation. A GAMET advisory board was established to structure and provide guidance across agencies. A country support team—a network of consultant experts (the majority from Africa) in monitoring and evaluation capacity building—made more than 70 visits to more than 20 countries active in the MAP. GAMET also supported the design and implementation of a new management development intervention, the Rapid Results Initiative in Eritrea. The initiative focuses on achieving highly visible and rapid results in AIDS prevention and treatment—and puts in place an accountability framework.

Each of the agencies participating in the GAMET initiative faces tensions between its internal requirements for monitoring and evaluation and its desire to facilitate a coordinated approach at the country level. Donors are committed to reducing the burden of multiple monitoring and evaluation requests and policies, but each is also under pressure to show impact in the near term, which can undercut even the best intentions to rely on country-based systems. Spending staff time coordinating approaches and building country capacity rather than fulfilling fiduciary responsibilities to monitor their own programs generates additional problems. Despite the obstacles, GAMET shows promise, especially as governments and agencies see the benefits of a common approach to monitoring and evaluating national HIV/AIDS programs.

Source: World Bank staff.

---

put together a mechanism for continuing consultation and for monitoring progress.

The *Framework for Action to Accelerate Progress on the Health, Nutrition, and Population Millennium Goals,* endorsed at the high-level policy meeting in May 2003 in Ottawa, Canada, holds promise for all stakeholders. The focus is on building stronger national health systems as a platform for delivering essential services to the poor. The framework lays out commonly held principles and describes a process for countries and donors to work together in expanding and improving the effectiveness of their investments in health systems (box 10.6). It requires country actions, such as incorporating analysis of Millennium Development Goal challenges and policy and funding gaps in poverty strategy papers, and simpler arrangements for donor coordination. It also calls for stronger global efforts to invest in key public goods with multicountry benefits, such as research and development for new drugs and vaccines for AIDS, tuberculosis, and malaria. And it promotes docu-menting and sharing successful cases of national efforts to achieve the malnutrition and maternal and child health goals.

At the first High-Level Forum on health MDGs, cohosted by the World Health Organization and the World Bank in Geneva, January 8–9, 2004, heads of development agencies, bilateral agencies, global health initiatives, and ministers of finance and health met to informally discuss concrete actions to accelerate and monitor progress toward the Millennium Development Goals for health and nutrition. The forum focused on major constraints to progress in three areas: financial resources and aid effec-tiveness, human resources, and monitoring performance. It highlighted the policy steps that developing countries need to implement to save lives—and the harmonized actions that donors must take to increase the impact of financial and technical support to developing countries. The key conclusions and actions agreed on at the High-Level Forum are presented in box 10.7.

Box 10.6 Key actions to accelerate progress on the health, nutrition, and population Millennium Goals: The Ottawa consensus

What donors should do

Create donor buy-in and coherence by subscribing to a country-based Millennium Development Goals for health strategy, includ-ing goals and targets, policy actions, financing proposals, and monitoring arrangements, within a framework guided by the Poverty Reduction Strategy Paper and associated sectoral strategies.

Build on existing mechanisms at the country level, including Poverty Reduction Strategy Papers and sectorwide approaches, bilateral and multilateral funding streams, and those emanating from the global health initiatives.

Harmonize efforts to overcome funding gaps, fungibility issues, rigidity in financing recurrent expenditures, and lack of predictability of aid flows.

Commit to providing additional long-term financial assistance disbursed through existing multilateral and bilateral channels and instruments. No new funding body is envisaged. Donors would move toward long-term assistance in a reliable and timely manner, including support for recurrent expenditures.

Increase efforts to work with NGOs and communities.

Reduce the transactions costs of development assistance to health, by seeking to harmonize reporting requirements, procurement rules, and financial management systems.

Support capacity building for results-oriented monitoring and evaluation. Donors would also commit to an independent review of their actions and to sharing the lessons of this review with other stakeholders.

What countries should do

Develop a credible strategy. Prepare as part of the Poverty Reduction Strategy Paper process a credible strategy and imple-mentation plan (or review gaps and opportunities in existing strategies and plans) for achieving faster progress toward the Millennium Development Goals for health, based on a solid analysis of impediments to faster progress and a thorough assessment of policy options.

Tackle key constraints, including the need for better human resources, safe and predictable supply of drugs, stronger man-agement systems, and more effective public-private interactions.

Adopt a strong multisectoral framework within and beyond the health sector. This framework would be explicit about policy changes beyond health, such as overall public administration reform, and about other multisectoral activities.

Make a commitment to improve governance and policies, including policies on decentralization, civil society participation and monitoring, public-private partnerships, and public expendi-ture allocation decisions.

Strengthen transparency, monitoring and evaluation, through commitment to open and transparent reporting.

Provide voice to citizens—especially poor people, in formulating and implementing strategy. Consultations would be undertaken as part of the Poverty Reduction Strategy Paper process and beyond and include NGOs and communities.

Source: Reference 14.

As a result of the Ottawa meeting, donors and leaders of devel-oping countries decided to create a High-Level Forum that would convene twice a year over a two-year period to review progress on the health goals, monitor changes in donor commit-ments and behaviors in moving toward stronger harmonization, and discuss and act on issues holding back faster progress.

References

1. OECD Development Assistance Committee. 2000. *Recent Trends in Official Development Assistance to Health.* Paris: OECD.

2. Michaud, C. 2003. *Development Assistance for Health (DAH): Recent Trends and Resource Allocation.* Harvard Center for Population and Development Studies, Cambridge, MA.

3. Feyzioglu, T.N., V. Swaroop, and M. Zhu. 1996. "Foreign Aid's Impact on Public Spending." Policy Research Working Paper 1610, World Bank, Washington, DC.

4. Burnside, C., and D. Dollar. 2000. "Aid, Growth, the Incentive Regime and Poverty Reduction." In *The World Bank: Structure and Policies,* eds. C.L. Gilbert and D. Vines, 210–27. Cambridge: Cambridge University Press.

5. World Bank. 1998. *Assessing Aid: What Works, What Doesn't, and Why.* Oxford: Oxford University Press.

6. World Bank. 2003. *Attaining the Millennium Development Goals in India: How Likely and What Will it Take?* Washington, DC: World Bank.

7. El-Saharty, S., E. Richardson, and S. Chase. 2003. *Egypt and the Millennium Development Goals.* World Bank, Washington DC.

8. Naimoli, J.F., T. Johnston, and M. Schneidman. 2003. "Reaching the MDGs in Burkina Faso. An Assessment of MDG #4: Reduce Child Mortality by Two-Thirds by 2015." Background paper for the MDG Economic Sector Work. World Bank, Health, Nutrition, and Population Department, Washington, DC.

9. World Bank and Ministry of Health of Guinea. *Guinea: A Country Status Report on Health and Poverty (Health, Nutrition and Population Inputs for the PRSP and HIPC Process).* World Bank, Africa Region Human Development Unit, Washington, DC.

10. Soucat, A., S. Bonu, and Y. Camara. 2003. "Guinea Case Study." Background paper for the Millennium Development Goal

Economic Sector Work. World Bank, Africa Region Human Development Unit, Washington, DC.

11. Soucat, A. 2003. "Mauritania Case Study: Poverty Reduction Strategy Leads to Dramatic Increase of Resources for Health and Nutrition Services." Background paper for the Millennium Development Goal Economic Sector Work. World Bank, Africa Region Human Development Unit, Washington, DC.

12. Abrantes, A. 2003. Personal communication. World Bank.

13. World Bank. 2002. *Annual Review of Development Effectiveness. Achieving Development Outcomes: The Millennium Challenge.* Washington, DC: World Bank.

14. "Framework for Accelerating Progress on Health, Nutrition, and Population MDGs 2003." Presented at Ottawa Policy Meeting on HNP MDGs.

15. High Level Forum on Health MDGs, Geneva. 2004. http://www.who.int/hdp/en/summary.

Data and Methods

Rates of change

Unless stated otherwise, rates of change are computed on the assumption that the indicator in question falls by the same proportion each year. Rates are computed using discrete growth formulae. If m_{1990} and m_{2015} are the rates of malnutrition in 1990 and 2015, the Millennium Development Target requires that $(m_{2015} - m_{1990})/m_{1990} = 0.5$, or equivalently $m_{2015} = 0.5 m_{1990}$. If m grows at an average (negative) rate r per year, $m_{2015} = m_{1990}(1 + r)^{25}$. Substituting $m_{2015} = 0.5 m_{1990}$ gives $r = -0.27$.

Malnutrition

Data on malnutrition (underweight among children) come from the World Health Organization's malnutrition database, available at **www.who.int/nutgrowthdb/**. The data comprise very incomplete series for the 1990s for a large number of developing countries. Many countries do not have data for adjacent years. For each country, a regression was estimated for this report for the 1990s, linking the natural logarithm of underweight to the year of the survey, the coefficient being interpretable as the average annual rate of reduction (or increase) over the period for which data are available. The coefficients were then averaged—using population sizes as weights—to obtain regional averages. This method is less restrictive than the method used in an earlier study,[1] where regressions were in effect estimated at the regional level. Although countries were allowed to have different intercepts, they were assumed to have the same slopes as other countries in the region (that is, common rates of change).

Under-five mortality

Data come from the United Nations Children's Fund child mortality database, available at **www.childinfo.org**. The data comprise mostly complete series for 1960, 1970, 1980, 1990, 1995, and 2000. Average growth rates for, say, the 1990s were calculated assuming constant proportionate growth using the formula $r = (m_{2000}/m_{1990})^{1/10} - 1$.

Maternal mortality

See Box 2.1 and appendix B.

Communicable disease mortality

See appendix B.

Modeling prospects for future progress on the health Millennium Development Goals

The modeling strategy is to ask how future changes will affect the growth rate of the Millennium Development Indicator in question. Mortality or malnutrition, m, is assumed to be related to a vector of determinants, x, in the following way:

$$\ln m = \alpha + \beta \ln x + \varepsilon$$

where ln denotes natural logarithm, α and β are coefficients, β is interpretable as an elasticity, and ε is an error term. Differentiating this expression with respect to time yields a growth equation of the form:

$$\dot{m} = \beta \dot{x} + \dot{\varepsilon}$$

where $\dot{m}$ is the rate of growth of m and so on. The change in the growth rate can be written:

$$\Delta \dot{m} = \beta \Delta \dot{x} + \Delta \dot{\varepsilon}$$

so that if the growth rates of each of the elements of x remain the same over time, m will continue to fall at the same rate. If, by contrast, there is a change in the growth rate of, say, x_1 (which might be per capita income) but all the other x's ($x_2, \ldots, x_K$) continue to grow at the same rate, the change in the rate of growth of m is given by:

$$\Delta \dot{m} = \beta_1 \Delta \dot{x}_1.$$

Given an estimate of the elasticity β_1 and an estimate of change in the growth rate of x_1, one can estimate the size of the change in the growth rate of m likely to result from a change in the growth rate of x_1. The same method can be used to assess the effects of changes in growth rates of several x's simultaneously.

Regression models for the growth simulations

Elasticities for the various country-level determinants of each of the Millennium Development Indicators are needed to operationalize this growth simulation approach. For this report, the study by Filmer and Pritchett[2] of country-level influences on child mortality was extended and replicated on more recent data and on other Millennium Development Indicators.

Regressions were estimated linking the Millennium Development Indicators to government health spending as a percent of GDP, income per capita, and variables capturing female education, access to drinking water, income inequality, ethnolinguistic fractionalization, and regional dummies. Regressions were also run including a measure of infrastructure in addition to these determinants. Regressions were run for under-five mortality (2000), maternal mortality (1995), underweight (2000), and tuberculosis mortality (2000) as the dependent variable. All variables were entered in logarithmic form to facilitate the growth accounting outlined above. As in Filmer and Pritchett's study, countries with missing values for variables other than health spending and income were retained in the sample by including in the regression a missing value dummy variable flag and setting the variable with the missing value equal to zero for the country in question. Table A.1 provides the variable definitions and the sources of the data.

As in Filmer and Pritchett's study, government health spending is treated as endogenous to eliminate any reverse causality—governments may choose their spending levels in the light of their mortality rates. As in Filmer and Pritchett's study, the instruments used were the average levels of defense and health spending by the country's neighbors (as

identified by Filmer and Pritchett). Also included in the instrument set was the average value of an index of "voice" among neighbors. In contrast to Filmer and Pritchett, but like Rajkumar and Swaroop,[1] this study allows for the possibility that the elasticity of government health spending may depend on the quality of governance, the hypothesis being that health spending will have a larger impact on health outcomes in better-governed countries. Governance is measured using the Bank's Country Policy and Institutional Assessment (CPIA) index, which is increasing in quality of governance and takes a minimum of 1 and a maximum of 6. Part I countries (the industrial countries), for which no CPIA score is available, were assigned a CPIA score of 5. The government spending variable is interacted with the CPIA score, and elasticities and t-statistics are computed for different values of the CPIA index. The interaction is also treated as endogenous, with the three original instruments interacted with the CPIA score serving as instruments for the spending-CPIA interaction.[3]

Per capita income is converted using purchasing power parity (PPP) dollars (as in Filmer and Pritchett) and official exchange rates. Using PPP dollars may be more appropriate, but since PPP dollars are not specific to the health sector (or more accurately to the goods and services that make for lower mortality and malnutrition), it is not obvious that the overall PPP is necessarily always a more appropriate converter than the exchange rate. The broad conclusions are unaffected, but some of the magnitudes involved are sensitive to the choice.

Female education is captured through variables that indicate the percentage of women 15 and over who have completed primary education, the percentage of women 15 and over who have completed secondary education, and the percentage of women 15 and over who have completed higher-level schooling. The "missing" category is women who have not completed any level of education. Including female education in this way allows investigation of the returns—in terms of better health outcomes—of increasing primary completion rates and of narrowing gender differentials in education enrolment, both of which are Millennium Development Goals in their own right. It also allows for the possibility that primary and secondary education have different effects on health outcomes. The water variable proved to be highly collinear with a sanitation variable originally included, so only the water variable was retained. In addition, as in Filmer and Pritchett, income inequality (measured through the Gini coefficient) and an index of ethnolinguistic fractionalization were included. The final variable—not included in the Filmer and Pritchett specification—is the length of the country's paved road network in kilometers (the number

Table A.1 Variable Definitions

Variable	Definition	Source
Log government health expenditures as a percentage of GDP	Government health expenditures as proportion of GDP	Reference 7
Log government health expenditures as a percentage of GDP interacted with CPIA	The CPIA (Country Policy and Institutional Assessment) assesses the quality of a country's policy and institutional framework. The index contains 20 items grouped into four categories: economic management, structural policies, policies for social inclusion and equity, and public sector management and institutions. The index ranges from a minimum of 1 (unsatisfactory for an extended period) to a maximum of 6 (good for an extended period).	World Bank (not public domain)
Log per capita income in U.S. dollars	Per capita income measured in US dollars at official exchange rates	Reference 7
Log per capita income in international dollars	Per capita income measured at PPP exchange rates	Reference 7
Log percentage of female population 15 and over that completed primary school	Proportion of females that completed primary school	Reference 5
Log percentage of female population 15 and over that completed secondary school	Proportion of females that completed secondary school	Reference 5
Log percentage of female population 15 and over that completed high school	Proportion of females that completed higher school	Reference 5
Log percentage of population with access to safe water	Proportion of population with improved drinking water sources and sanitation	Reference 6
Gini coefficient for income inequality	The Gini coefficient measures the proportional deviation of income distribution from perfect equality. A Gini coefficient of 0 represents perfect equality; a Gini coefficient of 1 means that one person receives 100 percent of income.	Reference 7
Index of ethnolinguistic fractionalization	Probability that two people speak the same native language	Reference 2
Kilometers of paved road as fraction of land area	Length of paved road in kilometers (number of kilometers of roads times the fraction of roads that are paved) as a proportion of the country's area (in square kilometers)	Reference 7
Regional dummies	One for industrial countries and one for each of the following World Bank regions: Europe and Central Asia, Latin America and the Caribbean, Middle East and North Africa, South Asia, and Sub-Saharan Africa (East Asia and the Pacific is omitted)	n.a.
Defense spending by neighbor	Average level of defense spending by the country's neighbors	Reference 7 Definition of neighbor: Reference 2
Health spending by neighbor	Average level of health spending by the country's neighbors	Reference 7 Definition of neighbor: Reference 2

n.a. Not applicable.

of kilometers of roads times the fraction of roads that are paved), expressed as a proportion of the country's area (in square kilometers). This variable captures infrastructure.

Table A.2 shows the results of the regressions. Equation 3 in each case is closest to the Filmer and Pritchett specification—per capita income is converted using PPPs, and the infrastructure variable is excluded. All equations differ from the Filmer and Pritchett specification in that the spending-CPIA interaction is included. In virtually all specifications, the interaction is negative, suggesting that better-governed countries have larger (in absolute size) elasticities of mortality and malnutrition with respect to government health spending. This result is consistent with the findings of Rajkumar and Swaroop. For a given value of the CPIA index, the spending elasticities are smallest for under-five mortality and become statistically significant for under-five mortality only at very high CPIA scores. The low elasticity of under-five mortality with respect to government health spending is consistent with Filmer and Pritchett, though somewhat at odds with Rajkumar and

Table A.2 Regression Results

	U5MR 2000				MMR 1995			
	[1]	**[2]**	**[3]**	**[4]**	**[1]**	**[2]**	**[3]**	**[4]**
	Coef. (ltl)	**Coef. (ltl)**	**Coef. (ltl)**	**Coef. (ltl)**	**Coef. (ltl)**	**Coef. (ltl)**	**Coef. (ltl)**	**Coef. (ltl)**
log govt hlth exps as % gdp	1.091 (2.13)	1.38 (2.70)	1.083 (1.95)	1.306 (2.39)	−0.589 (0.71)	0.064 (0.08)	−0.86 (0.67)	0.059 (0.05)
log govt hlth exps as % gdp interacted with cpia	−0.292 (2.92)	−0.328 (3.11)	−0.267 (2.57)	−0.286 (2.64)	−0.033 (0.21)	−0.170 (1.05)	0.035 (0.15)	−0.130 (0.63)
log per capita income US dollars	−0.325 (3.63)	−0.358 (4.00)			0.025 (0.62)	0.035 (0.86)		
log per capita income internat'l dollars			−0.484 (3.77)	−0.547 (4.63)			0.034 (0.48)	0.055 (0.80)
log % female pop aged 15+ completed primary school	0.009 (0.10)	−0.042 (0.44)	−0.009 (0.09)	−0.047 (0.50)	0.120 (0.76)	0.035 (0.23)	0.127 (0.72)	0.046 (0.28)
log % female pop aged 15+ completed secondary school	−0.054 (0.71)	−0.053 (0.67)	−0.053 (0.70)	−0.047 (0.59)	−0.353 (3.13)	−0.318 (2.89)	−0.328 (2.71)	−0.296 (2.55)
log % female pop aged 15+ completed higher school	0.056 (0.78)	0.053 (0.71)	0.060 (0.85)	0.058 (0.79)	0.052 (0.42)	0.025 (0.21)	0.007 (0.05)	−0.008 (0.07)
log % pop with access to safe water	−0.333 (1.59)	−0.473 (2.16)	−0.262 (1.23)	−0.339 (1.48)	−0.669 (1.87)	−0.969 (3.00)	−0.782 (1.89)	−1.144 (3.26)
Gini coefficient for income inequality	0.007 (1.10)	0.010 (1.49)	0.010 (1.50)	0.012 (1.93)	−0.015 (1.40)	−0.008 (0.83)	−0.021 (1.54)	−0.009 (0.81)
index of ethnolinguistic fractionalization	0.274 (0.97)	0.425 (1.56)	0.298 (1.01)	0.431 (1.58)	−0.240 (0.58)	−0.018 (0.05)	−0.374 (0.63)	0.072 (0.14)
kilometers of paved road as fraction of land area	−0.091 (2.16)		−0.072 (1.58)		−0.131 (2.35)		−0.159 (2.07)	
Europe & Central Asia	0.082 (0.38)	−0.072 (0.34)	−0.010 (0.04)	−0.139 (0.66)	−0.613 (1.50)	−0.895 (2.33)	−0.511 (0.95)	−0.910 (1.98)
Industrialized country	0.017 (0.06)	−0.097 (0.33)	−0.250 (0.94)	−0.363 (1.34)	−0.721 (1.43)	−0.705 (1.39)	−0.743 (1.27)	−0.840 (1.54)
Latin America & Caribbean	0.020 (0.08)	0.008 (0.03)	−0.192 (0.77)	−0.232 (0.88)	1.076 (2.51)	1.051 (2.45)	1.218 (2.28)	1.078 (2.11)
Middle East & North Africa	0.352 (1.28)	0.332 (1.13)	0.218 (0.79)	0.187 (0.64)	0.886 (1.85)	0.821 (1.72)	0.788 (1.30)	0.707 (1.18)
South Asia	0.532 (2.11)	0.427 (1.59)	0.517 (2.08)	0.428 (1.66)	1.132 (2.76)	0.971 (2.36)	1.137 (2.55)	1.036 (2.34)
Sub–Saharan Africa	0.662 (2.89)	0.582 (2.48)	0.498 (1.97)	0.401 (1.63)	1.828 (4.87)	1.783 (4.79)	1.819 (4.05)	1.696 (4.02)
constant	6.731 (6.99)	7.709 (8.16)	8.083 (7.59)	8.983 (9.50)	8.047 (4.88)	9.418 (6.21)	8.608 (4.59)	9.823 (5.44)
Additional variables	All equations include dummy variables for when schooling, water, Gini coefficient and road network are missing (in these cases the variable itself is set equal to zero).							
# countries	120	120	119	119	113	113	113	113
Adjusted R squared	0.912	0.898	0.913	0.903	0.883	0.883	0.866	0.872
Elasticity of dependent variable with respect to gov hlth exps as % gdp, evaluated at value of cpia indicated								
1.00	0.799 (1.87)	1.053 (2.51)	0.816 (1.75)	1.020 (2.26)	−0.622 (0.90)	−0.106 (0.16)	−0.824 (0.78)	−0.071 (0.08)
2.00	0.507 (1.46)	0.725 (2.16)	0.548 (1.43)	0.734 (2.02)	−0.654 (1.18)	−0.276 (0.51)	−0.789 (0.93)	−0.201 (0.27)
3.00	0.215 (0.77)	0.397 (1.49)	0.281 (0.89)	0.447 (1.54)	−0.687 (1.58)	−0.446 (1.06)	−0.754 (1.15)	−0.331 (0.58)
3.25	0.142 (0.53)	0.315 (1.24)	0.215 (0.71)	0.376 (1.36)	−0.695 (1.70)	−0.489 (1.24)	−0.745 (1.22)	−0.363 (0.68)
3.50	0.069 (0.27)	0.233 (0.96)	0.148 (0.51)	0.304 (1.15)	−0.703 (1.82)	−0.531 (1.42)	−0.736 (1.30)	−0.396 (0.79)
4.00	−0.077 (0.32)	0.069 (0.30)	0.014 (0.05)	0.161 (0.66)	−0.720 (2.07)	−0.617 (1.81)	−0.719 (1.46)	−0.460 (1.05)
4.50	−0.223 (0.96)	−0.095 (0.42)	−0.119 (0.46)	0.018 (0.08)	−0.736 (2.26)	−0.702 (2.16)	−0.701 (1.61)	−0.525 (1.32)
5.00	−0.369 (1.56)	−0.259 (1.09)	−0.253 (0.97)	−0.125 (0.51)	−0.752 (2.34)	−0.787 (2.38)	−0.683 (1.69)	−0.590 (1.55)

Table A.2 Regression Results (continued)

	Underweight 2000				TB mortality 2000			
	[1]	[2]	[3]	[4]	[1]	[2]	[3]	[4]
	Coef. (ltl)	Coef. (ltl)	Coef. (ltl)	Coef. (ltl)	Coef. (ltl)	Coef. (ltl)	Coef. (ltl)	Coef. (ltl)
log govt hlth exps as % gdp	0.348 (0.44)	−0.014 (0.02)	0.473 (0.51)	0.022 (0.02)	1.025 (1.34)	1.239 (1.67)	1.124 (1.33)	1.304 (1.61)
log govt hlth exps as % gdp interacted with cpia	−0.218 (1.26)	−0.154 (0.90)	−0.245 (1.24)	−0.166 (0.84)	−0.374 (2.42)	−0.412 (2.61)	−0.400 (2.43)	−0.421 (2.50)
log per capita income US dollars	−0.271 (2.14)	−0.232 (1.85)			−0.325 (2.36)	−0.322 (2.40)		
log per capita income internat'l dollars			−0.300 (1.89)	−0.243 (1.59)			−0.351 (1.77)	−0.392 (2.18)
log % female pop aged 15+ completed primary school	0.318 (1.98)	0.332 (2.10)	0.269 (1.65)	0.298 (1.86)	0.123 (0.79)	0.040 (0.26)	0.087 (0.53)	0.016 (0.10)
log % female pop aged 15+ completed secondary school	−0.046 (0.43)	−0.099 (0.90)	−0.062 (0.56)	−0.112 (0.99)	−0.035 (0.29)	−0.083 (0.69)	−0.067 (0.55)	−0.098 (0.81)
log % female pop aged 15+ completed higher school	−0.096 (0.81)	−0.062 (0.51)	−0.086 (0.71)	−0.057 (0.46)	0.091 (0.79)	0.126 (1.08)	0.109 (0.93)	0.136 (1.16)
log % pop with access to safe water	−0.262 (0.82)	−0.197 (0.62)	−0.273 (0.84)	−0.221 (0.64)	−0.162 (0.49)	−0.378 (1.14)	−0.178 (0.51)	−0.346 (0.97)
Gini coefficient for income inequality	0.009 (0.94)	0.007 (0.72)	0.009 (0.95)	0.007 (0.71)	0.007 (0.65)	0.008 (0.86)	0.007 (0.62)	0.009 (0.92)
index of ethnolinguistic fractionalization	0.111 (0.24)	−0.079 (0.17)	0.086 (0.18)	−0.127 (0.27)	0.129 (0.30)	0.179 (0.44)	0.080 (0.17)	0.156 (0.37)
kilometers of paved road as fraction of land area	0.030 (0.43)		0.041 (0.54)		−0.134 (2.05)		−0.126 (1.76)	
Europe & Central Asia	−1.246 (3.60)	−1.206 (3.77)	−1.334 (3.71)	−1.253 (3.79)	−0.456 (1.37)	−0.692 (2.17)	−0.549 (1.56)	−0.765 (2.33)
Industrialized country	0.347 (0.65)	0.250 (0.46)	0.011 (0.02)	−0.024 (0.05)	−0.320 (0.73)	−0.599 (1.37)	−0.619 (1.44)	−0.863 (2.02)
Latin America & Caribbean	−0.166 (0.48)	−0.189 (0.53)	−0.337 (0.96)	−0.321 (0.87)	−0.792 (2.09)	−0.796 (2.02)	−0.984 (2.41)	−0.999 (2.39)
Middle East & North Africa	−0.460 (1.15)	−0.465 (1.13)	−0.598 (1.47)	−0.570 (1.35)	−1.915 (4.42)	−1.951 (4.36)	−2.060 (4.59)	−2.091 (4.56)
South Asia	0.447 (1.24)	0.524 (1.48)	0.471 (1.29)	0.557 (1.56)	−0.079 (0.20)	−0.219 (0.54)	−0.031 (0.08)	−0.176 (0.43)
Sub–Saharan Africa	−0.053 (0.17)	−0.006 (0.02)	−0.125 (0.36)	−0.052 (0.15)	0.330 (0.93)	0.315 (0.89)	0.275 (0.69)	0.221 (0.58)
constant	5.156 (3.39)	4.790 (3.15)	5.969 (3.55)	5.426 (3.30)	5.465 (3.57)	6.919 (4.83)	6.350 (3.65)	7.817 (5.23)
Additional variables	All equations include dummy variables for when schooling, water, Gini coefficient and road network are missing (in these cases the variable itself is set equal to zero).							
# countries	85	85	85	85	118	118	117	117
Adjusted R squared	0.709	0.699	0.704	0.693	0.825	0.813	0.818	0.809
Elasticity of dependent variable with respect to gov hlth exps as % gdp, evaluated at value of cpia indicated								
1.00	0.130 (0.20)	−0.168 (0.26)	0.228 (0.30)	−0.144 (0.19)	0.651 (1.03)	0.827 (1.37)	0.724 (1.03)	0.883 (1.33)
2.00	−0.087 −0.305	−0.321 −0.475	−0.017 −0.262	−0.310 −0.476	0.276 −0.098	0.415 0.003	0.323 −0.077	0.463 0.042
3.00	(0.18) (0.82)	(0.64) (1.23)	(0.03) (0.61)	(0.52) (1.06)	(0.54) (0.24)	(0.87) (0.01)	(0.56) (0.17)	(0.87) (0.10)
3,.25	−0.360 (1.04)	−0.514 (1.41)	−0.324 (0.81)	−0.518 (1.24)	−0.192 (0.49)	−0.100 (0.28)	−0.177 (0.40)	−0.063 (0.16)
3.50	−0.414 (1.27)	−0.552 (1.60)	−0.385 (1.04)	−0.559 (1.43)	−0.285 (0.76)	−0.203 (0.59)	−0.277 (0.65)	−0.168 (0.44)
4.00	−0.523 (1.75)	−0.629 (1.95)	−0.508 (1.52)	−0.643 (1.82)	−0.472 (1.35)	−0.409 (1.25)	−0.478 (1.19)	−0.378 (1.06)
4.50	−0.632 (2.13)	−0.706 (2.19)	−0.630 (1.96)	−0.726 (2.13)	−0.659 (1.91)	−0.615 (1.87)	−0.678 (1.74)	−0.589 (1.66)
5.00	−0.740 (2.32)	−0.783 (2.29)	−0.753 (2.22)	−0.809 (2.28)	−0.847 (2.38)	−0.821 (2.36)	−0.878 (2.21)	−0.799 (2.16)

Swaroop, who found significant elasticities of government spending at the sample median level of governance. (Their index of governance was, however, different.)

The health spending elasticities for the Millennium Development Indicators other than under-five mortality are not only larger absolutely than those for under-five mortality, they also become statistically significant at lower CPIA scores. The results suggest that—whatever the Millennium Development Indicator—simply adding additional dollars to the budget of a ministry of health in a country with a CPIA index of less than 3 will not yield improvements in any Millennium Development Indicator. By contrast, in countries with CPIA scores of 3.25 and higher, additional dollars in the ministry of health budget could reduce rates of maternal mortality (see equation 1 in table A.2). The cut-off for malnutrition is somewhat higher—a CPIA of 3.5 or so (compare with equation 2), which given the insignificance of the road variable might be argued to be preferable to equation 1. In the case of tuberculosis mortality, the CPIA cut-off is about 4.25 (see equation 1). These elasticities indicate the effects at the margin of adding dollars to the ministry of health budget on the assumption that the additional dollars are allocated across programs and institutions in proportion to current allocations. Adding dollars specifically to a government tuberculosis program might yield a significant payoff in terms of reduced tuberculosis mortality at much lower CPIA levels than 4.25. The results cannot, however, tell us whether or not this is the case.

Under-five mortality appears to be more responsive to per capita income than the other Millennium Development Indicators, with the possible exception of tuberculosis mortality. Female education has a significantly negative effect only on maternal mortality—and even then only at the secondary level. The lack of any effect on under-five mortality is at odds with the Filmer and Pritchett results, which report a significant effect of years of education. Access to drinking water has a significant negative effect on maternal mortality in all specifications and on under-five mortality in the specifications in which exchange rates are used to convert per capita incomes. Income inequality has mostly an insignificant effect, though there is some suggestion it makes a difference to under-five mortality. The same is true of the index of ethnolinguistic fractionalization. The road infrastructure variable, by contrast, has a significant negative effect on under-five mortality, maternal mortality, and tuberculosis mortality.

Forecasting trends in economic growth and the nonhealth goals

Economic growth forecasts are taken from the Bank's *Global Economic Prospects.*[4]

For secondary school completion the extra growth required to achieve gender parity in the proportion of the population 15 and over that has completed secondary education is computed. In the absence of this extra growth, completion rates are assumed to grow linearly between 2000 and 2015, following the same trend as between 1995 and 2000. This yields the 2015 value for males that females will also need to reach to achieve the gender Millennium Development Goal. The forecast assumes that achievement of the goal occurs through accelerated linear growth for females from the female 2000 value to the male 2015 value. This gives the growth rate needed between 2000 and 2015 to achieve the gender goal. This rate is compared with the current growth rate to obtain the extra growth in secondary completion required to achieve the gender goal.

For access to drinking water, the extra growth required to halve the proportion of the population without access between 1990 and 2015 is computed. In the absence of this extra growth, the access rate is assumed to rise (or fall) between 2000 and 2015 linearly at the same rate as in the 1990s. The growth that would need to occur to achieve the goal is found by assuming access grows linearly between 2000 and 2015, starting from the 2000 value and ending in 2015 at the value implied by the Millennium Development Goal. The extra growth is the difference between the projected growth based on current trends and the growth required to achieve the goal.

References

1. Rajkumar, A., and V. Swaroop. 2002. "Public Spending and Outcomes: Does Governance Matter?" Policy Research Working Paper 2840, World Bank, Washington, DC.

2. Filmer, D., and L. Pritchett. 1999. "The Impact of Public Spending on Health: Does Money Matter?" *Social Science and Medicine* 49 (10): 1309–1323.

3. Wooldridge, J.M. 2002. *Econometric Analysis of Cross Section and Panel Data.* Cambridge, MA: MIT Press.

4. World Bank. 2003. *Global Economic Prospects and the Developing Countries.* Washington, DC: World Bank.

5. Barro, R.J., and J.W. Lee. 2000. "International Data on Educational Attainment: Updates and Implications." CID Working Paper No. 42, Harvard University, Center for International Development, Cambridge, MA.

6. UNICEF. 2003. Statistics Water and Sanitation Databases. www.childinfo.org/eddb/water.htm and millenniumindicators.un.org/unsd/mi/mi_indicator_xrxx.asp?ind_code=30.

7. World Bank. 2003. *World Development Indicators.* Washington, DC: Washington, DC.

Why Tracking Progress Toward the Health Goals Isn't Easy

Assessments of progress toward the Millennium Development Goals are subject to uncertainties because of differences in how the indicators are defined, which measurement instruments are used, how frequently the information is collected, and how much effort has been invested in the development of measurement systems.

Child malnutrition

The prevalence of underweight children is defined as the proportion of children under five whose weight for their age is less than two standard deviations below the median for an international reference population. Data collection is most often done with household surveys, which require that the interviewers measure children and obtain their age in months. Inaccuracies in this information, as well as other errors due to sampling errors, are the main reasons for the uncertainties about the estimated prevalence of malnutrition. Confidence intervals at the 95 percent level in the Demographic and Health Survey sample are typically about plus or minus two percentage points, but the interval varies depending on the size of the sample and the prevalence of underweight children.

Household surveys that measure malnutrition indicators are usually conducted several years apart, and several countries do not have baselines for the earlier years of the Millennium Development Goal period. In some countries, surveys are not nationally representative and may produce estimates that are not comparable with earlier or later estimates. Some countries have used different reference populations, which are not usable at all.

As with all indicators, measuring changes over time implies using at least two estimates that are subject to unknown biases, which makes establishing significant changes more difficult. The WHO has assembled a database of such data, available at **www.who.int/nutgrowthdb/**. For this report, a regression was estimated for each country for the 1990s, linking the natural logarithm of underweight children to the year of the survey. The coefficient can be interpreted as the average annual rate of decrease—or increase—over the period for which data are available. The coefficients were then averaged—using population sizes as weights—to obtain regional averages. This is less restrictive than the method used in an earlier study,[1] in which regressions were in effect estimated at the regional level. Although countries were allowed to have different intercepts, it was assumed they had the same slopes as other countries in the region (that is, the same rates of change).

Child mortality—infant and under-five mortality

Infant and child mortality are measured using vital registration systems and household surveys. Vital registration systems can provide detailed and precise annual statistics when all or nearly all births and deaths of children under five are registered. But many countries have vital registration systems that do not capture all births or deaths, making such systems of little use for estimating mortality indicators. When compared with other sources of information, estimates based on vital registration systems are frequently found to be too low.

Household surveys measure infant and child mortality by asking female respondents to report the number of children they have given birth to and the survival status of the children. Some surveys collect detailed information to construct full birth histories for each respondent, while others collect only enough information to estimate childhood mortality indicators with additional demographic models. Where both types of data are available, they frequently produce different estimates and trends in mortality. As with all household surveys, sampling and other errors produce uncertainty about the exact level of the indicators. Confidence intervals at the 95 percent level for under-five mortality in Demographic and Health Surveys vary from as low as plus or minus 5 per 1,000 (India 1998/99) to as high as plus or minus 11 per 1,000 (Ethiopia 2000). At any level of disaggregation, confidence intervals tend to be larger.

Because of the retrospective reporting on childhood deaths, survey-based estimates generally are not estimates for the year of the survey but are commonly presented as averages for the five-year period before the survey. Annual estimates are rarely available, as these would require very large sample sizes.

One advantage of collecting childhood mortality estimates with surveys is that one obtains estimates for as long as 15 years in the past, allowing trends to be estimated from a single survey. When multiple household surveys are available and estimates have been made from both birth histories and demographic models, additional analytical efforts are required to produce a consistent series. The latest exercise (available at www.childinfo.org) has produced data for 1960, 1970, 1980, 1990, 1995, and 2000.[2,3] The data for 1990 and 2000 were used to compute the average annual rate of decline (or increase) using the formula $r = (m_{2000}/m_{1990})^{1/10} - 1$, where m_{1990} and m_{2000} are the mortality rates for 1990 and 2000.

Maternal health—the maternal mortality ratio

The maternal mortality ratio is one of the more problematic indicators to monitor. The indicator is a ratio of the number of deaths directly or indirectly related to pregnancy and the number of live births in a given time period. Because not all pregnancies result in live births, the ratio always overestimates the true risk of dying of maternal causes. The use of births as the denominator makes it theoretically possible for the measure to be greater than one.

Maternal mortality ratios can be estimated with vital registration data, but the incompleteness of vital registration systems is a major obstacle to their use in epidemiology. Where vital registration is complete, both the numerator and denominator for the maternal mortality ratio can be obtained. But even in countries with relatively good overall cause of death data, maternal causes are generally not very accurate. Even in countries with complete coverage of deaths in vital registration, maternal deaths may be misclassified in as many as 50 percent of cases.

In other countries the cause of death is sometimes established through the "verbal autopsy" method, in which sur-

viving household members or others (such as health care workers) who were close to the deceased are interviewed to establish cause of death. The questionnaire used in such studies includes questions about signs and symptoms of illnesses at the time of death, medical history, and obstetrical history. The verbal autopsy methodology often fails to identify deaths early in pregnancy due to ectopic pregnancy or abortion or those occurring some time after delivery.

Household surveys are the main instrument for measuring maternal mortality indicators. The usual approach is based on the so-called sisterhood methods, in which female respondents are asked to report on the survival of sisters. These methods do not produce reliable results when fertility is low (a total fertility rate of about 3 or lower) or where fertility has changed a great deal in recent years. Depending on which questions are asked, the estimates generally refer to mortality that occurred several years before the survey (10–12 years in some cases). Sisterhood methods cannot reliably report on early pregnancy-related deaths, as pregnancy status will be less likely to be known to the respondents. Induced abortion–related deaths are likely to be underreported for the same reason. Even with large sample sizes, standard errors tend to be very large. For example, the Malawi Demographic and Health Survey in 1992 generated a maternal mortality ratio of 752, with a 95 percent confidence interval of 523–803, for the six years before the survey. Because of such large confidence intervals and the number of years before the survey to which the estimate refers, household surveys are not suitable for monitoring short-term trends in maternal mortality or assessing the impact of programs.

The cost and complexity of collecting data with these methods has led the WHO and UNICEF to develop models that predict maternal mortality indicators.[3] Such models use variables such as the proportion of births with a skilled attendant, fertility rates, variables indicating regions, and HIV/AIDS prevalence to model the maternal mortality ratio. These variables may not be good predictors of the maternal mortality indicators, and they may themselves be poorly measured. For these reasons, maternal mortality ratios estimated in this way have wide margins of uncertainty. This modeling approach was used to estimate changes in the maternal mortality ratios at the regional level in the 1990s.

Incidence, prevalence, and death from HIV/AIDS, tuberculosis, and malaria

Monitoring trends in communicable diseases requires surveillance for correct diagnosis of a disease through clinical diagnosis or laboratory confirmation.

Surveillance of HIV/AIDS prevalence has focused on testing pregnant women in antenatal clinics. Such surveillance is subject to various biases: the sites are more likely to be located in or near urban areas, pregnant women may have different risks of infection than the overall female population of reproductive age, and pregnant women are not likely to be representative of the entire adult population. A new approach to establishing adult HIV prevalence is being implemented as part of Demographic and Health Surveys by serosurveys of household members. But high levels of nonresponse may limit the usefulness of this approach.

For malaria, incidence is particularly difficult to establish, as the symptoms of malaria are similar to those of many other acute infectious diseases that affect children. Even when microscopy is available, the cause of fever in children will be difficult to determine, as malaria parasitaemia are frequently present in children in endemic areas, making it difficult to determine which organism is responsible for the fever. Measurement of malaria mortality is equally difficult in the absence of cause-specific informa-

tion recorded as part of vital registration systems. Too few children with severe malaria are admitted to hospitals to rely on hospital records: an estimated 90 percent of child deaths occur at home in Sub-Saharan countries. Given the difficulty of diagnosing malaria correctly in these circumstances, the best approach is believed to be monitoring all causes of under-five mortality in malarious areas.

References

1. de Onis, M., E.A. Frongillo, and M. Blossner. 2000. "Is Malnutrition Declining? An Analysis of Changes in Levels of Child Malnutrition Since 1980." *Bulletin of the World Health Organization* 78 (10): 1222–1233.

2. Hill, K., and A. Yazbeck. 1994. "Trends in Child Mortality, 1960–90: Estimates for 84 Developing Countries." Background Paper No. 6 to *World Development Report 1993: Investing in Health.* World Bank, Washington, DC.

3. Hill, K., R. Pande, M. Mahy, and G. Jones. 1999. *Trends in Child Mortality in the Developing World: 1960 to 1996.* New York: UNICEF.

Index

Cash transfer programs, 82, 83f
Child morbidity
    acute respiratory infection, 52f, 117f
    health care access and utilization and, 6, 49
    household health resources and, 70
    strategies for increasing use of household health
        interventions to reduce, 86–88t
    vaccination and immunization coverage, 49, 53f
Child mortality
    among poor populations, 36, 44–45
    causes of death, 48–49
    in developing world, 2
    educational attainment and, 40
    effective existing interventions, 48–49, 48t, 50f
    future prospects, 4, 31, 38, 39f, 41, 45
    government health spending and, 7, 56, 57, 58, 59, 60
    health care access and utilization and, 6, 26, 47
    human resources for health and, 112
    linkages with other Millennium Development Goals, 32
    management factors in prevention program
        effectiveness, 100–101f
    Millennium Development Goals, 35
    potential benefits of increased coverage of home-
        delivered interventions, 49–52
    progress toward Millennium Development
        Goals, 2, 31, 35–37, 45
    social fund investment and, 62
    utilization of existing interventions and, 49–52, 54f
    water access and, 40–41
    worldwide, 1, 25, 26
China, 45, 139, 142, 146
    child mortality, 49–52
    HIV/AIDS in, 131
Colombia, 35
Community context, 70, 79
Consumer information and education, 10, 82–87, 106
    medication use, 14–15, 118, 120
Contraception, 10, 87f
Contracting for health services, 12, 103–105
Cost of care, 79–80, 146
    medication costs, 15, 118–119, 122–124
Côte d'Ivoire, 38, 79f, 112, 117f
Cuba, 138

D

Debt relief, 28
Decentralization of health service delivery, 12–13, 102–103
Delivery of health services
    accountability in, 11–13, 93–94, 95
    actors, 94–95

autonomization, 101–102
decentralization, 12–13, 102–103
focus of Millennium Development Goals, 45
government contracting for, 12, 103–105
government role in, 132
household role, 49, 64, 69, 70
informal provider network, 106–107
management issues, 11, 93
management philosophies, 96–98
marginal budgeting for bottlenecks, 9, 61–64
opportunities for improving, 93–94, 107
ownership in, 94–95
potential benefits of increased coverage of home-
    delivered interventions, 49–52
potential challenges in, 93, 95–96
privatization, 102
rationale for government involvement,
    132–133, 140f
reforms to increase provider accountability, 98–107
regulation of private health care providers, 105–106
See also Human resources for health; Public health
    functions
Developing countries
    disease surveillance and monitoring, 138
    health care access and utilization, 6, 26, 49
    international health initiatives in, 1
    malnutrition patterns, 25, 26, 31–35
    maternal mortality patterns, 37
    mortality and morbidity patterns, 1, 25, 26
    policy reforms tied to, 157–158
    progress toward Millennium Development Goals, 2, 31,
        32–38, 45–46
    water access, 89
    See also specific country
Development assistance
    continuity issues, 19, 145, 152, 161
    coordination of donor actions in, 164–165
    effectiveness, 7, 156–157
    fungibility, 158–159
    government allocation and, 18, 152, 158–159
    international health initiatives and global partnerships,
        17, 18–19, 28, 29f, 159–160
    monitoring use of, 20
    obstacles to effectiveness, 17–18, 152–153, 155
    performance-based, 18
    as share of government spending, 151, 152f
    strategies for improving effectiveness, 18–19, 153, 155,
        159, 160–161
    transaction costs, 18, 159
    trends, 28, 145, 156

Guatemala, 104f, 123f
Guinea, 162f

H

Haiti, 12
Health care workers. *See* Human resources for health
Higher-income countries
    child mortality reduction in, 35–36
    health care access and utilization, 6, 49, 53f
    prevention and treatment strategies, 53f
HIV/AIDS, 49
    in China, 131
    core public health functions in preventing/treating,
        134–137t
    drug supply and distribution, 15
    economic development and, 1
    effective existing interventions, 48t
    effects on health worker supply, 114
    health care access and utilization, 6
    maternal mortality and, 43
    medications, 124f, 125f
    Millennium Development Goals, 37
    prevalence trends, 37–38
    program monitoring and evaluation, 164f
    progress toward Millennium Development
        Goals, 45–46
    public health functions to combat, 142f, 143
    vaccine development, 126f
    worldwide mortality and morbidity, 1, 25, 26, 37–38
Honduras, 45, 83f
Households
    bottlenecks in delivery of health interventions, 63–64
    child health interventions, 70
    community context, 70
    definition, 9n
    in delivery of health interventions, 49, 64, 69, 70
    determinants of health behavior, 28, 69, 70–71, 80,
        84–85, 86, 87
    health care spending, 16, 26, 79–80, 146
    health knowledge and beliefs, 82–87
    health resources of, 69
    health system role of, 9–11, 27, 45, 64, 69, 70, 132
    help-seeking behaviors, 70
    hygiene and sanitation behavior, 16
    indoor air pollution, 16, 141–142
    potential benefits of increased coverage of home-
        delivered interventions, 49–52
    reducing economic obstacles to health care, 71–82
    strategies for increasing use of health
        interventions by, 86–92t
Human resources for health
    birth attendants, 43–44, 49

    compensation, 13, 114–115
    cross-border flows, 114
    HIV/AIDS effects on, 114
    influence on consumer health behavior, 87
    patterns, 13
    performance and productivity, 13, 113
    policy issues, 111
    problems in, 111
    progress toward Millennium Development Goals
        and, 111, 112
    public *vs.* private, 93
    recruitment and training, 13–14, 65–66, 115–117
    skills, 13, 14, 27–28, 65, 111, 113, 117
    supply, 112–113, 114
    within-country differences, 113
    worker expectations, 14, 14f, 115, 116f
    worldwide disparities, 49, 112
Hungary, 123f
Hygiene and sanitation, 16, 89
    intersectoral synergies to improve, 141

I

India, 10, 16, 70, 79f, 84
    human resources for health, 13, 115, 116f
    immunization program, 84
    nutrition programs, 11, 99f
    private health care spending in, 146
    public health spending, 19, 61, 161
    Self-Employed Women's Association, 84f
    tuberculosis intervention, 65, 66
Indonesia, 9, 27, 45, 82, 93, 96–98, 123f
Infectious disease
    core public health functions in preventing/treating,
        134–137t, 137
    economic effects, 1
    linkages with other Millennium Development Goals, 32
    poverty and, 26–27
    progress toward Millennium Development Goals, 37–38
    public health system response to crisis outbreaks, 139
    surveillance and monitoring activities, 138
    utilization of current interventions to prevent, 6, 26, 49
    worldwide patterns, 1
    See also specific disease
Initiative for Public-Private Partnerships for Health, 160
Institutions and policies, government, 55
    accountability in, 11–13, 65, 96–105
    accreditation of hospitals, 103
    autonomization, 101–102
    community representation, 11–12
    decentralization, 12–13, 102–103
    development aid effectiveness and, 17–18, 19, 155,
        156–157

development assistance conditional upon
    reforms in, 157–158
drug supply and distribution, 14–15, 120–125
focus of Millennium Development Goals and, 45
human resources management, 111
influence of, in community health behavior, 70, 87
management issues in health service delivery, 11, 96–98
Millennium Development Goals and health goals of,
    42–44, 162–163
privatization, 102
progress toward Millennium Health Goals and quality
    of, 56–60, 64
regulation of private health care providers, 105–106
strategies for improving, 19, 64–66
structural problems of health service delivery
    system, 95–96
in support of core public health functions, 139, 140f
See also Public health functions
Insurance, 9–10, 80
    drug coverage, 15, 122, 123f
Integrated Management of Childhood Illness, 8, 10, 14, 49,
    61, 66, 80, 86, 98, 117
Integrated Management of Pregnancy and Childbirth, 49
Intellectual property regimes, drug development and, 15,
    119–120, 124–125
Intersectoral cooperation, 16, 139–142

J
Jamaica, 98

L
Latin America and Caribbean
    child mortality patterns, 59
    economic growth, 4, 40
    effects of government health spending, 59
    health services contracting, 12
    HIV/AIDS in, 124f
    maternal mortality patterns, 37, 43
    mortality patterns, 2
    progress toward Millennium Development Goals, 2
    water access, 41
    See specific country
Lesotho, 60
Liberia, 112
Lithuania, 123f

M
Madagascar, 12
Malaria, 46, 52, 138f
    core public health functions in preventing/treating,
        134–137t
    effective existing interventions, 48t

Malaysia, 45, 81, 96–98, 112
Mali, 9, 20, 63, 164
Malnutrition
    among poor populations, 35
    child mortality and, 48–49
    effective existing interventions, 48t
    food supply and access, 79f, 80
    government health spending and, 56, 57, 57t, 58, 59
    household-level interventions, 71f
    intersectoral strategies to improve, 16
    linkages with other Millennium Development Goals, 32
    management factors in nutrition program
        effectiveness, 99f
    Millennium Development Goals, 32
    national commitment to programs against, 157f
    progress toward Millennium Development Goals,
        2, 31, 32–35
    social costs, 26–27
    utilization of current interventions to prevent, 6
    within-country differences, 2
    worldwide, 1, 25, 26
Management of health service institutions, 93
    accountability, 11, 65, 93, 96–98
    government role in, 132
    performance-based approaches, 98–101
    philosophies and styles, 96–98
    strategies for improving drug availability and use, 120
    structure of health delivery system, 95–96
Marginal budgeting for bottlenecks, 9, 61–64
Mass media, 87
Maternal mortality
    determinants of, 43
    effective existing interventions, 48, 48t, 51f
    future prospects, 4, 31, 41–42, 43–44
    government health spending and, 57, 58, 59
    linkages with other Millennium Development Goals, 32
    Millennium Development Goals, 31, 37, 43
    progress toward Millennium Development Goals,
        2, 4, 31, 37
    trend data, 2, 43
    utilization of existing interventions and, 49, 52–53
    water access and, 40–41
    worldwide, 1, 25, 26
Mauritania, 162f
Measles, 134–137t
Medicines and health supplies, 66
    consumer information, 14–15, 85, 118, 120
    counterfeit drugs, 118f
    determinants of supply and distribution, 14
    government regulation, 15, 122–125
    inappropriate/irrational use, 118f
    intellectual property issues, 15, 119–120, 124–125

W

Water access
  accountability issues, 89
  future prospects, 41
  health outcomes and, 10–11, 16, 85, 89
  intersectoral synergies to improve, 141
  linkages with other Millennium Development Goals, 32
  Millennium Development Goals, 40–41
  privatization programs, 88*f*, 89
  progress toward Millennium Development Goals, 4, 31, 41–42, 58–59
Within-country differences
  child mortality, 36
  health care resource allocations, 8–9, 60–61
  health services access and utilization, 6, 49
  human resources for health, 113
  malnutrition, 2
  measurement of Millennium Development Goals, 4
  progress toward Millennium Development Goals, 44–45

Women's issues
  agricultural policies, 16, 142
  educational attainment, 4, 31, 40
  financial autonomy, 82, 84*f*
  health care access and utilization, 10
World Bank
  Comprehensive Rural Health Project, 70
  health lending, 20, 156–157, 163
  International Development Assistance grants, 17, 18
  International Development Association grants, 156, 158*f*
  Millennium Development Goals and, 19–21, 155, 161–164
  Poverty Reduction Strategy Papers, 18, 19, 20, 21, 28, 112, 142, 155
  social investment funds, 62
  staff, 164
World Trade Organization TRIPS Agreement, 124–125

Z

Zambia, 1, 13, 115
Zimbabwe, 12